The Boston IVF
Handbook of Infertility

A Practical Guide for Practitioners Who Care for Infertile Couples, Fourth Edition

REPRODUCTIVE MEDICINE AND ASSISTED REPRODUCTIVE TECHNIQUES SERIES

David Gardner
University of Melbourne, Australia

Zeev Shoham
Kaplan Hospital, Rehovot, Israel

The Boston IVF Handbook of Infertility

A Practical Guide for Practitioners Who Care for Infertile Couples, Fourth Edition

Edited by

Steven R. Bayer, MD
Reproductive Endocrinologist
Boston IVF
Clinical Instructor of Obstetrics, Gynecology and Reproductive Biology
Harvard Medical School

Michael M. Alper, MD
Medical Director and Reproductive Endocrinologist
Boston IVF
Associate Professor of Obstetrics, Gynecology and Reproductive Biology
Harvard Medical School

Alan S. Penzias, MD
Reproductive Endocrinologist
Boston IVF
Associate Professor of Obstetrics, Gynecology and Reproductive Biology
Harvard Medical School

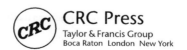

CRC Press
Taylor & Francis Group
Boca Raton London New York

CRC Press is an imprint of the
Taylor & Francis Group, an **informa** business

CRC Press
Taylor & Francis Group
6000 Broken Sound Parkway NW, Suite 300
Boca Raton, FL 33487-2742

© 2018 by Taylor & Francis Group, LLC
CRC Press is an imprint of Taylor & Francis Group, an Informa business

No claim to original U.S. Government works

Printed on acid-free paper

International Standard Book Number-13: 978-1-4987-8124-4 (Pack—Paperback and eBook)

Visit the Taylor & Francis Web site at
http://www.taylorandfrancis.com

and the CRC Press Web site at
http://www.crcpress.com

Contents

Preface

From its early inception over 30 years ago, the field of assisted reproductive technology (ART) and infertility has been rapidly changing. The field is one of the most innovative and fascinating areas of medicine. In order to keep up with the latest advances, it is critical for any textbook in the field to be up to date. Much has changed since our initial edition 15 years ago. Also, much has changed at Boston IVF as well—our group of fertility specialists has expanded from 4 to now more than 20, resulting in many more contributors sharing their expertise in the new edition.

In the new edition of the handbook, all of the core topics in the field of infertility have been updated, and several new chapters have been added. Genetics is playing a more and more important role in our specialty. The chapter on preimplantation genetic testing highlights the application of genetics in modern-day ART. The ability to screen embryos for their chromosomal status has led to improved implantation rates and efficiency in in vitro fertilization (IVF). Endometriosis remains an important cause of infertility, and a new chapter on this topic covers the diagnosis and current treatment paradigm. A chapter has been added on the treatment options for the LGBT community. Access to effective treatment for same-sex couples remains difficult in some areas because of legal, cultural, and logistical reasons. Some treatments for same-sex couples are simple (such as donor insemination for same-sex female couples), and some may be more involved such as donor egg/gestational surrogacy for same-sex male couples. The transgender community also deserves special attention to help these individuals pursue their gender identification and, at the same time, plan for their reproductive options as well. The advent of egg freezing and banking has revolutionized the donor egg field; in fact, vitrification techniques to freeze eggs is one of the most important advances in our field since intracytoplasmic sperm injection (ICSI) was introduced more than 20 years ago. A chapter on elective egg freezing presents the application of this new technology for those women who want to preserve their fertility. Finally, realizing the role of other key players in the delivery of quality care, we have added chapters highlighting our expertise in the areas of nursing, the IVF laboratory, and administration.

This fourth edition of *The Boston IVF Handbook of Infertility* represents the collective efforts of the many professionals at Boston IVF. It represents 30 years of our company's efforts to improve the care that we provide and help our patients resolve their fertility issues. We hope you enjoy our book and it helps you with the care of your patients.

Michael M. Alper, MD
Medical Director and President, Boston IVF

Acknowledgments

This book is dedicated to our patients, who display the utmost courage and determination in their journey to one day becoming parents.

About Boston IVF

Boston IVF was established in 1986 as one of the first freestanding IVF centers in the United States. Since its inception Boston IVF has been a leader in the cutting-edge reproductive technologies. The unique practice model and commitment to the highest quality medical care has resulted in continued growth and success of the organization. To this end, Boston IVF has established itself as one of the largest IVF centers in the United States and has been responsible for the birth of more than 30,000 babies. As a testament to its commitment to quality, Boston IVF became the first IVF center in North America to become ISO-9001 certified. The strong affiliation of Boston IVF with the Beth Israel Deaconess Medical Center and the Harvard Medical School has resulted in broad-based clinical and basic science research that has helped to advance the field of infertility. Boston IVF also has maintained a strong commitment to education. There is active teaching of nurses, medical students, physicians in training and fellows. Through its commitment to quality patient care, medical research, and education, Boston IVF is a recognized world leader in infertility.

Contributors

Michael M. Alper
Boston IVF
Harvard Medical School
Boston, Massachusetts

C. Brent Barrett
Boston IVF
Boston, Massachusetts

Steven R. Bayer
Boston IVF
Harvard Medical School
Boston, Massachusetts

Brian M. Berger
Boston IVF
Harvard Medical School
Boston, Massachusetts

Merle J. Berger
Boston IVF
Harvard Medical School
Boston, Massachusetts

Alice D. Domar
Boston IVF
Harvard Medical School
Boston, Massachusetts

Sharon Edwards
Boston IVF
Boston, Massachusetts

Sonia Elguero
Boston IVF
Albany, New York

Marsha Forman
Boston IVF
Albany, New York

Kathryn J. Go
Boston IVF/IVF New England
Lexington, Massachusetts

Susan Gordon-Pinnell
Boston IVF
Boston, Massachusetts

Daniel Griffin
Boston IVF
Evansville, Indiana

Jesse Hade
Boston IVF
Scottsdale, Arizona

Benjamin Lannon
Boston IVF
Harvard Medical School
Portland, Maine

Derek Larkin
Boston IVF
Boston, Massachusetts

Stephen Lazarou
Harvard Medical School
Boston, Massachusetts

Kerri L. Luzzo
Boston IVF/IVF New England
Lexington, Massachusetts

Kristin MacCutcheon
Boston IVF
Boston, Massachusetts

Lynn Nichols
Boston IVF
Boston, Massachusetts

Selwyn P. Oskowitz
Boston IVF
Harvard Medical School
Boston, Massachusetts

Samuel C. Pang
Boston IVF/IVF New England
Lexington, Massachusetts

Samuel A. Pauli
Boston IVF/IVF New England
Lexington, Massachusetts

Alan S. Penzias
Boston IVF
Harvard Medical School
Boston, Massachusetts

Nina Resetkova
Boston IVF
Harvard Medical School
Boston, Massachusetts

Terry Chen Rothchild
Boston IVF
Boston, Massachusetts

David A. Ryley
Boston IVF
Harvard Medical School
Boston, Massachusetts

Denny Sakkas
Boston IVF
Harvard Medical School
Boston, Massachusetts

Rita M. Sneeringer
Boston IVF
Harvard Medical School
Boston, Massachusetts

Kim L. Thornton
Boston IVF
Harvard Medical School
Boston, Massachusetts

Jeanie Ungerleider
Boston IVF
Boston, Massachusetts

Kristen Page Wright
Boston IVF/IVF New England
Lexington, Massachusetts

Alison E. Zimon
Boston IVF
Harvard Medical School
Boston, Massachusetts

1

Overview of Infertility

Alan S. Penzias

Significant advances have been made in the field of reproductive medicine over the past several decades. The knowledge that has been gained has provided a better understanding of the science of infertility and has resulted in the development of reproductive technologies that have greatly benefited infertile couples. However, with the introduction of these new therapies, there is a realization that infertility is not a simple medical problem, but there are legal, economic, moral, and ethical issues that must be addressed. This chapter will provide an overview of infertility and discuss its broader impact on society today.

Historical Perspective

Realizing the importance of reproduction, early scientists, philosophers, and others have ventured to gain an understanding of the human reproduction system and the disorders that alter its function. While most of our understanding of human reproduction has been gained over the past 50 years, this could not have been possible without the insight and knowledge from early investigation.

Infertility in the Bible

The earliest references to reproduction date back to antiquity with the biblical directive to "be fruitful, and multiply" [1]. In fact, those words are used three separate times in the book of Genesis [2,3]. It is no surprise therefore that fertility and procreation played a vital role in early life and beliefs. A woman was measured by her ability to bear children, and infertility was viewed as a punishment for wrongdoing, with God being the source of fertility.

Problems with infertility beset our ancestors from the start. Sarah and Abraham were unable to conceive [4]. Sarah considered the problem and asked Abraham to "go in unto my maid; it may be that I may obtain children by her" [5]. Abraham honored Sarah's request and Hagar conceived. We can probably view this as the first recorded test of male infertility but in retrospect confirmed that the infertility resided with Sarah.

Ancient Greece

Hippocrates (460–380 BC) was one of the first authors of various medical works dealing with gynecology. Six treatises that deal with reproduction were attributed to him. The diagnosis of infertility was based on the concept of free passage or continuity of the external genitalia and the vagina with the rest of the body. In *The Aphorisms of Hippocrates*, he wrote "If a woman do not conceive, and wish to ascertain whether she can conceive, having wrapped her up in blankets, fumigate below, and if it appear that the scent passes through the body to the nostrils and mouth, know that of herself she is not unfruitful" [6]. In the same treatise, Hippocrates speculated on the conditions needed to foster pregnancy. "Women who have the uterus cold and dense do not conceive; and those also who have the uterus humid, do not conceive, for the semen is extinguished, and in women whose uterus is very dry, and very hot, the semen is lost from the want of food; but women whose uterus is in an intermediate state between these temperaments prove fertile" [6].

Aristotle of Stagira (384–322 BC) was one of the greatest Greek philosophers of his time and was also one of the greatest zoologists and naturalists of antiquity. Although not a physician, he discussed many issues relating to reproduction in his thesis *The Generation of Animals*. Aristotle gave to medicine certain fundamentals such as comparative anatomy and embryology. A common ancient method of interfering with male fertility was castration. Aristotle knew that castration makes a male infertile despite his belief that the testes are only weights holding down the spermatic passages and not the source of the seed. "For the testes are no part of the ducts but are only attached to them, as women fasten stones to the loom when weaving" [7]. He was probably misled by his observation that a recently castrated bull succeeded in impregnating a cow: "a bull mounting immediately after castration has caused conception in the cow because the ducts had not yet been drawn up" [7].

The Renaissance

Andreas Vesalius (1514–1564), a Belgian physician and anatomist, published his revolutionary book *De Humani Corporis Fabrica* (On the Structure of the Human Body) in 1543. Vesalius contributed to an accurate description of the entire female genital system including ligaments, tubes, and blood supply. He was the first to use the terms pelvis and decidua. He also was the first to describe the ovarian follicle.

Gabrielle Fallopio (1523–1562) of Modena was a student of Vesalius. He described the oviducts and wrote further on the morphology of the ovaries. His name has been permanently connected with the oviduct or fallopian tube. He also named the clitoris, the vagina, and the placenta.

Lazzaro Spallanzani (1729–1799), though not a physician, made enormous contributions to our understanding of fertility. In his monograph, *Fecondazione Artificiale*, he showed that conception was achieved as a result of contact between eggs and sperm. He succeeded in fertilizing frog eggs by placing them in the immediate contact with the secretions expressed from the testicles of the male frog. He also performed some of the first successful artificial insemination experiments on lower animals and on a dog [8].

Modern Era

J. Marion Sims (1813–1883) is considered the father of American gynecology. Among his numerous contributions, Sims played an important role in establishing the role of cervical secretions in affecting sperm survival in the genital tract. On the basis of Sims' work, Max Huhner (1873–1947), in his 1913 book, *Sterility in the Male and Female and Its Treatment*, introduced the Sims–Huhner test (later termed the post-coital test).

I.C. Rubin introduced the first clinical test to determine tubal patency. Initially, he started by using a radioactive material but realized that this approach had its limitations. He then turned to tubal insufflation using oxygen in 1920. This was later changed to carbon dioxide as it was reabsorbed more easily, caused less discomfort, and avoided the danger of embolism. In the test, the insufflation is usually carried out at a gas pressure of less than 120 mm of mercury. The manometer reading decreases to 100 or less if the tubes are clear; if between 120 and 130, there is probably partial stricture; if it rises to 200 and above, it is suggestive that the tubes are obstructed [9]. This test is no longer performed as there are many more accurate tests of tubal patency available.

In 1935, Stein and Levanthal described a series of patients with amenorrhea, hirsutism, and obesity. They named the condition the Stein–Levanthal syndrome (later termed polycystic ovarian syndrome). They noted that several of these women started to menstruate after they underwent an ovarian biopsy. This led to the development of the wedge resection as a treatment for this condition which proved to be quite effective in the restoration of menstrual function. To this day, we still do not have an understanding as to why an ovarian wedge resection or the modern-day ovarian drilling procedure is effective.

1950s: The Development of the Radioimmunoassay (RIA)

In the 1950s, the RIA was developed by Solomon Aaron Berson and Rosalyn Sussman Yalow. The RIA allowed the detection and measurement of steroid and peptide hormones that are present in the serum and urine in very low concentrations. As a result of this monumental work, Yalow received the Nobel Prize in physiology in 1977. The introduction of RIA was pivotal and developed the foundation to modern-day endocrinology. The information gained helped us to understand the steroid pathways in endocrine organs and also helped with the diagnosis and characterization of endocrine disorders. The RIA also provided an important tool in monitoring the patient undergoing ovulation induction.

1960s: The Introduction of Fertility Medications

Clomiphene citrate (CC) was an oral medication introduced in 1962. It was the first medical therapy developed to correct ovulatory dysfunction secondary to anovulation. To this day, it continues to be the most commonly prescribed medication for the infertile female.

In the 1960s, FSH and LH were extracted from the urine of menopausal women, which gave rise to the development of an injectable medication called human menopausal gonadotropins. This medication was used for ovulatory dysfunction that was refractory to CC. It was a much stronger agent and required closer monitoring of serum estradiol levels, which could now be measured by RIA. In 1962, Dr. Bruno Lunenfeld in Israel reported the first pregnancy achieved with the use of human menopausal gonadotropins.

1980s: Reproductive Surgery

During the 1980s, there was an emphasis on reproductive surgery to correct tubal/peritoneal factors that were causing infertility. Laparoscopy was becoming increasingly popular and evolved into a routine part of the infertility evaluation. Laparoscopy was first introduced in the United States in 1911 by Bertram Bernheim at the Johns Hopkins Hospital. It wasn't until the introduction of the automatic insufflator in 1960 and the development of a fiber optic light source did the procedure become practical. Initially, laparoscopy was only a diagnostic tool and the surgeon would have to resort to a laparotomy to correct altered pelvic anatomy. In the ensuing years with the advent of laparoscopic instrumentation, operative laparoscopy was born, which allowed the surgeon to not only diagnose but also treat most abnormalities that were encountered. However, in the 1990s, rising in vitro fertilization (IVF) success rates soon surpassed the success rates resulting from corrective surgery. Presently, there are fewer indications to resort to surgery.

1990s: The IVF Revolution

On July 25, 1978, Louise Joy Brown, the world's first successful "test-tube" baby, was born in Great Britain. This marvelous achievement earned Robert Edwards the 2010 Nobel Prize in Physiology or Medicine. The first IVF success was a culmination of decades of work. In 1944, along with Harvard scientist Miriam F. Menkin, John Rock fertilized the first human egg in a test tube. On February 6, 1944, they produced the first laboratory-fertilized, two-cell human egg [10].

Author Martin Hutchinson summarized the chronology of IVF technology when he wrote:

> The idea of in vitro fertilisation had first been put forward as early as the 1930s, but it was not until the 1950s that anyone managed to fertilise a mammal egg in a test tube. Rabbits were one thing, but, as scientists were finding out, the secrets of the human reproductive system proved to be hard-won indeed. Professor Edwards said: "By 1965 I'd been trying to mature human eggs for the past five years." There was nobody racing against us—nobody had figured any of the ideas of this concept. It took further years of effort to produce a magical figure—37 hours—the length of time it took for a human egg to become ready for fertilisation after a particular point in a woman's cycle [11].

The establishment of the first IVF pregnancy was truly amazing and the initial experience was detailed in a publication by Edwards et al [12]. The initial cycles involved women who were followed during their natural cycle. The LH surge was identified with 3 hourly LH determinations and the laparoscopic egg retrieval was scheduled accordingly. More than 30 cycles were initiated before success was achieved, which led to the birth of Louise Brown. Since the inception of IVF, many modifications have been instituted in every step of the treatment, which has resulted in increased success. Following this first success, IVF programs were established all throughout the world. Presently, approximately 1.5 million ART cycles are now performed globally each year, producing 350,000 babies. It is estimated that more than 5,000,000 children have been born through this technique [13,14].

Today, advances in IVF technology enable conception and childbirth in couples with conditions that were previously thought to be uncorrectable. Direct aspiration of sperm from the testes, uterine transplant for women born without a uterus, and transplantation of frozen ovarian tissue were beyond anyone's wildest imagination in 1978. Further advances in the field of molecular genetics and the ability to biopsy a blastocyst in the laboratory have created new opportunities for couples who are carriers of genetic conditions as well as those who wish to reduce the risk of miscarriage.

The Definition of Infertility

There has been considerable debate about an acceptable definition of infertility. First, there is confusion about the use of the word itself—_infertility_—which, upon translation, means "not fertile" and therefore would be synonymous with sterility. While it is true that all women who are sterile would be considered infertile, the contrary is not true—not all women who are infertile are sterile. Therefore, many women would be better categorized as being "subfertile" instead of infertile. Despite these shortcomings, the all-inclusive term _infertility_ is here to stay and there is little that can be done to change it.

The most succinct definition of infertility has been published and recently updated by the _American Society for Reproductive Medicine_ [15].

> Infertility is a disease* defined by the failure to achieve a successful pregnancy after 12 months or more of appropriate, timed unprotected intercourse or therapeutic donor insemination. Earlier evaluation and treatment may be justified based on medical history and physical findings and is warranted after 6 months for women over age 35 years.
> *Disease is "any deviation from or interruption of the normal structure or function of any part, organ, or system of the body as manifested by characteristic symptoms and signs; the etiology, pathology, and prognosis may be known or unknown."
>
> Dorland's Illustrated Medical Dictionary, _31st edition, 2007:535._

The time threshold of 12 months for women under the age of 35 is relatively arbitrary. Of those pregnancies that do occur, 78%–85% are achieved in the first 6 months of trying. With this in mind, one could argue that an evaluation is warranted for every couple that has failed to achieve a pregnancy after 6 months of trying or therapeutic donor insemination. Other reasons to move up the time of the evaluation is when the woman is over the age of 35 or when there is a known or suspected cause of infertility (i.e., anovulation, a known tubal factor, endometriosis, etc.).

Epidemiology

Infertility continues to be a prevalent problem in our society today. Over the past few years, the many issues surrounding infertility have become popular topics in the lay press. This has resulted in an increased awareness of infertility, but has also given the impression that we are amid an epidemic of this problem. The National Survey of Family Growth performed by the National Center for Health Statistics has provided insight into the prevalence of infertility in the United States. This survey has been performed several times since 1965, and the most recent survey was published in 2013 on data collected between 2006 and 2010 [16]. More than 12,000 women between the ages of 15 and 44 were surveyed about fertility issues. Highlights of the survey are as follows:

- 12.3% of married women or 7.5 million women had impaired fecundity (impaired ability to get pregnant or carry a baby to term).
- 6.1% of married women, or approximately 1 million women were infertile (unable to get pregnant after at least 12 consecutive months of unprotected sex with husband).
- The rate of infertility in null gravida women is correlated with age:
  - 15–29 years   7.3%
  - 30–34 years   9.1%
  - 35–39 years   25%
  - 40–44 years   30%
- The rate of infertility is impacted on by parity (Figure 1.1).
- The overall rate of infertility has decreased over time (Figure 1.2).
- 38% of nulliparous infertility women have used fertility services.

Infertility continues to be a persistent problem in the United States, but it has implications worldwide as well. The World Health Organization has estimated that infertility affects 50–80 million women worldwide, and this may be an underestimate [17]. In developing countries, the incidence of infertility has been estimated to be as high as 50% [18]. One reason for the higher rate of infertility in developing countries is reduced access to medical treatments including antibiotics to reduce the transmission and consequences of sexually transmitted diseases. The ramifications of infertility in these populations are far reaching. Many societies depend on their offspring for survival. In addition, the inability to bear children for some cultures results in a social stigma that can result in a loss of social status and violence. The challenge is how to provide infertility services in a cost-effective and accessible way to all women. However, many countries are less apt to provide infertility services since their ultimate goal may be to control population growth.

Economics

The total expenditure on infertility services in the United States is estimated to be $3 billion per year. While this initially appears to be a significant amount of health care dollars, it represents 0.1% of the total money expended on health care in the United States, which, in 2014, was estimated to be $3 trillion. Many countries provide infertility services within their national health care system. However, insurance

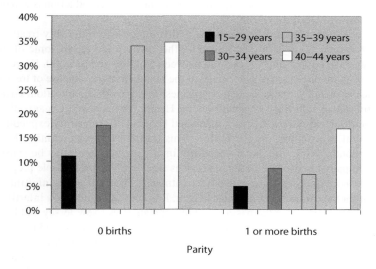

FIGURE 1.1 Percentage of married women 15–44 years of age with 12 months infertility, by parity and age: United States, 2002. Note: the calculation of percentage of infertility in age groups did not include women who had undergone a sterilization procedure. (Data obtained from the National Survey of Family Growth, 2002 [14].)

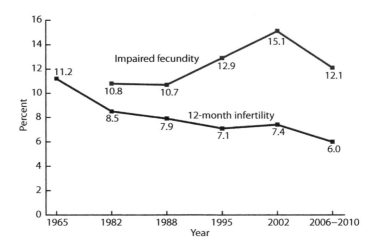

FIGURE 1.2 This figure shows the percentage of married women 15–44 years of age with 12 months infertility, from 1965 to 2010. The rate of infertility has decreased over time (from 8.5% in 1982 to 6.0% in 2006–2010). Impaired fecundity increased from 11% in 1982 to 15% in 2002 but decreased to 12% in 2006–2010. Those women who were surgically sterile were not included in the final calculation. (Data obtained from the National Survey of Family Growth, 1982–2010 and the National Fertility Study, 1965 [16].)

coverage for infertility treatment in the United States is left up to employers and insurance plans, which can be influenced by state insurance mandates. Unfortunately, most American women do not have insurance coverage for this medical problem.

How do we achieve more wide-scale coverage for infertility services? First, the stigma of infertility must be overcome. Society does not view infertility as a medical problem and considers the treatment to be elective, likened to plastic surgery. It is paradoxical that, as a society, there are no qualms about paying for the medical expenses for individuals who have been irresponsible and caused themselves harm with smoking or alcohol abuse. In contrast, for the majority of infertile couples, irresponsible behavior is not a cause of their plight. The solution is to establish infertility as a medical diagnosis. Some states have already done this to some degree but we have to get other states to follow suit. The federal government has also taken a stand—in 1998, the Supreme Court ruled that reproduction is a major life activity under the Americans with Disabilities Act.

The other misconception that must be overcome is that the costs of infertility treatment are a drain on the health care system. This is in part fueled by the costly price tag of some of the treatments. For instance, the average cost of an IVF cycle is between $12,000 and $15,000. However, since those seeking IVF treatment are only a small percentage of the population, the expense of treatment has minimal impact on society, namely, the insurance companies. In a previous publication, Griffin and Panak reported on the impact of infertility expenditures on Health Maintenance Organizations (HMOs) in Massachusetts where infertility coverage is a mandated benefit [19]. Infertility expenditures amounted to only 0.41% of total expenditures by the HMOs. This translates into an additional cost of $1.71 to each member per month. While this is an added minimal expense, there may be substantial savings to the insurance company to cover IVF-related services since high-order multiple pregnancies that are extremely costly are more likely to occur with other treatments. The truth is that infertility coverage is an inexpensive benefit for the insurance companies to bear. Presently, 15 states have infertility mandates in place, but it has been 15 years since the passage of the last state laws (New Jersey and Louisiana, 2001). Unfortunately, as a society, we are dealing with escalating health care costs, and individual states and insurance companies may be reluctant to expand services to the infertile couple.

The consequences of fertility treatments, namely, multiple pregnancies, also pose a cost to society. The utilization of fertility treatments including ovulation induction drugs (with and without inseminations) and IVF has resulted in a significant increase in the number of multiple pregnancies. There is special concern over high-order multiple pregnancies (triplets and more), which have a higher rate of

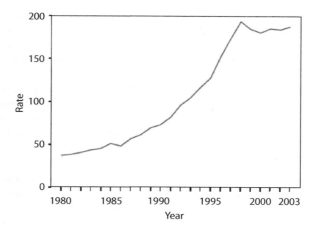

FIGURE 1.3 Rate (per 100,000 live births) of triplet and other higher-order multiple births—United States, 1980–2003. (From CDC, *MMWR* 2005;54(41):1058.)

complications. The rate of high-order multiple pregnancies quadrupled from 1980 to 1997 (37 vs. 174 per 100,000 live born infants) [20]. There is no doubt that this is the result of an increased number of patients seeking infertility treatments. Fortunately, as IVF success rates have continued to increase, most practices are starting to encourage elective single-embryo transfer. Pressure to transfer more than one embryo is more likely to occur if the couple is paying out of pocket for the treatment, which will limit the number of cycles they can afford. A previous report demonstrated that the multiple pregnancy rates were lower in states that had laws in place to provide IVF coverage (38% vs. 43%) [21].

The impact of high-order multiple pregnancies is immense. There is an increased risk of maternal and fetal complications, with the most significant complication being prematurity and its attended consequences. Babies born from triplet pregnancies have a 20% chance of a major handicap, a 17-fold increase in cerebral palsy, and a 20-fold increase in death during the first year after birth (as compared to a singleton pregnancy) [22]. There is a substantial cost to care for these premature infants; the approximate cost estimates in 2010 U.S. dollars for a twin, triplet, and quadruplet pregnancy are $90,000, $260,000, and $400,000 respectively [23]. In the 1990s, there was a concerted effort from the American College of Obstetricians and Gynecologists and the American Society for Reproductive Medicine to develop guidelines to help reduce the number of embryos transferred [24,25]. These efforts have been effective, and since 1997, there has been a plateau in the number of high-order multiple pregnancies (Figure 1.3). In addition, the continued progress in the field has produced higher implantation rates, which also has provided a further impetus to reduce the number of embryos transferred without impacting on pregnancy rates [26]. A change in the way the Centers for Disease Control and Prevention (CDC) reports outcomes of IVF cycles, highlighting the birth of a single, normal-weight term baby, has provided further motivation to consider transferring a single embryo in most cases as the new goal begins to shape public perception.

Ethics

The right to procreate is an undeniable human right. This is not refuted, but the major question in society today is how far are we willing to go with technology to produce an offspring? The surge of ethical issues no doubt has resulted following the advent of IVF and IVF-related procedures. The first IVF success in 1978 was the result of historic work by Drs. Patrick Steptoe and Robert Edwards that spanned almost an entire decade. When it became apparent where they were heading with their research, two notable ethicists, Leon Kass and Paul Ramsey, voiced vehement objections over the direction and ultimate goal of their work [27,28]. The ethical concerns primarily focused on the potential harm to offspring that would be born as a result of IVF. The momentum of their work progressed and ultimately resulted in the birth of Louise Brown in 1978. Soon after, hundreds of IVF centers have opened up in the United States and abroad. It has been estimated that 5 million babies have been born as a result of IVF technology. There have been multiple studies reporting on the babies born from IVF and there is no conclusive evidence that IVF increases the risk of birth defects. Therefore, as we look back, the previous ethical concerns about IVF were unfounded. However, IVF was only the beginning and has been a platform for other treatments including egg donation, gestational surrogacy, and preimplantation genetic diagnosis (PGD), which has resulted in new ethical dilemmas.

There are ongoing ethical concerns about third-party reproduction arrangements, the most common of which is egg donation. The majority of egg donation arrangements are with anonymous donors. While there may be an element of altruism, the main reason why women donate eggs is financial. Egg donors need to be paid for their services, but how much is too much? Advertisements have appeared in college newspapers recruiting prospective donors with a certain level of intelligence, physical characteristics, and athletic ability—with price tags up to $50,000–$100,000. These high prices devalue the whole process and likens egg donation to the trading of a commodity. Most in the field regard these practices as unacceptable. Furthermore, the financial enticement significantly weakens the informed consent process of the egg donor. In addition, it may affect the donor in being forthright in providing important aspects of her medical and family history that could disqualify her. When two professional societies weighed in with guidance to clinicians on what they felt were reasonable fees that could be paid to egg donors without crossing the murky border of trading eggs as a commodity, they were subject to a class action lawsuit. The suit, settled in 2016, caused the societies to remove guidance on compensation to donors from their published guidelines.

PGD and preimplantation genetic screening (PGS) are other developments in IVF and are now being offered by most IVF centers. The first case of PGD was performed on human embryos in 1992 to screen the embryos for cystic fibrosis [29]. The number of genetic conditions that can be tested for by using PGD is virtually limitless. There is no disagreement that PGD should be performed to prevent the transmission of a serious disease, but what is the role of PGS? Presently, we can assess embryos for their chromosomal makeup, which may be beneficial for the woman with repeated miscarriages, the older woman undergoing IVF, or one who is a carrier of a balanced translocation. How do we manage the fertile couple who request PGS for the purposes of sex selection? This brings up several ethical concerns, and while many IVF centers have taken the stand that they will not perform PGS for this purpose, others will offer this service.

Other ethical questions surround IVF when it is not used for reproductive purposes. We have the ability to support the development of the human embryo in the laboratory to the blastocyst stage. At this stage of development, differentiation of the embryo has occurred into the inner cell mass and trophectoderm. Within the inner cell mass are totipotent cells that have the ability to develop into any cell type within the body. In 1998, the first embryonic stem cell line was developed following the isolation of cells from a blastocyst. The possibilities are immense and hundreds if not thousands of cell lines have been established worldwide. Where do these embryos come from? A common source is spare embryos that are already frozen but which couples do not wish to use for further procreative purposes. It is estimated that nearly 1 million cryopreserved human embryos are stored by IVF programs throughout the United States. The fate of most of these embryos is uncertain, but most will not be used by the couple for reproductive purposes. In 2000, Boston IVF was approached by scientists at Harvard University about developing human embryonic stem cell lines from blastocysts. The goal of the work was to better understand the pathogenesis and develop new therapies for type 1 diabetes. The research was privately funded because at that time federal sanctions prohibited the National Institutes of Health from funding this type of research. The research was approved by the Institutional Review Board. Patients who made a decision to discard their embryos were contacted to see if they would be interested in donating them for this research. The response was overwhelming, and many couples donated their spare embryos for this research. Dozens of stem cell lines have been developed, and the research is ongoing. There is ongoing debate in society as to when life begins and whether the use of embryos in this fashion breaches ethical boundaries.

The manipulation of human gametes in the laboratory as part of IVF has also created another possibility, which is cloning. Cloning is not a new concept. In the 1950s, scientists used this technology to successfully clone salamanders and frogs. In the years that followed, the technique was attempted with mammals but was fraught with failure, and it was concluded at that time that mammalian cells were too specialized to clone. However, progress in the area continued, and in 1996, Campbell et al. successfully cloned the first mammal, an adult sheep [30]. To accomplish this feat, these researchers took mammary gland cells from an adult sheep and placed them in a culture solution with only minimal nutrients, essentially starving the cells and caused shutdown of major genetic activity. With an electrical current, they were able to fuse a mammary cell with an enucleated egg cell, which was then transferred into a host uterus. The initial attempts were met with failure, and some abnormal lambs were born and died. Finally, after 300 attempts, they were successful and "Dolly" was born. Other mammals have been cloned since, including cows, mice, pigs, and horses. There are many benefits to cloning. In the agriculture industry, cloning animals allows the creation of better livestock for food production. Cloning animals that have been genetically altered allows the production of human proteins and organs that are suitable for transplantation.

Cloning humans may also be beneficial in fighting disease. The term *therapeutic cloning* refers to a situation where it is possible to differentiate normal heart cells from a stem cell line and inject them back into the diseased heart of an affected individual. This may also prove successful in treating those with spinal cord injuries, leukemia, kidney disease, and other disorders. However, there is concern that human cloning may be used for reproductive purposes. There are many ethical concerns about human reproductive cloning; many find it simply appalling. Several years ago, plans were announced to proceed with human cloning for reproductive purposes. In response, many countries throughout the world have placed a ban on this research. To date, there is no federal legislation in the United States placing a ban on the practice, but many states have enacted their own legislation.

Regulation

There has been a call for the government to step in and regulate the infertility field. One piece of regulation that has been enacted in the United States is the Fertility Clinic Success Rate and Certification Act of 1992. The objective behind the bill and ultimately the law was to make IVF units accountable for their statistics and make the statistics available to the consumers. It is now mandatory for all IVF units to submit their statistics to the CDC on a yearly basis. The impetus behind this legislation is that these published statistics will allow consumers to compare "quality" between centers and help them with their selection. Unfortunately, it does everything but accomplish this goal. By the time the statistics are published, they are 2–3 years old and do not necessarily reflect the practices of any clinic in present time. The outcomes are affected by any clinic's inclusion and exclusion criteria used for patient selection. For instance, a center can increase its success rate by moving patients more quickly to IVF or discouraging those with a lower than average success rate from undergoing the treatment. In addition, clinics are encouraged to transfer more embryos to increase their rate but of course this increases the chance of a multiple pregnancy. Furthermore, some IVF centers are misusing their statistics for self-promotion and advertising. Quite amazingly, statistics are even being used by insurance companies to determine which centers they will contract with. This is a very poor decision and encourages physician practices that are not in the best interest of the patient or the insurance company. Unfortunately, the law is here to stay. There has been a move for states to regulate IVF units especially after the birth of octoplets in California in 2009. Many have previously enacted legislation dealing with embryo research and cloning and there is reason to believe that they will broaden their regulation in other areas of the specialty. Regulation is common abroad as well. Many countries limit the number of embryos that are transferred and some have banned egg donation, sperm donation, and gestational surrogacy.

Conclusion

With the advent of reproductive technologies, infertility has become a complex medical problem with legal, moral, ethical, and financial implications that relate to the infertile couple and society at large. We have come so far and who knows where we will be 20–30 years from now.

REFERENCES

1. Genesis 1:28.
2. Genesis 9:1.
3. Genesis 9:7.
4. Genesis 16:1.
5. Genesis 16:2.
6. *The Aphorisms of Hippocrates*. Translated by Francis Adams. Retrieved May 5, 2006 from: http://etext .library.adelaide.edu.au/mirror/classics.mit.edu/Hippocrates/aphorisms.5.v.html
7. Aristotle. *On the Generation of Animals*. Translated by Arthur Platt. Retrieved May 5, 2006 from: http://etext.library.adelaide.edu.au/a/aristotle/generation/genani1.html
8. Lazzaro Spallanzani. Retrieved May 5, 2006 from: http://www.whonamedit.com/doctor.cfm/2234.html
9. Rubin's Test. *Encyclopedia Britannica*. Retrieved May 5, 2006 from: http://www.britannica.com/eb /article-9064325
10. *Today in Science*. Retrieved May 5, 2006 from: http://www.todayinsci.com/cgi-bin/indexpage.pl?http:// www.todayinsci.com/2/2_06.htm
11. Edwards: The IVF Pioneer. Martin Hutchinson. BBC News online staff. Retrieved May 5, 2006 from: http://news.bbc.co.uk/1/hi/health/3093429.htm
12. Edwards RG, Steptoe PC, Purdy JM. Establishing full-term human pregnancies using cleaving embryos grown in vitro. *Br J Obstet Gynaecol* 1980;87:737–56.
13. International Committee for Monitoring Assisted Reproductive Technologies (ICMART) press release. ESHRE Istanbul; Turkey: July 2012. Assisted Reproductive Technology Success Rates: National Summary and Fertility Clinic Reports. Atlanta: U.S. Department of Health and Human Services; 2010.
14. European Society of Human Reproduction and Embryology (ESHRE). 5 Million Babies. European Society of Human Reproduction and Embryology (ESHRE); 2012. [updated 2012; cited 2015 31.8]; Available from: http://www.eshre.eu/Press-Room/Press-releases/Press-releases-ESHRE-2012/5-million -babies.aspx.
15. Definition of infertility and recurrent pregnancy loss. The Practice Committee of the American Society for Reproductive Medicine. The American Society for Reproductive Medicine, Birmingham, Alabama. *Fertil Steril* 2013;99:63.
16. Chandra A, Copen C, Stephen EH. Infertility and Impaired Fecundity in the United States, 1982–2010: Data from the National Survey of Family Growth. National Center for Health Statistics Report number 67. August 14, 2013. http://www.cdc.gov/nchs/data/nhsr/nhsr067.pdf.
17. World Health Organization. Infertility: A tabulation of available data on prevalence of primary and secondary infertility. Geneva, WHO, Programme on Maternal and Child Health and Family Planning, Division of Family Health, 1991.
18. Cates W, Farley TM, Rowe PJ. Worldwide patterns of infertility: Is Africa different? *Lancet* 1985;2:596–8.
19. Griffin M, Panak WF. The economic cost of infertility-related services: An examination of the Massachusetts infertility insurance mandate. *Fertil Steril* 1998;70:22–9.
20. Martin JA, Park MM. Trends in twin and triplet births: 1980–97. National Vital Statistics Report; vol. 47, no. 24. Hyattsville, Maryland: US Department of Health and Human Services, CDC, National Center for Health Statistics, 1999.
21. Reynolds MA, Schieve LA, Jeng G, Peterson HB. Does insurance coverage decrease the risk for multiple births associated with assisted reproductive technology? *Fertil Steril* 2003;89:16–23.
22. American College of Obstetricians and Gynecologists. Clinical Management Guideline for Obstetricians and Gynecologists. Multiple gestation: Complicated twin, triplet and high order multifetal pregnancy. Number 56, October 2004.
23. ESHRE Capri Workshop Group. Multiple gestation pregnancy. *Hum Reprod* 2000;15:1856–64.
24. American Society for Reproductive Medicine. Guidelines on number of embryos transferred. A Practice Committee Report—A committee Opinion. (Revised). American Society for Reproductive Medicine. 1999.
25. American College of Obstetricians and Gynecologists. Nonselective embryo reduction: Ethical guidance for the obstetrician-gynecologist ACOG Committee Opinion 215. Washington: American College of Obstetricians and Gynecologists, 1999.

26. Tepleton A, Morris JK. Reducing the risk of multiple births by transfer of two embryos after in vitro fertilization. *N Engl J Med* 1998;339(9):573–7.
27. Kass LR. Babies by means of in vitro fertilization: Unethical experiments on the unborn? *N Engl J Med* 1971;285(21):1174–9.
28. Ramsey P. Manufacturing our offspring: Weighting the risks. *Hastings Cent Rep* 1978;8(5):7–9.
29. Handyside AH, Lesko JG, Tarin JJ et al. Birth of a normal girl after in vitro fertilization and preimplantation diagnostic testing for cystic fibrosis. *N Engl J Med* 1992;327:905–9.
30. Campbell KHS, McWhir J, Ritchie WA, Wilmut I. Sheep cloned by nuclear transfer from a cultured cell line. *Nature* 1996;380:64–6.

2

Factors Affecting Fertility

Steven R. Bayer and Merle J. Berger

There are known and unknown factors that affect the human reproductive system. Of the known factors, some can be altered, thereby increasing the chances of pregnancy, while others cannot. An understanding of these factors is important when counseling the infertile couple. Some of the more important factors that have been studied are discussed below.

Maternal Age

The single most important factor that influences a couple's chance of conceiving either naturally or following treatment is the woman's age. This has become more of an issue since many women are delaying their childbearing, which has been a trend noted over the last several decades [1]. In the United States from 1979–2014, the average age of first time mothers has steadily increased by 4.9 years from 21.4 years to 26.3 years [2]. First time mothers that are in the 35- to 39-year age group have increased sixfold over the same time frame [3]. This trend has not only occurred in the United States but has been reported in other developed countries as well. There are many contributory factors to offer an explanation of this trend. Women (including teenagers) are better educated about contraceptive options, are pursuing higher education and careers, and are getting married later. A major problem is that many women are unaware of the age factor and wait until it is too late to pursue a pregnancy. The media has not helped with the reporting of Hollywood celebrities many in their late 40s and even 50s that have achieved pregnancy "on their own" when in fact these pregnancies were achieved with egg donation. For those women who want to delay pregnancy, the advent of egg freezing now allows them to preserve their fertility.

A woman's fertility generally begins to decline after the age of 24, and there is an acceleration of the decline after the age of 37 (Figure 2.1). The frequency of intercourse decreases with age, but this does not solely account for the decline. In the past, there were two theories proposed to explain the decreased fertility, including an age-related uterine dysfunction and reduced egg quality. There was support for the former theory in the animal model. However, the overwhelming success of egg donation in older women has established that the age-related decrease in fertility is the result of declining egg quality.

In one respect, a woman's future fertility is in progressive decline since birth when one considers the contingent of oocytes that reside in the ovaries. Every female is endowed with the highest number of oocytes (6–7 million) in utero at 20 weeks of gestation. The eggs are present in the primordial follicles and arrested in prophase of meiosis I. From this time forward, atresia sets in and the number of oocytes is reduced to 2 million at birth and 600,000–700,000 at puberty. At age 37, a woman has approximately 25,000 eggs—just over 1% of the eggs that she was born with. There are data that suggest that the process of atresia is accelerated after the age of 37 [4]. While there is evidence in the mouse model that oocytes postnatally can undergo mitosis and be replenished, there is no evidence that this occurs in the human [5]. Up until the time of menopause, follicular development is a continuum. The only chance that any follicle will progress to ovulation is that it must be at a critical stage of maturation and rescued by rising FSH levels that only occur for a short period during the early follicular phase.

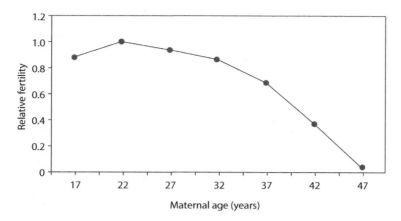

FIGURE 2.1 Relative fertility is graphed according to maternal age. An odds ratio of 1.0 was assigned to the 20- to 24-year age group that has the highest fertility rate. (Modified from Coale AJ, Trussell TJ. *Popul Indes* 1974;40:185–256.)

In addition to the reduced number of eggs that occur with aging, there is reduced quality of the eggs as well. With aging, there is a greater chance that the egg released at ovulation has an abnormal chromosomal contingent that results from faulty meiosis. The actual cause of the aneuploidy is poorly understood but could be the result of dysfunction with the mitotic spindles or a loss of adhesion between sister chromosomes, which would interfere with their alignment during meiosis. These chromosomal imbalances can prevent normal fertilization or halt early embryonic development. Chromosomal abnormalities explain between 70% and 80% of first-trimester losses. Studies performed on embryos resulting from in vitro fertilization (IVF) have confirmed an increased incidence of aneuploidy in embryos arising from older women. In a previous study, the rate of aneuploidy in embryos from women ages 30, 35, 40, and 45 was 23%, 34%, 58%, and 84%, respectively [6]. The increased chance of chromosomal errors with advanced maternal age is further supported by the increased rate of spontaneous abortions and chromosomal anomalies in babies born to older women [7].

Paternal Age

Like their female counterparts, many males are also delaying their time in becoming a father. The impact of paternal age on fertility has been subject of continued debate and the topic of two reviews [8,9]. As do their female counterparts, men experience decreased gonadal function with advancing age. Testosterone production begins to decrease around the age of 40 [10]. A male at age 75 has about half of the circulating free testosterone as a male does in his 20s [11]. Semen parameters also change with aging—there is a decrease in the semen volume, motility, and normal morphology. In review of prior studies, it has been suggested that the aging male has reduced fertility that begins in the late 30s and early 40s. Despite these changes, the reduction in a man's fertility is subtle and, in some men, may be insignificant. While a woman's fertility drops precipitously in the fourth decade, men can maintain their fertility into their 60s and even later. A significant number of pregnancies are fathered by men over the age of 50 in Japan and Germany (Figure 2.2). The oldest father on record is 94 years of age [12]. Further, a review by Dain et al. of 10 studies that examined the impact of paternal age on ART outcome concluded that there were insufficient data to suggest that paternal age altered outcome of IVF treatment [13].

The rate of aneuploidy in oocytes increases with a woman's age and is the cause of most pregnancy losses. Aneuploidy or disomy in sperm may explain some pregnancy losses. The rate of aneuploidy in sperm is 2%, and there is no evidence to support an increased rate of aneuploidy involving autosomes in men with advanced age [14]. However, there are data to support that, with advanced paternal age, there is an increased risk of disomy involving the sex chromosomes [15].

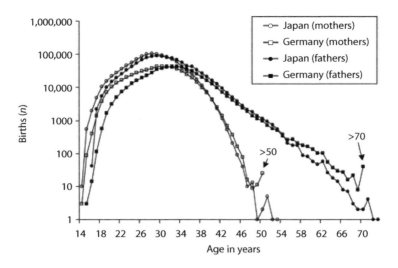

FIGURE 2.2 Maternal and paternal age at the time of birth of offspring born in Germany (2001; n = 550,659) and in Japan (2002; n = 1,135,222). (Reprinted from Kühnert B, Nieschlag E. Reproductive functions of the ageing male. *Human Reproduction Update* 2004 10(4):327–39. Copyright European Society of Human Reproduction and Embryology. Reproduced by permission of Oxford University Press/Human Reproduction.)

Timing of Intercourse

The establishment of pregnancy is dependent on properly timed intercourse around the time of ovulation. Our patients are always asking about the optimal time and frequency of intercourse to maximize their chances. A previous study by Wilcox et al. helps to shed light on this issue [16]. The investigators followed 221 women who were attempting pregnancy. All women kept track of the days they had intercourse and collected daily urine samples, which were then analyzed to determine the day of ovulation. Conception only occurred when intercourse occurred in a 6-day window that ended with the day of ovulation. The investigators confirmed that the greatest chance of pregnancy was when intercourse occurred beginning 2 days before ovulation (Figure 2.3). However, some pregnancies occurred when a single act of intercourse took place 5 days before ovulation. No pregnancies were

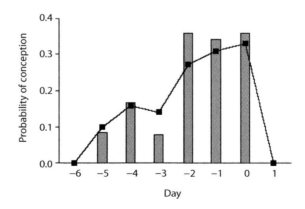

FIGURE 2.3 The conception rates for 129 menstrual cycles were recorded when intercourse occurred on a single day. The day of ovulation is Day 0. No pregnancies resulted when intercourse took place 7 or more days before ovulation or after ovulation. The solid line is an estimate by the model for all 625 cycles. (Reprinted with permission from Wilcox AJ, Weinberg CR, Baird DD. Timing of sexual intercourse in relation to ovulation. *N Engl J Med* 1995;23:1517–21. Copyright 1995 Massachusetts Medical Society. All rights reserved.)

achieved if intercourse only took place after ovulation occurred. The investigators also looked at how the frequency of intercourse affected conception. The greatest chance of pregnancy was when intercourse occurred two to three times during the 6-day time frame. Of interest is that lower pregnancy rates were noted when the frequency of intercourse was between four and six times during the fertile period.

Duration of Attempting Pregnancy

The monthly fecundity rate in the general population has been estimated to be between 15% and 20%, which is influenced by age. In a previous study, Schwartz and Mayaux reported on the cumulative pregnancy rates in 2193 women undergoing donor insemination [17]. The cumulative pregnancy rates after 12 months in the <31, 31–35, and >35 age groups were 73%, 61%, and 54%, respectively [15]. Between 78% and 85% of pregnancies that are achieved occur in the first 6 months of trying [18]. Taking this into consideration, if a couple has failed to achieve pregnancy after 6 months, it seems justified to perform an infertility evaluation and even consider treatment, especially if the woman is over the age of 35. An evaluation may be indicated sooner if there is an obvious or known cause of the infertility (i.e., anovulation, previous ectopic pregnancy, etc.).

Other Factors That Affect Fertility

Previous Contraception

Between 2011 and 2013, the contraceptive agents used by US women (excluding sterilization) were as follows: oral contraceptives, 26%; condoms, 15%; and long-acting reversible agents, 12% [19]. The intrauterine device (IUD) was a popular method of contraception in the 1970s, but one IUD in particular, the Dalkon shield, was linked to a higher risk of pelvic inflammatory disease (PID), which increased the chance of tubal factor infertility. The design of the Dalkon shield was the problem, and it was subsequently taken off the market, and the popularity of the IUD waned at least for the short term. Since safer IUDs have become available, the use of the IUD for contraception has had a resurgence. Between 2002 and 2011, the use of reversible contraceptive agents (IUD, implant) have increased fivefold. A previous meta-analysis concluded that the risk of PID after insertion of the new version IUDs was low but was more prevalent during the first month after insertion when there was a sixfold increase [20].

The impact of the previously used contraceptive agents on future fertility has been a topic of debate. Hassan and Killick reported on the results of a survey of 2841 who presented to antenatal clinic [21]. They analyzed in the study population the time to pregnancy (TTP) for different contraceptive agents that were discontinued. They concluded that TTP was affected by the type of contraception that was previously used. The TTP for the condom, oral contraceptives, IUD, and injection was 4.6, 7.6, 7.5, and 13.6 months, respectively. The TTP results were also affected by the length of use of the oral contraceptive agents and the injectable progestational agent. For women who used oral contraceptives, the TTP was increased to 8.9 months if it was used for >4 years. For those women who used the injectable contraceptive agents, the TTP if the agent was used for <1, 1–2, and 2–4 years was 4.5, 11.2, and 19.1 months, respectively.

Occupational Hazards

Chemical exposures can either result from an environmental exposure or more likely exposure in the workplace. The Occupational Safety and Health Administration (OSHA) regulates the workplace to ensure safety for all employees. Their primary focus is on potential exposures as they relate to general health but they have identified a number of agents that affect reproductive health as well. Of the countless chemical exposures in the workplace, only 1000 chemicals have been evaluated for their reproductive toxicities. It is well established that exposure to nitrous oxide (N_2O) is associated with reduced fertility and spontaneous abortion [22]. Since dental offices are less likely to have scavenging equipment in

TABLE 2.1

Chemical Agents That Have Been Shown to Alter Sperm Production

Chemical Spermatotoxins	
Lead	Dibromochloropropane (DBCP)
Carbaryl	Toluenediamine
Dinitrotoluene	Ethylene dibromide
Welding vapors	Ethylene glycol monoethyl ether
Perchloroethylene	Kepone
Bromine vapor	2,4-Dichlorophenoxy acetic acid

their offices, dental hygienists may be at particular risk [23]. Exposure to other work-related chemicals (i.e., cadmium, mercury, and dry cleaning chemicals) has also been reported to decrease fertility in women.

The male is more susceptible to environmental toxins since spermatogenesis is an ongoing and dynamic process. The first report of an occupationally related spermatotoxin appeared in the mid-1970s [24]. It showed that men who worked at factories that produced DBCP (a pesticide) had an increased incidence of infertility—the severity being dependent on the dose and length of exposure. Since this report was released, other spermatotoxins have been identified, which are listed in Table 2.1.

OSHA requires that all employers must have Material Safety Data Sheets (MSDS) available at the workplace for all exposures that the worker comes in contact with and they are readily available to the worker. The MSDS detail all known risks of the exposure on general health and reproductive health.

Diet

There are no data to suggest that any particular diet per se can affect fertility. However, the consequences of an inadequate diet with extremes of body weight can alter ovarian function and predispose women to infertility. Women with a body mass index (BMI) <19 or body fat content <22% are at risk for hypothalamic dysfunction affecting ovulation. At the other extreme, women with increased body weight may have associated polycystic ovarian syndrome, which can cause ovulatory dysfunction as well. There is growing evidence that increased body weight itself may reduce fertility aside from its impact on ovulatory function. In a study published by Boston IVF, Ryley et al. performed a retrospective study of more than 6000 IVF cycles [25]. When controlling for other factors, the conclusion was that, with advanced body weight, there is a statistically significant drop in implantation and pregnancy rates. Males with an elevated BMI have been confirmed to have a greater chance of altered sperm parameters and reduced fertility. Unfortunately, there is an epidemic of obesity in the United States, which is a contributory factor to the incidence of infertility. All patients should be encouraged to have a well-balanced diet, engage in regular exercise, and try to achieve a target BMI between 20 and 25.

Lifestyle Habits

There are many lifestyle habits that can affect our general health, and there is reason to believe that they may also have an impact on fertility.

Smoking

Of all of the lifestyle issues, smoking is the most significant. Smoking is a confirmed reproductive toxin. The deleterious effects of smoking during pregnancy are well established. Several published studies have demonstrated that smoking in women is associated with decreased fertility [26,27]. Smoking reduces a woman's chances of conceiving by almost half. Smoking can alter ovarian function in a number of ways [28]. The chemicals in smoke stimulate the hepatic metabolism of steroid hormones, thereby reducing their levels in the bloodstream. In vitro studies have demonstrated that the chemicals in smoke alter the enzymes that are necessary for ovarian hormone production. Finally, women who smoke generally go through an earlier menopause by 1–2 years, suggesting that the chemicals in smoke may be directly toxic to the ovaries. It is not known whether this is attributed to a direct action on the ovaries or indirectly through an alteration of the blood flow to the ovary. The published data are compelling enough to advise all women who smoke to stop to improve their fertility. Electronic cigarettes are advertised as a safer alternative to traditional smoking since they only contain nicotine and are devoid of all the other deleterious chemicals. However, there are no published data to support its safety while attempting pregnancy.

Caffeine Intake

The impact of caffeine on fertility and pregnancy outcome has been debated for years. Daily intake of caffeine at high doses (>500 mg; >5 cups of coffee/day) has been associated with reduced fertility [29]. During pregnancy, moderate caffeine intake (<200 mg/day) does not increase the risk of miscarriage, preterm labor, or intrauterine growth restriction (IUGR) [30]. The quantity of caffeine in beverages is variable. The average amount in a cup of coffee, tea, and a can of soda is approximately 100, 50, and 50 mg, respectively. Chocolate is another source of caffeine and contains 12 mg of caffeine per ounce. Daily intake of caffeine <200 mg/day appears to be safe during the preconception period and pregnancy.

Alcohol

The ill effects of alcohol on pregnancy are well established. However, the influence of alcohol on fertility has not been well studied. In 1998, two separate studies that examined the impact of alcohol on the establishment of pregnancy were published [31,32]. Both studies arrived at the same conclusion that alcohol, in a dose-dependent fashion, reduced the chance of a conception in the study populations. In a previous study of women undergoing IVF treatment, it was shown that those who had four or more alcoholic drinks per week had a reduced chance of achieving pregnancy (odds ratio, 0.86; confidence interval, 0.71–0.99), which was statistically significant [33]. Women undergoing fertility treatment should avoid alcohol once the treatment cycle is begun. There are no published data that suggest that moderate alcohol use affects male reproduction.

A previous study by Hassan and Killick lends further support to the idea that a healthy lifestyle improves fertility [34]. The investigators looked at the combined effects of lifestyle issues on the establishment of a pregnancy. More than 2000 women who presented for prenatal care were asked about lifestyle issues and then the investigators determined the TTP. The investigators confirmed that the TTP was delayed if the woman or her partner smoked, the partner consumed >20 units of alcohol per week, caffeine intake was >6 drinks per day, and the woman's BMI was >25 kg/m^2. Since many couples had multiple factors, the authors calculated the cumulative pregnancy rate when more than one factor was present (Figure 2.4).

Stress and Anxiety

There continues to be an ongoing debate about the role of stress in infertility. Lingering questions continue: Is stress a cause of infertility? Can stress decrease a woman's chance of pregnancy while undergoing treatment? For those patients who are stressed, what interventions are effective? There is no doubt that most patients that are seen at fertility clinics are stressed. For some patients, the stress and anxiety preceded their desire for pregnancy, whereas for others, it worsened or newly developed as a reaction to the disappointment of their situation. The stress associated with infertility is intense and is similar to the stress associated with a serious medical condition, such as cancer or HIV. In a previous study, it was reported that up to 40% of infertile women had anxiety or depression [35]. This is significant when one considers the incidence of anxiety/depression in the general population, which is 3%. Does stress prevent a woman from achieving pregnancy? Many of us have firsthand stories about the patient who conceives after a relaxing vacation or the woman who has battled years of infertility and then proceeds with a successful adoption then is surprised to learn she has achieved pregnancy on her own. These situations no doubt raise suspicion about the role of stress. While it may be difficult to prove that stress is a cause of infertility, there are data to suggest that it may reduce the chance of success with treatment.

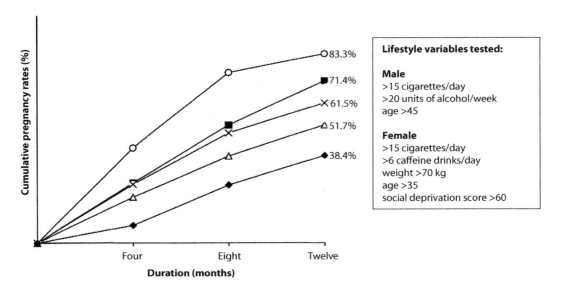

FIGURE 2.4 The effect of increasing numbers of lifestyle issues on the cumulative pregnancy rates within 1 year for a pregnant population. The lifestyle variables are presented in the box adjacent to the graph. Each line is the cumulative pregnancy rate for subgroups with different numbers of negative lifestyle variables: ○, No negative variables; ■, 1 negative variable; ×, 2 negative variables; △, 3 negative variables; ♦, 4 or more negative variables. (Reprinted from Hassan MAM, Killick SR. Negative lifestyle is associated with a significant reduction in fecundity. *Fertil Steril* 2004;81:384–92, with permission from the American Society for Reproductive Medicine.)

In a previous review, the majority of the published studies examining this issue concluded that anxiety and stress reduced a patient's chance of success with treatment [36]. In another publication, the largest investigation to date reported on a prospective study that involved 818 couples who were screened with a stress inventory at the start of treatment and then 12 months later treatment outcomes were determined. After controlling for female age and years of infertility, the authors concluded that female and male stress affected outcome of the treatment. There are different interventions we can offer our patients to counter the stress. Those that offer cognitive–behavioral intervention seem to be the most effective in decreasing anxiety and improving success rates [37,38]. While significant progress has been made, further research is needed to provide a better understanding of the role of stress and fertility.

Conclusions

There are many factors that ultimately affect a couple's chances of conceiving naturally or with reproductive technology. While some factors can be altered, thereby increasing the chances of pregnancy, others cannot. The single most important factor that affects a couple's chance of conceiving is the woman's age. A major challenge we face in reproductive medicine is to educate the populace about the impact of age, thereby preventing some women from delaying childbearing too long.

REFERENCES

1. Mathews TJ, Hamilton BE. Delayed childbearing: More women are having their first child later in life. NCHS Data Brief no. 21, August, 2009.
2. National Center Health Statistics Data Brief No. 232, January 2016.
3. National Center Health Statistics CHS Data Brief No. 152, May 2014.
4. Faddy MJ, Gosden RG, Gougeon A et al. Accelerated disappearance of ovarian follicles in mid-life: Implications for forecasting menopause. *Hum Reprod* 1992;7:1342–6.

5. Johnson J, Canning J, Kaneko T et al. Germline stem cells and follicular renewal in the postnatal mammalian ovary. *Nature* 2004;428:145–50.

6. Franasiak JM, Forman EJ, Hong KH. The nature of aneuploidy with increasing age of the female patner: A review of 15,169 consectutive trophectoderm biopsies evalauted with comprehensive chromosomal screning. *Fertil Steril* 2014;101:656–63.

7. Hook EB, Cross PK, Schreinemachers DM. Chromosomal abnormality rates at amniocentesis and in live-born infants. *J Am Med Assoc* 1983;249:2034–8.

8. Sartorius GA, Nieschlag E. Paternal age and reproduction. *Hum Reprod Update* 2010;16:65–79.

9. Kühnert B, Nieschlag E. Reproductive functions of the ageing male. *Human Reproduction Update* 2004;10(4):327–39.

10. Vermeulen A. Androgens in the aging male. *J Clin Endocrinol Metal* 1991;73:221–4.

11. Goemaere S, Van Pottelbergh I, Zmierczak H et al. Inverse association between bone turnover rate and bone mineral density in community-dwelling men >70 years of age: No major role of sex steroid status. *Bone* 2001;29:286–91.

12. Seymour FI, Duffy C, Koerner A. A case of authenticated fertility in a man, aged 94. *J Am Med Assoc* 1935;105:1423–4.

13. Dain L, Auslander R, Dirnfeld M. The effect of paternal age on assisted reproduction outcome. *Fertil Steril* 2011;95:1–8.

14. Luetjens, CM, Rolf C, Gassner P et al. Sperm aneuploidy rates in younger and older men. *Hum Reprod* 2002;17:1826–32.

15. Lowe X, Eskenazi B, Nelson DO et al. Frequency of XY sperm increase with age in fathers of boys with Klinefelters syndrome. *Am J Hum Genet* 2001;69:1046–54.

16. Wilcox AJ, Weinberg CR, Baird DD. Timing of sexual intercourse in relation to ovulation. *N Engl J Med* 1995;23:1517–21.

17. Schwartz D, Mayaux MJ. Female fecundity as a function of age: Results of artificial insemination of 2193 nulliparous women with azoospermic husbands. Federation CECOS. *N Engl J Med* 1982;306(7):404–6.

18. Ford WCL, North K, Taylor H et al. Increasing paternal age is associated with delayed conception in a large population of fertile couples: Evidence for declining fecundity in older men. *Hum Reprod* 2000;15:1703–8.

19. Use of Contraception in the United States: 2011–2013. Center for Disease Control (CDC). *Vital & Health Statistics*; Series 173; December 2014.

20. Grimes DA, Schulz KF. Antibiotic prophylaxis for intrauterine contraceptive device insertion. Cochrane Review. In: *The Cochrane Library*, Issue 3, 2004. Chichester, UK: John Wiley & Sons, Ltd.

21. Hassan MAM, Killick SR. Is previous use of hormonal contraception associated with a detrimental effect on subsequent fecundity? *Hum Reprod* 2004;19:344–51.

22. Cohen EN, Gift HC, Brown BW et al. Occupational disease in dentistry and chronic exposure to trace anesthetic gases. *J Am Dent Assoc* 1980;101:21–31.

23. Rowland AS, Baird DD, Weinber CR et al. Reduced fertility among women employed as dental assistants exposed to high level so nitrous oxide. *N Engl J Med* 1992;327(14):993–7.

24. Cohen EN, Bellville JW, Brown BW Jr. Anesthesia, pregnancy and miscarriage: A study of operating room nurses and anesthetists. *Anesthesiology* 1971;35:343–7.

25. Ryley DA, Bayer SR, Eaton A et al. Influence of body mass index (BMI) on the outcome of 6,827 IVF cycles. *Fertil Steril* 2004;82:S38–S39.

26. De Mouzon J, Spira A, Schwartz D. A prospective study of the relation between smoking and fertility. *Int J Epidemiol* 1988;17:378–84.

27. Bolumar F, Olsen J, Boldsen J. Smoking reduces fecundity: A European multicenter study on infertility and subfecundity. European Study Group on Infertility Subfecundity. *Am J Epidemiol* 1996;143:578–87.

28. Smoking and Women's Health. Education Bulletin, Number 240. American College of Obstetricians & Gynecologists, 1997.

29. Bolumar F, Olsen J, Rebagliato M, Bisanti L. Caffeine intake and delayed conception: A European multicenter study on infertility and subfecundity. European Study Group on Infertility Subfecundity. *Am J Epidemiol* 1997;15:324–34.

30. The American College of Obstetricians and Gynecologists. Committee Opinion; Moderate caffeine consumption during pregnancy. Number 462, 2015.

31. Jensen TK, Hjollund NHI, Henriksen TB et al. Does moderate alcohol consumption affect fertility? Follow up study among couples planning first pregnancy. *Br Med J* 1998;317:505–10.

32. Hakim RB, Gray RH, Zacur H. Alcohol and caffeine consumption and decreased fertility. *Fertil Steril* 1998;70:632–7.

33. Rossi BV, Berry KF, Hornstein MD et al. Effect of alcohol consumption on in vitro fertilization. *Obstet Gynecol* 2011;117:136.

34. Hassan MAM, Killick SR. Negative lifestyle is associated with a significant reduction in fecundity. *Fertil Steril* 2004;81:384–92.

35. Chen TH, Chang SP, Tsai CF, Juang KD. Prevalence of depressive and anxiety disorders in an assisted reproductive technique clinic. *Hum Reprod* 2004;19:2313–8.

36. Domar AD. Infertility and the mind/body connection. *The Female Patient* 2005;30:24–8.

37. Tuschen-Caffier B, Florin I, Karuse W, Pook M. Cognitive–behavioral therapy for idiopathic infertile couples. *Psychother Psychosom* 1999;68:15–21.

38. Domar AD, Clapp D, Slawsby EA et al. Impact of group psychological interventions on pregnancy rates in infertile women. *Fertil Steril* 2000;73:805–11.

3

The Infertility Workup

Jesse Hade

Introduction

The decision to seek medical attention occurs when a couple or an individual chooses to conceive but fails to do so in a timely manner. Some who seek care may consider themselves infertile but actually do not meet the criteria for immediate testing or treatment. It is necessary to understand the underlying concerns and nature of the patient's complaint and problem in order to best counsel, test, and render treatment when necessary.

Traditionally, women 35 years and younger, who fail to achieve pregnancy within 1 year of regular unprotected intercourse or therapeutic donor insemination, are considered infertile. However, this threshold is lowered to only 6 months of unprotected intercourse or therapeutic donor insemination, for women over the age of 35. Urgent attention is advised for women over the age of 40 who deserve immediate evaluation and treatment regardless of the duration of unprotected intercourse or use of donor insemination [1].

This change in threshold for evaluation and treatment based on female age is attributed to the change in fecundity. Fecundity is the monthly pregnancy or fertility rate. In humans, this rate declines with advancing female's age. For women under the age of 35, a monthly fecundity of 25% to 35% is expected within the first 6 months of conception, but women 40 years of age will expect only a 5% to 10% monthly pregnancy rate during this same time frame. The fecundity rates decline at an accelerated rate with each year of life beyond age 40 and will be 1% or less by age 45.

Not only does age affect fertility rates but so does the duration of failed conception. It is known that the monthly fecundity and probability of pregnancy are greatest within the first 3 months of coitus or insemination and decline precipitously with the increased duration of failed conception [2]. For young women, this translates into an 80%–90% chance of pregnancy within 1 year of unprotected intercourse with only an additional 5% to 15% chance of conceiving within the next 12 months of unprotected intercourse or donor insemination [3]. It is estimated that nearly 11% of all women age 15–44 in the United States have impaired fecundity and less than half ever seek out care and treatment [4].

Therefore, it is critical to understand that the above guidelines do not justify withholding needed care to those patients who may require earlier evaluation and treatment when physical findings and medical history warrant it.

Causes of Infertility

It has been estimated that one-third of all causes of infertility originate in the female, one-third in the male, and the remaining third are attributed to combined female and male factors. For the woman, contributing aspects include diminished ovarian reserve, endometriosis, disorders of ovulation, uterine abnormalities, tubal disease, and unexplained infertility. Men may experience spermatogenic problems related to both hypothalamic–pituitary impairment and anatomic testicular abnormalities and dysfunction. The role of the physician is to carefully assess the couple to determine which of any of the above are relevant and target treatment to the identified impairment.

Initial Consultation and Physical Exam

The initial consultation between the physician and the patient is the crucial first step in understanding the needs of the individual seeking your advice and care. An extensive history and physical examination for both the patient and her partner are necessary. A detailed history and focused review of systems should take between 30–80 minutes with an average of 60 minutes. Findings suggestive of an endocrine disorder should be sought. Screening for thyroid disease, hyperprolactinemia, galactorrhea, and hirsutism should be scrutinized and addressed in all patients. During the initial consultation, the clinician should attempt to define if the patient suffers from pelvic pain, dysmenorrhea, dyspareunia, or vaginismus since they all may have an impact on the likelihood of conception. It is for this reason that even women who desire to achieve pregnancy using donor sperm deserve a detailed evaluation before treatment.

A relevant history should contain information regarding all known medical problems including current and past medication usage, drug, latex, and food allergies as well as prior screening or treatment for a suspected clotting or thromboembolic disorder. Chemotherapy and radiation exposure for the treatment of a known malignancy should also be addressed at this time.

A gynecologic history encompassing the timing of puberty and menstrual cycle frequency with length and amount of flow is an essential component to identify. Details regarding ovulatory dysfunction, polycystic ovarian syndrome (PCOS), endometriosis, uterine leiomyomas, tubal disease, pelvic infection, and information pertaining to past abdominal, pelvic, and uterine surgeries should be documented. Although it may be intuitive to the clinician, coital frequency, number of prior sexual partners, and details pertaining to past fertility testing and treatments are all essential components to the infertility workup.

Obstetrical information regarding all prior pregnancies with known complications should be recorded. Details such as cervical incompetence, preterm labor or delivery, preeclampsia, gestational diabetes, ectopic pregnancy, multiple gestation, and prior miscarriages are also important facets to help the clinician determine relevant testing and treatment options of care.

A comprehensive family history should detail information regarding known cancers or inheritable malignancies. Family members with mental retardation, autism, or other known genetic, congenital, or inheritable conditions should be identified. In addition, personal information pertaining to the patient's ethnic background will help the clinician determine which preconception tests are appropriate to order. Social and dietary habits including alcohol and caffeine consumption, cigarette and illicit drug use, and body mass index (BMI) calculations, along with exercise and lifestyle choices all have an impact on a patient's fertility and ability to conceive. The psychological well-being of the patient is critical to a successful outcome. Thus, risk factors including stress, depression, and anxiety should be evaluated and addressed before pregnancy.

When applicable, all male partners should be questioned to determine their ability to achieve a successful erection with ejaculation during coitus. Information pertaining to a prior exposure to mumps as well as sexually transmitted diseases should be established. The use of specific medications known to interfere with male fertility including testosterone, 5-α reductase inhibitors, β-blockers, and phosphodiesterase inhibitors should be documented and possibly discontinued when appropriate [5]. Prior testicular and pelvic surgeries as well as chemotherapy and radiation exposure are critical pieces of information to obtain during the history. All prior sperm tests or relationships resulting in pregnancy should be divulged.

A complete physical and gynecologic examination should be performed after the initial consultation. The exam should contain a complete set of vital signs including blood pressure, pulse rate, and respiratory rate, as well as measurements of both weight and height to calculate BMI. The clinician should describe all thyroid, breast, cardiac, and respiratory abnormalities. When nipple discharge is present, simple microscopy may help determine if it is galactorrhea. Nearly 70% of women with galactorrhea will have hyperprolactinemia. Conversely, only 30% to 40% of women with hyperprolactinemia will have galactorrhea [6]. Vaginal and cervical discharge as well as uterine size, shape, and position should be noted when abnormal. If possible, adnexal tenderness, masses, and pelvic or vaginal nodules should be identified, since these may be signs of underlying endometriosis.

Patients with complaints of hirsutism and ovulatory dysfunction should have a thorough exam to describe the extent of their androgen excess. The clinician should focus attention to findings such as hair coarseness, distribution, and density pertaining to patient's face, body, and extremities and document symptoms of male pattern hair loss on the head when present. Signs of virilization include increased muscle mass and cliteromegaly. For those patients suspected of cortisol excess, denote the color, size, and location of abdominal striae, and indicate if fat disposition around the neck, face, and extremities has changed.

Men suspected of having spermatogenic, urogenital, or pelvic problems should have their examination performed by a trained professional. An individual with expertise in urology should perform the exam and focus on the presence or absence of varicoceles, document testicular location and size using an orchidometer, and identify congenital malformations of the epididymis, vas deferens, phallus, and meatal opening. A prostate examination may also be necessary for men with low or absent ejaculate.

Overall, the infertility evaluation can be initiated by a less experienced provider, but once an abnormal test is identified, the referral to a specialist with an infertility background is strongly recommended. It is known that the immediate referral of these patients to a physician with infertility training and expertise can reduce the overall emotional stress, cost, and time to conception [7]. The physical, psychological, and emotional well-being of both the patient and partner are all essential parts of the infertility process, and the practitioner should be a cognoscente of these factors when creating an appropriate plan of care.

Testing

Testing for both the patient and partner should be focused and streamlined to identify only the relevant factors necessary to render treatment. The practitioner should refrain from ordering redundant and superfluous tests and should make every effort to reduce both the emotional and financial burdens associated with this phase of the evaluation. For the female partner, a multitude of testing is performed during specific intervals of the menstrual cycle. Testing often begins with the onset of menses and usually takes one full menstrual cycle to complete. Once completed, the patient and her partner should return for a consultation to discuss realistic goals and expectations regarding their overall chance of pregnancy and delivery. After all options of care are reviewed, a treatment plan should be created and enacted in both a judicious and expedited manner.

It is critical to understand that test results do not predict outcome. Regardless of a test's sensitivity or specificity, or how encouraging or discouraging a result may be, the chance of delivering a live born child cannot be determined by any single or combination of tests. Testing can only determine what therapeutic options the patient or couple has (all options vs. limited or no options) and if the patient has an average or less than average probability of conception compared to age-matched peers. Religious, ethical, psychological, and physiologic factors are all influential aspects in the decision-making process. It is for this reason that test results should not be used in a punitive manner and deny patients the opportunity to undergo treatment when deemed applicable. Rather, study results should be used to inform patients of their treatment options and inform them when a lower than predicted chance of success is anticipated and what, if anything, could be done to improve outcome.

Ovarian Function

Ovarian function and ovarian reserve testing are each performed at specific intervals during the menstrual cycle. Ovarian function tests are used to determine if and when ovulation occurs and ovarian reserve testing is used to determine the density of remaining oocytes available to compete for ovulation.

A variety of methods are available to assess the timing of ovulation. Low-tech methods include daily basal body temperature (BBT) charting or mid-cycle luteinizing hormone (LH) urinary predictor kit testing. A more sophisticated higher-cost strategy involves both blood work and pelvic ultrasound to evaluate follicular growth and function. A day 16 to 24 progesterone level can also be obtained to confirm that ovulation occurred. This last step is valuable for patients with irregular menstrual cycles and chronic anovulation. However, ovulation can be inferred to occur in women who have regular menstrual cycles, with lengths ranging from 21 to 35 days and who have intercycle variability of less than 5 days between menses.

BBT Charting

BBT charting is the simplest and least expensive method to evaluate and determine if ovulation has occurred. For consistency, temperature measurements are recorded daily, upon awakening and before any physical activity, eating, or drinking. These temperature determinations can be recorded at other times during the day, but they need to be obtained at the same time daily. The follicular or pre-ovulatory phase of the menstrual cycle can vary in length from one menstrual cycle to the next. However, the luteal phase should constantly last 14 days from the time of ovulation to menses (assuming that pregnancy has not been achieved). After ovulation, the patient's body temperature will be between 0.4°F to 1.1°F higher than what was recorded before ovulation. This phenomenon in temperature change is directly related to the secretion of progesterone from the corpus luteum. Progesterone acts directly on the temperature, regulating neurons within the hypothalamus and CNS to increase thermogenesis and increase body temperature [8]. In ovulatory women, this post-ovulation spike in temperature will persist until menses and forms what is called a "biphasic" pattern in the patient's temperature log. Anovulatory women will not see this biphasic pattern in temperature change, nor will they report any significant change in daily temperature throughout their observations. BBT charting requires a minimum of 3 to 4 months of measurements to determine a patient's fertile period and only retrospectively predicts ovulation within a 3-day window [9].

Home Ovulation Predictor Kits

Most home ovulation predictor kits measure urinary concentrations of LH only. The LH surge is necessary to induce ovulation and usually occurs 24 to 36 hours before ovulation [10]. However, the timing of the LH surge and measurement of peak values vary based on assay quality and are often difficult to interpret and unfortunately inaccurate in their predictive usefulness. In an effort to improve the accuracy of these home tests, some predictor kits measure other hormones such as estrone-3-glucuronide (E3G) in addition to peak LH levels. E3G is a metabolite of estrogen formed after oxidation within the liver and peaks 12 to 24 hours before ovulation. This weak form of estrogen begins to rise approximately 3 days before ovulation but then declines to negligible levels 5 days later [11]. The hypothalamic–pituitary–ovarian axis is tonically under negative feedback control. Just before ovulation, a transformation occurs, inducing a positive feedback system. This phenomenon transpires when 17β-estradiol (E2) levels are sustained for at least 36 hours, with peak values ranging from 150 pg/mL or greater. Once released from its follicle, the oocyte has only 12 to 24 hours to be fertilized. If fertilization does not occur, then the process of apoptosis will begin and the demise of the egg will be inevitable [12]. It is for this reason that home ovulation predictor kit accuracy is essential to help predict the appropriate time for fertilization after ovulation.

Pelvic Ultrasound and Blood Work

A more precise predictor of ovulation can be achieved with the use of both blood work and a pelvic ultrasound. Unlike LH urinary predictor kits, blood measurements of E2, LH, and progesterone can be compared with findings observed on a pelvic ultrasound to best predict the occurrence of ovulation. Patients who have an ovarian follicle with a diameter greater than 18 mm associated with an E2 level over 150 pg/mL and LH level over 15 mIU/mL with a progesterone value of under 2.0 ng/mL have a high probability of ovulation within 24 to 48 hours after the documentation of those observations. This method of testing is expensive but useful for patients with PCOS and chronic anovulation. These patients typically have LH values near or at the pre-ovulatory range but without meeting any of the other findings typical of the mid-cycle.

Day 16–24 Progesterone Levels

Before ovulation, the ovary secretes primarily estrogen in the form of estradiol. After ovulation, the secretory environment of the ovary changes from that of estrogen to one dominated by the secretion of progesterone. This change is attributed to a loss in the population of cells during ovulation, which contain the enzyme necessary for estradiol production. Progesterone levels above 3 ng/mL are most commonly associated with ovulation and then progressively increase to peak 7 days later [13]. Following the peak, progesterone levels continually decline over the next 7 days until levels again fall to pre-ovulatory values and menses ensues.

Endometrial Biopsy

Endometrial biopsy is a simple and minimally invasive office procedure used to evaluate the endometrial cavity for both histologic and pathologic changes. Women experiencing abnormal vaginal bleeding often undergo this procedure to determine if an underlying infectious, premalignant or malignant process is occurring. Dating of the endometrium has long been the gold standard in evaluating infertile women for a suspected luteal phase defect [14]. More recently, this process has been replaced by the endometrial receptivity array (ERA) test. This is because histologic dating lacks the ability to distinguish fertile from infertile women [15]. The ERA test can more precisely determine an individual's window of implantation [16]. The ERA test accomplishes this by evaluating the mRNA levels within endometrial tissue to identify a specific molecular profile known as a "Transcriptomic Signature" [17]. Overall, 25% of patients undergoing in vitro fertilization (IVF) with recurrent failed embryo transfers will have an endometrium deemed "out of phase" when compared to the exact day of progesterone exposure. To improve pregnancy rates, the ERA test evaluates endometrial transcriptomic signatures and then recommends a new personalized change in the day of embryo transfer in relation to the day of progesterone exposure.

Ovarian Reserve Testing

The assessment of ovarian reserve begins with the onset of menses and is generally performed during day 2 to day 4 of bleeding. Reserve testing usually entails both blood work and a pelvic ultrasound. Hormonal levels from the pituitary gland and ovary are evaluated and correlated with the total antral follicle count (AFC) obtained during the pelvic ultrasound. Collectively, an estimate of the patient's reproductive potential can be made [18]. A patient's ovarian reserve best describes oocyte quantity and a patient's age best depicts oocyte quality. For young women under the age of 35, each oocyte has roughly a 10% probability of pregnancy and live birth. However, this rate declines rapidly with advancing age with pregnancy and delivery rates declining to 5% per oocyte by age 40 and to 1% or less by age 45 [19,20]. It is for this reason that young patients with diminished ovarian reserve have a better chance of pregnancy and live birth compared to women with advanced maternal age and a robust ovarian reserve [21].

Antral Follicle Count

The AFC is determined at the time of the initial pelvic ultrasound, and every follicle with a diameter between 2 and 10 mm is counted. Each ovary should contain at least 5 to 11 follicles. Young patients and patients with PCOS typically have high AFCs, with a minimum of 12 or more follicles per ovary. Women with diminished ovarian reserve usually have four or fewer antral follicles visualized per ovary. Some studies suggest that the AFC is the best predictor of an age-related decline in ovarian reserve and overall oocyte production during an IVF cycle [22,23].

Day 3 Hormone Testing

Another strategy regularly used to predict ovarian reserve is the serum measurement of specific pituitary and ovarian hormones on day 2 to day 4 of the menstrual cycle. Hormones commonly measured include anti-Müllerian hormone (AMH), follicle-stimulating hormone (FSH), estradiol (E2), and Inhibin-B. All four of these hormones independently reflect the follicular pool and can predict ovarian response to gonadotropins better than age alone.

AMH is a dimeric glycoprotein and a member of the transforming growth factor-β superfamily. It is directly secreted from ovarian granulosa cells located on preantral and antral follicles. AMH levels tend to be more consistent between menstrual cycles and are in dependent of the cycle day obtained. In young women, AMH values are normally above 2 ng/mL, but overtime, they progressively decline to become undetectable, approximately 5 years before menopause (Figure 3.1). Values of less than 1 ng/mL indicates a diminished ovarian reserve and are associated with both a poor response to ovarian stimulation and a lower likelihood of pregnancy after oocyte retrieval and embryo transfer [24].

Factors known to have a detrimental effect on ovarian reserve include chemotherapeutic drugs, ionizing radiation, and endometriosis [25]. Operative procedures involving the ovary or its blood supply can also impact and lower reserve. The surgical resection of an ovarian endometrioma permanently results in a post-procedural decrease in ovarian reserve with up to a 66% drop in serum AMH levels after the procedure. However, other surgeries including bilateral salpingectomy or routine ovarian cystectomy (for a cyst other than an endometrioma) have no lasting effect on AMH values after the procedure [26]. Paradoxically, low AMH values can be observed in some women with a normal ovarian reserve. The clinician should be aware that obesity, hypothalamic failure, use of oral contraceptive pills, and prolonged exposure to gonadotropin-releasing hormone agonists all artificially lower serum AMH levels [27,28]. For these women, AMH alone does not accurately reflect ovarian reserve and actions should be taken to either correct the underlying pathophysiologic problem or discontinue the offending medical therapy, before retesting or starting treatment.

Other common endocrine markers used to assess ovarian reserve include a day 3 serum FSH and an estradiol level. Despite their capricious cycle-to-cycle variability, these two hormones when measured together are useful prognostic indicators of low ovarian reserve and reduced response to ovarian stimulation [29]. Single measurements of either FSH or E2 alone are unreliable and not predictive and should not be routinely obtained. Women who have a normal ovarian reserve demonstrate FSH levels below

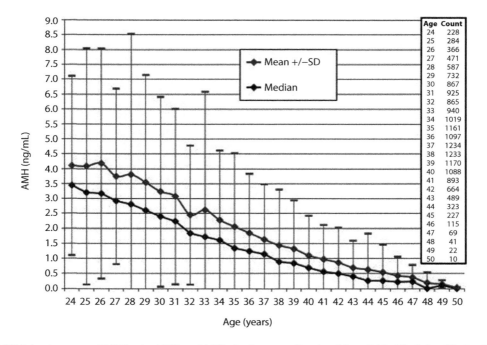

FIGURE 3.1 Age versus AMH levels. AMH, anti-Müllerian hormone. (Reprinted from Seifer DB, Baker VL, Leader B. Age-specific serum anti-Müllerian hormone values for 17,120 women presenting to fertility centers within the United States. *Fertil Steril* 2011;95:747–50, with permission from the American Society for Reproductive Medicine.)

10 mIU/mL and E2 levels below 60 pg/mL during the early follicular phase of the menstrual cycle. As women age and ovarian reserve diminishes, the mechanism controlling the communication and regulation of ovulation breaks down. As a result, an acceleration of follicular development during the late luteal into the early follicular phase of the succeeding menstrual cycle occurs. Eventually, the hypothalamus and pituitary gland become insensitive to rising E2 levels and the pituitary gland becomes uninhibited and releases increasing amounts of FSH into the circulation. Day 3 FSH levels will often rise above 10 mIU/mL despite having E2 levels greater than 70 pg/mL. This lack of negative feedback control of E2 on the release of FSH from the pituitary gland is an impending sign of low ovarian reserve and a lower reproductive potential.

Overall, anti-Müllerian hormone appears to be the best endocrine marker for assessing an age-related decline in ovarian reserve and can strongly predict a poor response to ovarian stimulation [30]. However, nearly 20% of women who have a reassuring day 3 FSH value under 10 mIU/mL will have a worrying AMH value below 1 ng/mL. Conversely, 5% of women with a normal AMH value will have an elevated and concerning day 3 FSH level. This discordance in values between a day 3 FSH and AMH clearly justifies measuring both day 3 FSH and E2 in addition to a serum AMH level to better predict and detect patients with a diminished ovarian reserve [31].

Clomiphene Citrate Challenge Test

Clomiphene citrate (CC) is a selective estrogen receptor modulator and is composed of a mixture of the two geometric isomers En-clomiphene (*trans*-isomer) and Zu-clomiphene (*cis*-isomer). Since both isomers have different half-lives and affinities for the various estrogen receptors within the tissues of the body, a mixed estrogenic and antiestrogenic reaction is often observed. CC exerts its functions through competitive inhibition of estrogen for its receptor. When administered, CC blocks the negative feedback effect of estrogen on both the hypothalamus and pituitary gland, which, in turn, increases the secretion of LH and FSH.

The clomiphene citrate challenge test (CCCT) utilizes this inhibitory effect of CC to identify women at risk of having a low ovarian reserve. A day 3 serum FSH is obtained before the administration of 100 mg of oral CC on menstrual cycle days 5–9. A second FSH level is obtained on cycle day 10 after the completion of the medication. An elevated FSH value above 10 mIU/mL obtained on either cycle day 3 or cycle day 10 indicates a diminished ovarian reserve. Women with abnormally elevated FSH values demonstrate a dramatically lower ovarian response to medical stimulation and a lower pregnancy and live birth rate when compared to women with a normal FSH after the CCCT [32]. However, fewer physicians use this test to predict ovarian reserve and now increasingly rely on serum AMH and ovarian AFCs to manage patient expectations.

Testing for Uterine and Fallopian Tube Abnormalities

Collectively, uterine and fallopian tubal problems comprise 25% of all causes of infertility, with the majority of these cases being tubal in origin [33]. Anatomic, congenital, pathologic, and infectious abnormalities can affect conception by altering the normal interaction between the sperm and oocyte. Basic screening tests include a vaginal pelvic ultrasound and a hysterosalpingogram (HSG) or saline infusion sonohysterogram (SIS). Abnormal findings are often too unreliable to predict a negative outcome and consideration to perform a more definitive diagnostic test should be made.

Pelvic Ultrasound

The safest, least invasive, and most cost-effective imaging modality routinely employed to visualize and examine the pelvic anatomy is vaginal ultrasonography. Both 2-D and occasionally 3-D images are required to evaluate for suspected abnormalities within the uterus and ovaries. Uterine leiomyomas and polyps as well as ovarian cysts and masses can be easily observed, characterized, and even followed over time. Although uterine anomalies account for only 5% of all causes of infertility, they are more often associated with recurrent pregnancy loss and miscarriage. The best time to perform the vaginal ultrasound is during the first 4 days of the menstrual cycle. At this time, the endometrium is thin and both ovaries are resting and no cysts or follicles larger than 10 mm in diameter should be noticed. Any variation from normal should prompt an investigation to identify the underlying pathologic process and determine if treatment is required.

Hysterosalpingogram

The HSG is the best test to evaluate the constitution of the endometrial cavity and patency of both fallopian tubes. It can reveal anatomic distortions created by submucous leiomyomas, uterine synechia, and endometrial polyps. Congenital malformations including septate, bicornuate, and unicornuate uteri are easily discerned but often require a pelvic magnetic resonance imaging or even laparoscopy to confirm the diagnosis. To identify a tubal anomaly, the HSG has a sensitivity and specificity of 65% and 83%, respectively, and, surprisingly, only a 30% positive predictive value to correctly identify pathologies of the endometrial cavity [34,35].

Fallopian tube abnormalities account for 20% of all infertility-related issues. As a screening test, the HSG is invaluable and can eliminate tubal disease as the root cause of infertility. It can distinguish proximal from distal tubal disease as well as identify infectious and inflammatory etiologies such as hydrosalpinx, peritubal adhesions, and fimbria occlusion when present. The HSG requires an iodide-based radiopaque contrast as the infusion media. This contrast media can be oil-soluble (OSCM) or water-soluble (WSCM) in nature. Nearly all procedures performed today use WSCM rather than OSCM. WSCM is less expensive, has better imaging resolution, and harbors less risk of a complication. Problems including allergic reactions, anaphylactic shock, and pelvic lipogranuloma formations are more common with OSCM because of its higher viscosity and slower reabsorption rate [36]. The most dangerous risk associated with OSCM occurs when the contrast intravasates into the pelvic vasculature, leading to fat embolism formation, circulatory collapse, and, eventually, death. Women with occluded fallopian tubes and submucous myomas are at greatest risk of this problem.

Multiple studies suggest that pregnancy rates increase immediately following the HSG. This increase in pregnancy rate is highest within the first 4 months after the HSG and then progressively declines over time, to have no impact by 8 months later [37]. Interestingly, this effect on pregnancy rate is only observed in patients who receive OSCM but not for those who receive WSCM [38,39]. One possible explanation on how OSCM improves pregnancy rates is through its ability to dislodge and clear mucous plugs formed within the fallopian tubes [40]. However, a more likely explanation lies with oil's ability to alter the local pelvic immunity to primarily reduce inflammatory and autoimmune reactions that impact sperm, egg, and embryo survival [41]. This phenomenon is best observed in patients diagnosed with endometriosis, unexplained infertility, and male factor infertility. For this reason, some authorities advocate that once tubal patency is established, 3 mL of OSCM should be injected into the endometrial cavity and fallopian tubes as a means to increase fertility rates in subsequent cycles [42] (Figures 3.2 through 3.10).

Saline Sonohysterogram

Saline infusion sonohysterogram (SIS) is a valuable diagnostic tool used to evaluate women with infertility and abnormal vaginal bleeding. It is commonly performed on patients with an iodine sensitivity or allergy, who would otherwise undergo an HSG procedure. The SIS is safer and has less patient discomfort compared to the HSG. Sterile normal saline (NS) is used as the infusion media. NS is better tolerated than iodine because of its neutral PH with the tissues of the body. Ultrasound waves are used to evaluate the pelvic anatomy, thus reducing the patient's exposure to the effects of harmful radiation.

The SIS can reveal detailed information regarding the endometrial cavity as well as determine fallopian tube patency. However, unlike the HSG, the SIS is highly sensitive for detecting endometrial cavity abnormalities and has a positive predictive value of >90% for detecting pathologies such as submucous leiomyomas, polyps, and synechia [43]. Traditionally, the SIS was considered less helpful in

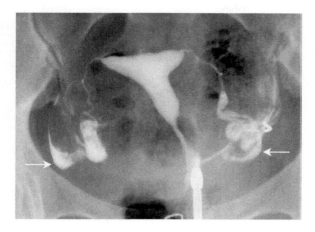

FIGURE 3.2 Normal HSG. This HSG demonstrates a uterine cavity that has a normal shape, and there are no filling defects noted within the cavity. Both fallopian tubes have filled and the arrows point to the dye that has exited the ends of both tubes into the abdominal cavity. HSG, hysterosalpingogram.

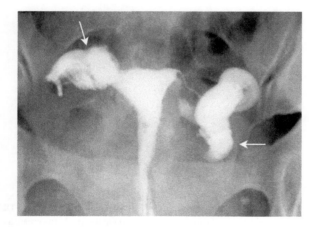

FIGURE 3.3 Distal tubal obstruction. In this x-ray, both fallopian tubes are filled, but their distal ends are dilated and no dye is seen escaping into the abdominal cavity. The ends of the tubes are indicated by the arrows. This finding is most likely the result of a pelvic infection.

documenting fallopian tube patency. However, newer techniques using Femvue (Femasys Inc.) employ a simultaneous mixture of air and saline to create a bubble mixture. On ultrasound, these air bubbles can be visualized traveling through the fallopian tubes to demonstrate areas of patency and occlusion (Figures 3.11 and 3.12).

Hysteroscopy and Laparoscopy

Hysteroscopy and laparoscopy are the gold standard diagnostic procedures performed after an abnormal screening or imaging test. These procedures allow the physician to correct underlying uterine and pelvic pathologies as well as visualize congenital and acquired anatomic abnormalities. Factors that contribute to infertility include endometriosis, peritoneal adhesions, and congenital tubal and uterine malformations. All of these disease processes can contribute to anatomic tubal distortions and even complete obstruction. When tubal patency is unclearly documented after an HSG or SIS procedure, laparoscopy with chromopertubation can discern fallopian tube patency from proximal and distal occlusion. Hysteroscopy with

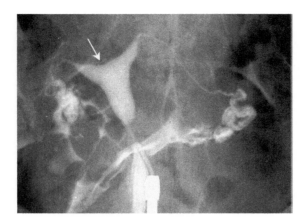

FIGURE 3.4 Arcuate uterus. In this otherwise normal study, a depression can be seen indenting the superior aspect of the uterine cavity (arrow). This is compatible with an arcuate uterus and is considered a normal variant. No additional workup is indicated. For comparison, a normal uterine cavity can be seen in Figures 3.2 and 3.3.

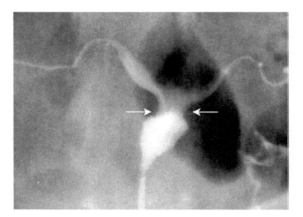

FIGURE 3.5 A DES uterus. The shape of this uterine cavity is compatible with previous DES exposure that causes impingement of the lateral walls as indicated by the arrows. The prominent uterine horns create a bicornuate shape as well. Overall, the uterine cavity has a "T shape" that is classic for previous DES exposure. DES, diethylstilbestrol.

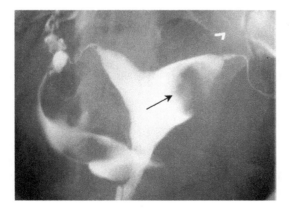

FIGURE 3.6 Submucosal fibroid. This hysterosalpingogram demonstrates a large filling defect in the left uterine horn, which was later found to be a submucosal fibroid. Also note the depression in the superior aspect of the cavity, which is an arcuate deformity.

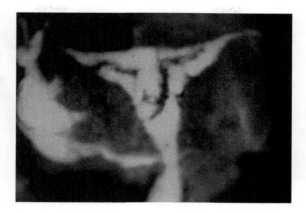

FIGURE 3.7 Asherman's syndrome. This HSG demonstrates multiple filling defects compatible with Asherman's syndrome. The patient is dilation and curettage (D&C) and underwent hysterscopic lysis of adhesions with restoration of the uterine cavity. HSG, hysterosalpingogram.

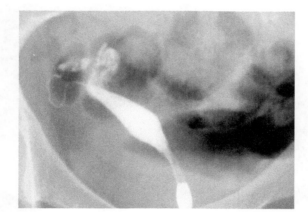

FIGURE 3.8 Unicornuate uterus. During this x-ray, only the right horn of the uterine cavity filled. This is compatible with a unicornuate uterus. A unicornuate uterus increases the risk of premature labor and fetal malpresentations. It can be accompanied by renal abnormalities.

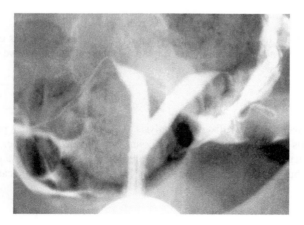

FIGURE 3.9 Uterine septum. This x-ray demonstrates a division in the uterine cavity, which was confirmed to be a uterine septum.

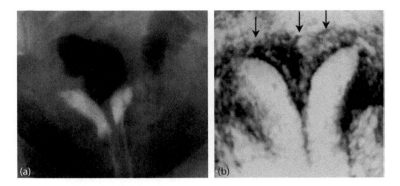

FIGURE 3.10 Is this uterine anomaly a septate or bicornuate uterus? (a) A uterine duplication anomaly confirmed by an HSG. Two separate cervices were cannulated and two separate uterine horns were noted. (b) A three-dimensional ultrasound image of the uterus of the same patient. The black arrows note the border of the outer extent of the myometrium of the uterine fundus. Conclusion: the anomaly is a uterine septum. HSG, hysterosalpingogram.

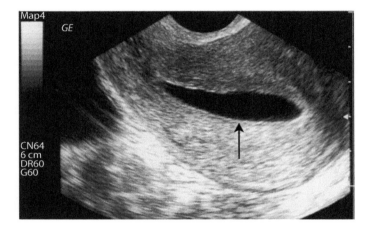

FIGURE 3.11 Sonohysterogram (normal cavity). This is a longitudinal image of the uterus taken at the time of a sonohysterogram. The black area (arrow) is the image of the saline that has been injected into the uterine cavity. Note that the borders of the uterine cavity are sharp and no masses are noted to be entering into the cavity. This study confirms a normal uterine cavity.

polypectomy, myomectomy, metroplasty, and resection of intrauterine adhesions can quickly and easily restore the anatomy back to normal and improve implantation, pregnancy, and live birth rates [44].

Evaluating Male Fertility

The evaluation of the male begins with semen analysis. This analysis identifies problems pertaining to the ejaculate and details findings regarding sperm count, movement, and shape. Anatomic, hormonal, genetic, and lifestyle factors all can contribute to a male's fertility. Overall, 40% of couples will have a male component contributing to their infertility, but for 20%, it will be the sole cause [45].

Semen Analysis

Semen analysis is a simple and relatively inexpensive test used to evaluate for male infertility. Although tests with abnormal findings clearly lead to failed fertilization and conception, male infertility can still

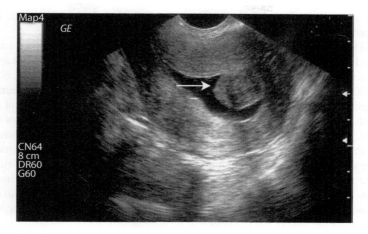

FIGURE 3.12 Sonohysterogram (abnormal cavity). In this image, the injected fluid in the cavity (appearing black) outlines an intracavitary mass, which was later confirmed to be a uterine fibroid.

be found in some men with completely normal sperm parameters. The semen analysis is a standardized test and requires that the patient abstain from ejaculation between 2 and 4 days before collection. The sperm sample should be produced in the facility processing and performing the analysis, but it can also be transported by the patient to that facility under proper conditions and within 60 to 90 minutes after home collection. Most patients produce the sample for testing through masturbation. However, for those men who cannot masturbate, the option of collecting a sample via intercourse can be offered. Special condoms, designed specifically for collecting sperm for analysis, must be purchased and used by the patient. These collection condoms are formulated differently from traditional condoms and do not disrupt or kill the sperm after ejaculation.

Once the sperm sample is collected and analyzed, the provider can determine if further testing or treatment is required. Most authorities use the World Health Organization's reference for defining the lower limits of the parameters of a normal semen analysis [46] (Table 3.1). These values have changed throughout the years and reflect the change in sperm parameters observed in men worldwide. This reference range includes values for overall ejaculate volume, sperm concentration, count, motility, and morphology. It is important to realize that the semen analysis is a quantitative assessment of the semen sample. Further, the normal ranges established for the various parameters are somewhat arbitrary and a previous study confirmed overlap between the semen parameters in a fertile and infertile population (Table 3.1).

Spermatogenesis occurs in the testicular tubules and requires a normal secretion of the hormone testosterone for maximum productivity. Varicoceles are dilated veins within the pampiniform plexus and internal spermatic veins located within the spermatic cord. It is the most common anatomic abnormality associated with male subfertility. More than 40% of all men with abnormal semen samples will have at least one varicocele identified on exam. Varicoceles exert their effect by raising testicular temperature, which then alters the production and quality of sperm. Eventually, all parameters including movement, shape, count, and function are effected. This can be corrected by surgery or with angiographic

TABLE 3.1

Normal Sperm Parameters of Semen Analysis

Liquefaction time	15 to 30 minutes
Ejaculate volume	1.5 mL to 5 mL
Sperm concentration	15×10^6 spermatozoa/mL
Total sperm count	>39 million sperm
Motility	>40% total motility
	>32% progressive motility
Morphology	>4% normal forms

embolization but, either way, requires the expertise of a trained urologist to examine the patient and determine if a benefit can be achieved [47].

Azoospermia is the term given to samples lacking any visible sperm. Both obstructive and nonobstructive causes can be implicated. Obstructive azoospermia commonly results from a blockage or congenital absence of the vas deferens. The vas deferens connects the testes with the urethra and is easily palpable during the physical exam or observed during a pelvic and testicular ultrasound. Between 1% and 2% of men have a congenital bilateral absence of the vas deferens (CBAVD), and they account for almost 25% of all patients with obstructive azoospermia [48]. These men likely have a cystic fibrosis transmembrane receptor mutation, which leads to defective Wölffian duct formation. This causes a failure of the vas deferens to connect the testes to the urethra, ultimately preventing the delivery of sperm into the ejaculate.

Nonobstructive azoospermia is caused by either an extremely low level or a complete lack of sperm production by the testes. These men typically have low levels of circulating testosterone and are thus unable to achieve normal spermatogenesis. Regardless if the insult is hypergonadotropic, eugonadotropic, or hypogonadotropic in origin, the end result of impaired spermatogenesis is the same. However, the treatment to correct the underlying disorder will be altered.

Hypergonadotropic hypogonadism results from overt testicular failure. This is often associated with either acquired or congenital anatomic defects of the testicles or from chromosomal abnormalities and rearrangements found during karyotype testing. Genetic deletions within specific regions of the Y-chromosome is another common cause of failed spermatogenesis in the presence of normal testosterone levels. As a result, all men with sperm counts of under 5 million should undergo both karyotype and Y-chromosome microdeletion testing. Conversely, hypogonadotropic hypogonadism is common among men with eating and body dysmorphic disorders. Men who routinely overexert themselves with strenuous exercise or those who have central nervous system tumors affecting hypothalamic and pituitary function may have a reversible cause of their azoospermia. Abuse and use of specific medications known to impact spermatogenesis include anabolic steroids, chronic opioids exposure, and past or present use of certain chemotherapeutic agents. Eighty percent of all men treated for testicular cancer will resume spermatogenesis within 5 years after completion of chemotherapy, and only 20% will have permanent azoospermia.

Other diseases and injuries to the testicles that can compromise testicular function include mumps orchitis, testicular torsion, cancer, and uncontrolled long-standing diabetes. The latter is more often associated with retrograde ejaculation rather than a reduction in spermatogenesis and sperm can often be retrieved from the bladder during a post-void collection. Testicular sperm aspiration and testicular

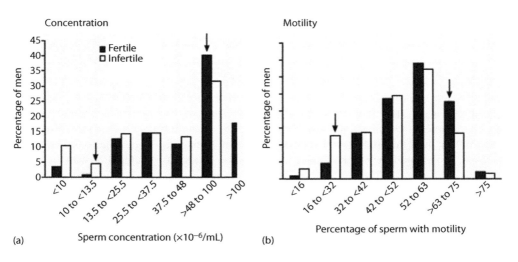

FIGURE 3.13 Comparison of semen parameters [concentration (a) and motility (b)] between men of fertile and infertile couples. In each panel, the left arrow separates infertile and indeterminate groups and the right arrow separates indeterminate from fertile groups. (Reprinted with permission from Guzick DS, Overstreet JW, Factor-Litvak P et al. Sperm morphology, motility, and concentration in fertile and infertile men. *N Engl J Med* 2001;345:1388–93. Copyright 2001 Massachusetts Medical Society. All rights reserved.)

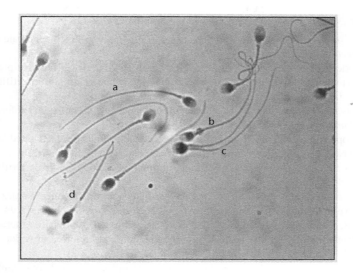

FIGURE 3.14   Examples of varied sperm morphology: (a) normal, (b) midpiece defect, (c) tail defect, and (d) tapered head.

sperm extraction are two common methods employed to retrieve sperm for men with azoospermia. Even men with overt testicular failure have a 50% chance of retrieving viable sperm for use during an IVF cycle.

All men found to have an abnormal semen analysis should have a repeat semen analysis to confirm the finding. Men with repeatedly abnormal semen samples should undergo hormonal evaluation for FSH, LH, TSH, PRL, total testosterone, and estradiol. When sperm counts are continuously below 5 million, genetic testing including a karyotype, cystic fibrosis (CF) with 5T-allele polymorphism analysis, and Y-chromosome microdeletion testing should also be offered. Other tests including DNA fragmentation testing and sperm decondensation testing should be ordered and interpreted with extreme caution since the predictive reliability of these two tests is unclear (Table 3.1; Figures 3.13 and 3.14).

Postcoital Test

The postcoital test (PCT) is usually performed several days before ovulation and, under microscopy, reveals a minimum of five moving sperm per high power field. The lifespan of sperm ranges from 1 to 5 days with a median survivability of 1.5 days. Aside from sperm quality and quantity, a multitude of factors dictate their durability. Influential facets regarding their longevity include cervical mucus elasticity, vaginal and cervical mucus PH, findings of coexisting infections, and known pathologic processes that alter the normal anatomy and ecosystem of the cervix and vagina [49]. It is estimated that abnormalities of cervix and its mucus secretions account for almost 3% of all the cases of infertility [50]. However, PCT analysis is inconsistent and nonpredictive in determining either cervical or spermatic problems and is therefore useless in its utility. The PCT is not recommended and should not be a part of the initial workup or evaluation of the patient [51].

Conclusion

The causes of infertility can be varied and the infertility evaluation will provide a better understanding of the potential causes. Up to 25% of couples will have a combination of factors. Therefore, it is important that a complete evaluation is performed and the evaluation is not halted after a single abnormal test is encountered. After the evaluation is completed, the couple should be seen in consultation to discuss the results and formulate a treatment plan.

REFERENCES

1. The Practice Committee of the American Society for Reproductive Medicine. Female age-related fertility decline. *Fertil Steril* 2014;101:633–34.
2. Gnoth C, Godehardt D, Godehardt E, Fank-Herrmann P, Freundi G. Time to pregnancy: Results of the German prospective study and impact on the management of infertility. *Hum Reprod* 2003;18:1959–66.
3. Slama R, Hansen OK, Ducot B et al. Estimation of the frequency of involuntary infertility on a nation-wide basis. *Hum Reprod* 2012;27:1489.
4. Chandra A, Copen CE, Stephen EH. Infertility and impaired fecundity in the United States. 1982–2010: data from the National Survey of Family Growth. *Natl Health Stat Report* 2013;1.
5. Samplaski MK, Nangia AK. Adverse effects of common medications on male fertility. *Nat Rev Urol* 2015 Jul;12(7):401–13.
6. Romero Gutierrez G, Aguirre Beltran AF, Figueroa Solana MI, Malacara Hernandez JM. Correlations between hyperprolactinemia and galactorrhea. *Ginecol Obstet Mex* 1989 Nov;57:294–7.
7. VanderLaan B, Karande V, Krohm C et al. Cost considerations with infertility therapy: Outcome and cost comparisons between health maintenance organization and preferred provider organization care based on physician and facility cost. *Hum Reprod* 1998;13:1200.
8. Charkoudian N, Stachenfeld NS. Reproductive hormone influences on thermoregulation in women. *Compr Physiol* 2014 Apr;4(2):793–804.
9. Kippley J, Kippley S. *The Art of Natural Family Planning* (4th ed.). Cincinnati, OH: The Couple to Couple League. 1996. pp. 72,298–299.
10. Ferreira-Poblete A. The probability of conception on different days of the cycle with respect to ovulation: An overview. *Adv Contracept* 1997 Jun;13(2–3):83–95.
11. Johnson S, Weddell S, Godbert S, Freundl G, Roos J, Gnoth C. Development of the first urinary reproductive hormone ranges referenced to independently determined ovulation day. *Clin Chem Lab Med* 2015 Jun;53(7):1099–108.
12. Miao YL, Kikuchi K, Sun QY, Schatten H. Oocyte aging: Cellular and molecular changes, developmental potential and reversal possibility. *Hum Reprod Update* 2009 Sep–Oct;15(5):573–85.
13. Wathen NC, Perry L, Lilford RJ, Chard T. Interpretation of single progesterone measurement in diagnosis of anovulation and defective luteal phase: Observations on analysis of the normal range. *Br Med J (Clin Res Ed)* 1984;288:7.
14. Noyes RW, Hertig AT, Rock J. Dating the endometrial biopsy. *Am J Obstet Gynecol* 1975;122:262–3.
15. Murray MJ, Meyer WR, Zaino RJ, Lessey BA, Novotny DB, Ireland K et al. A critical analysis of the accuracy, reproducibility, and clinical utility of histologic endometrial dating in fertile women. *Fertil Steril* 2004;81:1333–43.
16. Nalini M. Endometrial receptivity array: Clinical application. *J Hum Reprod Sci* 2015 Jul–Sep; 8(3):121–129.
17. Nevins JR, Potti A. Mining gene expression profiles: Expression signatures as cancer phenotypes. *Nat Rev Genet* 2007 Aug;8(8):601–9.
18. Practice Committee of the American Society for Reproductive Medicine. Testing and interpreting measures of ovarian reserve. *Fertil Steril* 2015;103:e9–17.
19. Lemmen JG, Rodríguez NM, Andreasen LD, Loft A, Ziebe S. The total pregnancy potential per oocyte aspiration after assisted reproduction—In how many cycles are biologically competent oocytes available? *J Assist Reprod Genet* 2016 Jul;33(7):849–54.
20. Serour G, Mansour R, Serour A, Aboulghar M, Amin Y, Kamal O, Al-Inany H, Aboulghar M. Analysis of 2,386 consecutive cycles of in vitro fertilization or intracytoplasmic sperm injection using autologous oocytes in women aged 40 years and above. *Fertil Steril* 2010 Oct;94(5):1707–12.
21. Demko ZP, Simon AL, McCoy RC, Petrov DA, Rabinowitz M. Effects of maternal age on euploidy rates in a large cohort of embryos analyzed with 24-chromosome single-nucleotide polymorphism-based preimplantation genetic screening. *Fertil Steril* 2016 May;105(5):1307–13.
22. Bozkurt B, Erdem M, Mutlu MF, Erdem A, Guler I, Mutlu I, Oktem M. Comparison of age-related changes in anti-Müllerian hormone levels and other ovarian reserve tests between healthy fertile and infertile population. *Hum Fertil (Camb)* 2016 Aug;8:1–7.

23. Kotanidis L, Nikolettos K, Petousis S, Asimakopoulos B, Chatzimitrou E, Kolios G, Nikolettos N. The use of serum anti-Mullerian hormone (AMH) levels and antral follicle count (AFC) to predict the number of oocytes collected and availability of embryos for cryopreservation in IVF. *J Endocrinol Invest* 2016 Jul 2.

24. Ebner T, Sommergruber M, Moser M, Shebl O, Schreier-Lechner E, Tews G. Basal level of anti-Mullerian hormone is associated with oocyte quality in stimulated cycles. *Hum Reprod* 2006;21:2022–6.

25. Gracia CR, Sammel MD, Freeman E, Prewitt M, Carlson C, Ray A, Vance A, Ginsberg JP. (Children's Hospital of Philadelphia). Measures of ovarian reserve are impaired in a dose-dependent manner. Reproductive hormone levels in menstruating survivors exposed to high-dose therapy are similar to those in late-reproductive-age women. *Fertil Steril* 2012 Jan;97(1):134–40.

26. Rustamov O, Krishnan M, Roberts SA, Fitzgerald CT. Effect of salpingectomy, ovarian cystectomy and unilateral salpingo-oopherectomy on ovarian reserve. *Gynecol Surg* 2016;13:173–8.

27. Kallio S, Puurunen J, Ruokonen A, Vaskivuo T, Piltonen T, Tapanainen JS. Antimullerian hormone levels decrease in women using combined contraception independently of administration route. *Fertil Steril* 2013;99:1305–10.

28. Chan C, Liu K. Clinical pregnancy in a woman with idiopathic hypogonadotropic hypogonadism and low AMH: Utility of ovarian reserve markers in IHH. *J Assist Reprod Genet* 2014;31:1317–21.

29. Jirge PR. Ovarian reserve tests. *J Hum Reprod Sci* 2011 Sep;4(3):108–13.

30. Meczekalski B, Czyzyk A, Kunicki M, Podfigurna-Stopa A, Plociennik L, Jakiel G, Maciejewska-Jeske M, Lukaszuk K. Fertility in women of late reproductive age: The role of serum anti-Müllerian hormone (AMH) levels in its assessment. *J Endocrinol Invest* 2016 Jun 14.

31. Leader B, Baca Q, Seifer D, Bake VL. High frequency of discordance between antimüllerian hormone and follicle stimulating hormone levels in serum from estradiol-confirmed days 2 to 4 of the menstrual cycle from 5,354 women in U.S. fertility centers. *Fertil Steril* 2012;98(4):1037–42.

32. Csemiczky G1, Harlin J, Fried G. Predictive power of clomiphene citrate challenge test for failure of in vitro fertilization treatment. *Acta Obstet Gynecol Scand* 2002 Oct;81(10):954–61.

33. Yen SS, Jaffe RB, Barbieri RL (1999). *Reproductive Endocrinology* (4th ed.). W.B. Saunders.

34. Broeze K et al. Are patient characteristics associated with the accuracy of hysterosalpingography in diagnosing tubal pathology? An individual patient data meta-analysis. *Hum Reprod Update* 2011 May–Jun;17(3):293–300.

35. Soares SR, Barbosa dos Reis MM, Camargos AF. Diagnostic accuracy of sonohysterography, transvaginal sonography, and hysterosalpingography in patients with uterine cavity diseases. *Fertil Steril* 2000;73:406–11.

36. Johnson NP et al. The FLUSH Trial—Flushing with Lipiodol for Unexplained (and endometriosis-related) Subfertility by Hysterosalpingography: A randomized trial. *Hum Reprod* 2004;19(9):2043–51.

37. Steiner AZ, Meyer WR, Clark RL, Hartmann KE. Oil-soluble contrast during hysterosalpingography in women with proven tubal patency. *Obstet Gynecol* 2003 Jan;101(1):109–13.

38. Rasmussen F, Lindeguist S, Larson C, Justesen P. Therapeutic effect of hysterosalpingography: Oil-versus water-soluble contrast media—A randomized prospective study. *Radiology* 1991 Apr;179(1):75–8.

39. Watson A, Vandekerckhove P, Lilford R, Vail A, Brosens I, Hughes E. A meta-analysis of the therapeutic role of oil soluble contrast media at hysterosalpingography: A surprising result? *Fertil Steril* 1994 Mar;61(3):470–7.

40. Vandekerckhove P, Watson A, Lilford R, Harada T, Hughes E. Oil-soluble versus water-soluble media for assessing tubal patency with hysterosalpingography or laparoscopy in subfertile women. *Cochrane Database Syst Rev* 1996; Issue 4. Art No.:CD000092. doi: 10.1002/14651858. CD000092.

41. de Pablo MA, Alvarez de Cienfuegos G. Modulatory effects of dietary lipids on immune system functions. *Immunol Cell Biol* 2000 Feb;78(1):31–9.

42. DeCherney AH, Kort H, Barney JB, DeVore GR. Increased pregnancy rate with oil-soluble hysterosalpingography dye. *Fertil Steril* 1980 Apr;33(4):407–10.

43. Seshadri S, El-Toukhy T, Douiri A, Jayaprakasan K, Khalaf Y. Diagnostic accuracy of saline infusion sonography in the evaluation of uterine cavity abnormalities prior to assisted reproductive techniques: A systematic review and meta-analyses. *Hum Reprod Update* 2015 Mar–Apr;21(2):262–74.

44. Jan Bosteels et al. The effectiveness of hysteroscopy in improving pregnancy rates in subfertile women without other gynaecological symptoms: A systematic review. *Hum Reprod Update* 2010;16(1):1–11.

45. Thonneau P, Marchand S, Tallec A, Ferial ML, Ducot B, Lansac J et al. Incidence and main causes of infertility in a resident population (1,850,000) of three French regions (1988–1989). *Hum Reprod* 1991;6:811–6.

46. World Health Organization. *WHO Laboratory Manual for the Examination and Processing of Human Semen.* 5th ed. 2010 WHO press, World Health Organization, Switzerland.

47. Nieschlag E, Behre HM, Schlingheider A, Nashan D, Pohl J, Fischedick AR. Surgical ligation vs. angiographic embolization of the vena spermatica: A prospective randomized study for the treatment of varicocele-related infertility. *Andrologia* 1993 Sep–Oct;25(5):233–7.

48. Oates RD, Amos JA. The genetic basis of congenital bilateral absence of the vas deferens and cystic fibrosis. *J Androl* 1994;15:1–8.

49. Wilcox AJ, Weinberg CR, Baird DD. Timing of sexual intercourse in relation to ovulation: Effects on the probability of conception, survival of the pregnancy, and sex of the baby. *N Engl J Med* 1995 Dec 7;333(23):1517–21.

50. Hull MG, Glazener CM, Kelly NJ, Conway DI, Foster PA, Hinton RA, Coulson C, Lambert PA, Watt EM, Desai KM. Population study of causes, treatment, and outcome of infertility. *Br Med J (Clin Res Ed)* 1985;291:1693–7.

51. Oei SG, Helmerhorst FM, Bloemenkamp KW, Hollants FA, Meerpoel DE, Keirse MJ. Effectiveness of the postcoital test: Randomized controlled trial. *BMJ* 1998;317:502–5.

4

Preconceptional Counseling

Steven R. Bayer

The goal of treatment of the infertile woman goes beyond just simply helping her achieve a pregnancy, but rather the ultimate goal is the establishment of a pregnancy that ends with a healthy mother and a healthy baby. An important prerequisite to infertility treatment is preconceptional counseling. Preconceptional counseling is an assessment of the medical, social, genetic, environmental, and occupational factors that can affect fertility and the health of a pregnancy (Figure 4.1). In this chapter, a comprehensive summary and framework for preconceptional care is presented.

Lifestyle Habits

A social history with an assessment of lifestyle habits is an important part of the medical history that should be obtained from the male and female partners. The use of tobacco, alcohol, and recreational drugs should be ascertained and the couples should be appropriately counseled. These habits may not only be harmful during pregnancy but could also impair conception.

Smoking

Smoking continues to be a major public health care issue that continues to challenge the medical community. According to the Centers for Disease Control and Prevention (CDC), there continues to be an encouraging downward trend of smoking in the United States. At the time of the initial CDC data collection in 1965, 42.4% of US adults smoked, and the incidence has since decreased year by year to an all-time low of 16.8% in 2014 [1]. Approximately 14.8% of women in the reproductive age group continue to smoke [1]. The ill effects of smoking on general health are well known. There are substantial data to support that smoking compromises reproductive health and is considered a reproductive toxin [2]. Women who smoke are at greater risk of having infertility, a spontaneous abortion, and a tubal pregnancy. During pregnancy, maternal smoking increases the chances of abruptio placenta, premature rupture of the membranes, and impaired fetal growth. Maternal smoking during pregnancy also increases the chance of the sudden infant death syndrome. Smoking may impair meiotic spindle function, which can lead to aneuploidy. Maternal smoking has been shown to increase the risk of trisomy 21 [3,4]. It is clear that any woman who smokes and is contemplating a pregnancy should be strongly encouraged to stop. It is encouraging that 70% of active smokers would like to stop but nicotine is a strong addiction and simple counseling will not prove effective in most cases. Referring the patient back to her primary care physician is prudent for counseling and intervention. Strategies for smoking cessation include behavioral modification, over-the-counter nicotine replacement products, and pharmacologic agents including bupropion and varenicline tartrate. The CDC has been very active in smoking cessation, and for additional information, visit the website: www.cdc.gov/tobacco/quit_smoking/.

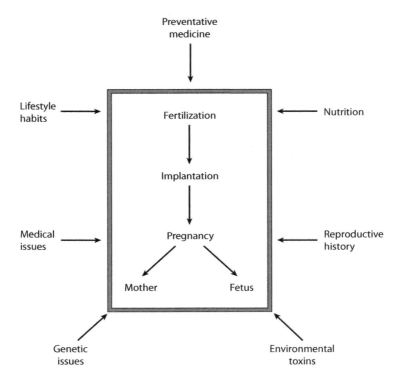

FIGURE 4.1   Factors that can affect fertility and pregnancy.

Alcohol

Alcohol use during pregnancy is problematic for the developing fetus, which can cause sequelae in the child after the delivery. Fetal alcohol spectrum disorders (FASD) are a group of conditions that can occur in children exposed to in utero alcohol [5]. The risk of fetal alcohol exposure is related to the degree and timing of alcohol intake but no level of alcohol intake is considered safe. At the extreme is the fetal alcohol syndrome with associated low birth weight, dysmorphic features, and mental retardation. Other signs and symptoms of FASD include attention-deficit disorders, learning disabilities, poor memory, speech/language delay, and poor coordination, among others. It has been confirmed that maternal alcohol intake can decrease the chances of conception [6]. Therefore, any woman who is trying for a pregnancy should limit alcohol intake and avoid it altogether once pregnancy is established. Finally, heavy alcohol intake may suggest an addiction and a history of other drug use should be ascertained. In some cases, referral for counseling may be indicated before the couple attempts a pregnancy.

Recreational Drug Use

The use of recreational drugs is absolutely contraindicated while a couple is attempting to conceive and during pregnancy. Males who use marijuana on a regular basis have lower serum testosterone levels and decreased sperm counts. Other drugs used by the mother, such as cocaine and heroine, may lead to a severe neonatal withdrawal reaction. Further, the use of intravenous drugs increases the risk of human immunodeficiency virus (HIV) and hepatitis infections.

Body Weight/Nutrition

There is no doubt that our general health is influenced by what we eat, how much we eat, and how much energy we expend with activity and exercise. In addition, nutrition impacts on reproductive health can influence the establishment and maintenance of a pregnancy. There is growing concern about the increased incidence of obesity (body mass index [BMI] > 30) in the United States. There is evidence to suggest that we are in the midst of an epidemic of this problem. From the most recent CDC published report inclusive of data from 1988 to 2014, the incidence of obesity (BMI > 30) increased 1.6-fold from 23.2% to 38.2% and the incidence of extreme obesity (BMI > 40) increased 2.7-fold from 3.0% to 8.1% [7]. The incidence of obesity is higher in women than in men (41% and 35.5%, respectively). The rate of obesity is also disparate among different ethnic populations. The incidence of obesity was 11.9% in non-Hispanic Asian, 35.5% in non-Hispanic white, 45.7% in Hispanic, and 56.9% in non-Hispanic black women. While there may be a genetic or medical explanation for some, the majority of cases of obesity are preventable and simply the result of a sedentary lifestyle and an unhealthy diet. All-cause mortality is increased in obese individuals, and if the trend does not change, obesity may become one of the leading causes of death.

A major concern about increased body weight is the increased incidence of complications that may occur during pregnancy including spontaneous abortion, gestational diabetes, hypertension, thromboembolism, congenital anomalies, and stillbirth [8,9]. Women who are overweight tend to have babies with macrosomia, which increases the chance of shoulder dystocia and the need for a Cesarean section. A Cesarean section that is performed on a woman who is overweight is associated with a higher incidence of anesthetic and surgical complications. In a previous report, obesity was responsible for 18% of maternal mortalities and 80% of anesthesia-related mortalities [10]. Guidelines that provide a strategy for the clinician in dealing with obesity in the patient population have been published [11,12].

In response to the growing obesity problem, the US Department of Agriculture recently has published the *2015–2020 Dietary Guidelines for Americans* (www.cnpp.usda.gov/2015-2020-dietary-guidelines-americans). As a general recommendation, adults should be encouraged to maintain a balanced diet of grains, vegetables, fruits, meats, and dairy products. Foods with a high content of saturated and *trans* fats and oils and carbohydrates should be used sparingly. In addition to a healthy diet, engagement in aerobic exercise on a regular basis is recommended.

Assessing the Body Habitus

The BMI or the Quetelet's index is a determination of whether an individual's weight is appropriate (Table 4.1). It is a calculation that takes into account the weight and height (weight [kg]/height [m^2]). The BMI is a quantitative measure that helps to put into perspective the individual's weight. There are online calculators to determine the BMI.

Recommendation before conception:

- BMI > 30 refer to a nutritionist
- BMI > 35 refer to a nutritionist and high-risk obstetrician
- BMI > 40 defer treatment.

TABLE 4.1

BMI Classification

Weight Classification	**BMI**
Underweight	<20
Normal	20–25
Overweight	25–30
Obesity	>30
Class I	30–35
Class II	35–40
Class III	>40

Caffeine Intake

Daily intake of caffeine at high doses (>500 mg; >5 cups of coffee/day) has been associated with reduced fertility [13]. The impact of lesser amounts of caffeine on fertility has been the subject of debate. During pregnancy, moderate caffeine intake (<200 mg/day) does not increase the risk of miscarriage, preterm labor, or intrauterine growth restriction [14]. The quantity of caffeine in beverages is variable. The average amount in a cup of coffee, tea, and a can of soda is approximately 100, 50, and 50 mg, respectively. Chocolate is another source of caffeine and contains 12 mg of caffeine per ounce. Daily intake of caffeine <200 mg/day appears to be safe during the preconception period and pregnancy.

Vitamin Supplementation

Women who take folic acid before pregnancy reduce their chance of having a baby with a neural tube defect (NTD). NTDs are birth defects associated with abnormal developments of the spine and skull. The most common types of NTDs are anencephaly and spina bifida. In the United States, the occurrence of NTDs is approximately 1 per 1500 deliveries. Previous studies have reported that women who supplemented their daily diet with folic acid experienced a reduction in the frequency of NTDs [15–17]. Some studies have suggested that folic acid may prevent the development of other birth defects including cardiac, renal, cleft lip/palate, and limb abnormalities [18,19]. In the United States, considering that many pregnancies are unintended, all cereal grain products were fortified with 140 µg per 100 g. The CDC has reported a 28% reduction in NTDs between the pre-fortification period (1995–1996) and post-fortification period (1999–2011) [20]. It is now recommended that all women of childbearing age who are capable of becoming pregnant should consume 0.4 mg of folic acid per day. This can be accomplished either through dietary supplementation or by taking an over-the-counter multivitamin preparation, which contains 0.4 mg of folic acid.

Women who are overweight (BMI > 30) have an increased chance of having a baby with an NTD [9,21]. In this population, it is prudent to prescribe a daily supplement of 1.0 mg of folic acid or a prenatal vitamin. It is recommended that a woman who has had a previous pregnancy complicated by an NTD or a family history of this defect should be treated with 4.0 mg of folic acid daily [22–24].

While vitamin supplementation is helpful, excessive vitamin intake can prove to be harmful to the developing fetus. Published data have confirmed that excessive intake of vitamin A increases the chance of congenital anomalies involving craniofacial, cardiac, thymus, and central nervous system organ systems [25]. Isotretinoin, a derivative of vitamin A, is used to treat severe acne. Women who take this drug orally during pregnancy have a 25% chance of congenital anomalies [26]. Prenatal vitamins contain safe amounts of vitamin A (<4000 IU). However, daily intake of vitamin A should not exceed 10,000 IU. Excessive intake of animal liver, a food that is rich in vitamin A, should also be avoided.

RECOMMENDATIONS FOR FOLIC ACID SUPPLEMENTATION TO PREVENT NTD*

- Routine—0.4 mg daily
- Obesity (BMI > 30)—1.0 mg daily (a prenatal vitamin or a 1.0-mg folic acid tablet)
- Previous history or family history of NTD—4.0 mg folic acid daily[†]

---

* For adequate prevention of an NTD, the folic acid supplement should be started 1 month before conception and continued during pregnancy.

† This level of intake can be achieved either by taking folic acid alone or folic acid tablets plus a prenatal vitamin that contains 0.8–1.0 mg of folic acid. To achieve this level of supplementation, more than one multivitamin (or prenatal vitamin) should not be taken on a daily basis. This will increase the intake of vitamin A over the safe level, which could increase the chances of birth defects.

Herbal Remedies

Over the past several years, there has been an increase in the use of alternative medical therapies including herbal remedies. Herbal remedies are advertised as "natural" but many have strong medicinal qualities. However, one must exercise caution in their use since there are very few published studies analyzing the effectiveness and safety of these agents especially during pregnancy [27]. In a previous study, three commonly used herbs including St. John's Wort, *Echinacea purpurea*, and *Ginkgo biloba* were demonstrated to be detrimental to egg and sperm function [28]. It is important to ask patients about the use of all medications, including herbal remedies. Many patients do not view herbal or over-the-counter medications as "true" medications. Until published studies confirm the safety of herbal remedies, women should be encouraged to discontinue these agents before and after pregnancy is established.

Routine Gynecological Care

Every woman should have a yearly blood pressure check, physical examination, pelvic examination, and Pap smear. The American College of Obstetrics and Gynecology (ACOG) recommendations regarding the frequency of Pap smear screening are as follows:

- Women aged 21–29 years should have a Pap test alone every 3 years. HPV testing is not recommended.
- Women aged 30–65 years should have a Pap test and an HPV test (co-testing) every 5 years (preferred). It is also acceptable to have a Pap test alone every 3 years.

ACOG also recommends an annual mammogram for women 40 and older. Earlier screening may be indicated if there is a family history of breast cancer.

Laboratory Testing

Routine laboratory studies are an essential part of preconceptional care. In essence, the same tests that are routine for any pregnant woman should also be performed on the woman who is contemplating a pregnancy. The tests that we recommend are presented below. A complete blood count may identify a woman who has anemia or some other abnormality that needs attention. A blood type and screen may uncover the presence of an antibody that could increase the chance of isoimmunization. In addition, knowledge of the blood type is also advantageous when a patient is experiencing bleeding during the early part of pregnancy and the clinician needs to know whether anti-D immunoglobulin (RhoGAM) is indicated.

PRECONCEPTIONAL BLOOD WORK

- TSH
- CBC
- Blood type and screen
- RPR
- Antibody screens for
  - Rubella
  - Varicella
  - Hepatitis—Hep B Antigen, Hep C Antibody
  - HIV
- Genetic screening (if indicated)

Thyroid function should be assessed with a serum TSH determination. Thyroid dysfunction is present in 3%–10% of women. Since thyroid disorders can be genetic, any woman who has a family history of thyroid dysfunction should be screened with a TSH level along with thyroid peroxidase antibodies. Despite a normal TSH level, if a woman has positive thyroid antibodies, she is at risk for thyroid dysfunction in the future, especially during pregnancy. Borderline hypothyroidism during the early stage of pregnancy has been reported to have an impact on fetal neuropsychological development [29,30]. A previous study confirmed that 85% of patients receiving treatment for hypothyroidism required an increase in thyroid replacement during the first trimester of pregnancy; thus, close vigilance is indicated [31]. During the post-partum period, thyroid antibodies can further alter thyroid function and place the woman at increased risk of postpartum depression. There is a great deal of controversy as to what is the upper limit of normal for the TSH level. Many laboratories use 4.0–5.0 mIU/L as the upper limit of normal but many medical endocrinologists consider 2.5 mIU/L to be the upper limits of normal since 95% of women will have a TSH level between 0.4 and 2.5 mIU/L. The Endocrine Society has taken the position that a normal TSH level should be less than 2.5 mIU/L, whereas the position of the American Association of Clinical Endocrinologists is that the upper limit of normal for the TSH level is 3.0 mIU/L. Since the upper normal limit of TSH is uncertain, when to institute thyroid replacement is the subject of debate. One approach is to treat all women when the TSH level is >2.5 mIU/L. Another approach is to not treat when the TSH level is in the stated upper normal range for the laboratory (2.5–4.0 mIU/L) as long as the thyroid peroxidase antibodies testing shows negative results and to only treat when the TSH level is >4.0 mIU/mL. When the thyroid peroxidase antibodies are positive, it is prudent to institute treatment when the TSH level is >2.5 mIU/mL.

Certain infections during pregnancy can pose a health risk to the mother and fetus. During childhood, it is public policy to administer immunizations that provide protection against many of these infections. Despite these efforts, a segment of the population remains at risk because of failure to receive the vaccine or failure to convert to immunity following a vaccination. Determining the immune status to certain infections including rubella, varicella, and hepatitis should be considered a routine part of pre-conceptional care. Screening for other infectious diseases may be indicated depending on the clinical circumstances.

Rubella (German Measles)

Rubella is a self-limited viral infection that is associated with a characteristic rash. A maternal infection during the first trimester of pregnancy can result in fetal death or cause severe damage to the fetal cardiac, neurological, ophthalmologic, and auditory organs. Since the introduction of the rubella vaccine in 1969, there has been a significant reduction in rubella infections and babies born with congenital rubella syndrome. However, in a previous study, one in nine women was not immune to rubella [32]. Screening for rubella immune status should be routinely performed on any woman who is contemplating pregnancy. Those women who are non-immune should be encouraged to receive the vaccine. The rubella vaccine is a live-attenuated virus, and the CDC recommendations are that a woman should avoid pregnancy for 1 month after receiving the vaccine.

Varicella (Chicken Pox)

Varicella is a highly contagious viral infection that is caused by a herpes virus. Many individuals experience a memorable varicella infection during their childhood, which provides lifelong immunity. It is now standard practice that children are vaccinated, which confers 90% immunity. A non-immune individual can acquire the infection after exposure to an individual who has a primary varicella infection or herpes zoster (a latent form of varicella). Symptoms of an infection include malaise, fever, and the development of characteristic vesicular lesions. Approximately 5% of individuals are non-immune to varicella [33]. There are concerns about a primary varicella infection that develops in an adult. Up to 20% of adults who acquire a primary varicella infection will develop a concomitant pneumonia, which is fatal in 40% of cases [34]. If a pregnant woman develops the infection during the first trimester, there is an increased risk of congenital anomalies [33]. Immunity to varicella can be assessed by blood testing for the presence of the varicella IgG antibody. A varicella vaccine is available and should be offered to non-immune individuals. The vaccine is administered in two doses 4–8 weeks apart. It is recommended that pregnancy be avoided during the vaccination period and until 1 month after the last injection.

Hepatitis Screening

Screening for hepatitis B and C is recommended for all pregnant women and those contemplating a pregnancy. While those with documented immunity to hepatitis pose no risk to the fetus, chronic carrier states do exist that can be associated with liver dysfunction and vertical transmission of the infection to the fetus. Women who have chronic active hepatitis should be appropriately counseled. Individuals who work with blood products or who are at high risk for a hepatitis B infection should be offered immunization. Male partners should also be screened for hepatitis B and C infections because of the potential transmission of an infection to their partner during intercourse or fertility treatments. For additional information on this topic, the reader is referred to a published review [35].

HIV Testing

An HIV infection can lead to acquired immunodeficiency syndrome. Many people who do not know that they are infected can infect others mainly through sexual contact. Of concern, is that an asymptomatic woman who is infected with the virus can pass the infection to her unborn child. HIV testing should be performed on all couples trying to conceive. In the past, HIV was considered to be a contraindication to pregnancy because of vertical transmission. However, with the advent of highly active antiretroviral therapy, which involves the administration of three or more drugs, the risk of vertical transmission is <1%–2%. Clearly, before any HIV-infected woman considers a future pregnancy, she should consult with an infectious disease expert and a maternal fetal medicine specialist.

Medical History

An important aspect of preconceptional care is an in-depth medical history to identify medical problems that could complicate a pregnancy. A medical condition or the medications used to treat the condition can have an impact on the establishment and health of a pregnancy. Another concern is that the pregnancy can worsen the medical condition and affect the health of the mother. In some cases, obtaining medical clearance may be indicated from the treating physician or a high-risk obstetrician before initiating treatment. Some of the more common medical problems that can be encountered are discussed below.

Diabetes Mellitus

Diabetes mellitus is a commonly encountered medical problem during pregnancy. It has been estimated that approximately 8.3% of the general population and between 2–5% of pregnant women have diabetes. Diabetes is associated with an increased incidence of congenital anomalies, which is directly related to the control of the diabetes before conception. A blood glucose level gives the clinician an idea of the glucose control at that point in time. The hemoglobin (Hgb) A1C level is an indicator of how well the diabetes has been controlled over the previous 3–4 months. If the HgbA1C is in the normal range (<6%), then the incidence of congenital anomalies approaches the incidence in the general population. In addition to the increased risk of congenital anomalies, poorly controlled diabetes during pregnancy is associated with increased fetal and maternal wastage. Therefore, the objective in diabetic women is to establish tight control of glucose levels before conception. Vascular disease can complicate diabetes and warrants an assessment of renal function and an ophthalmologic examination (to rule out a retinopathy) before pregnancy.

According to the American Diabetes Association 2017 recommendations, screening for diabetes should be considered in any woman who is overweight (BMI ≥ 25 kg/m^2) and any one or more of the following:

- Physical inactivity
- A first-degree relative with diabetes
- A high-risk race/ethnicity (e.g., African American, Latino, Native American, Asian American, Pacific Islander)
- Women who delivered a baby >9 lb or a history of gestational diabetes
- Hypertension
- HDL cholesterol level <35 mg/dL (0.90 mmol/L) and/or a triglyceride level >250 mg/dL (2.82 mmol/L)
- PCOS
- Severe obesity
- History of CVD
- Over the age of 45 years

Screening for diabetes can be accomplished by an HgbA1C, fasting plasma glucose test, or the 75-g oral glucose tolerance test (which includes a fasting plasma glucose test and a 2-hour glucose determination). For interpretation of the screening tests, refer to Table 4.2. Patients diagnosed with diabetes should be referred for further evaluation and treatment.

Hypertension

Chronic hypertension is a commonly encountered medical problem and, if left untreated, can cause irreparable damage to the kidneys and heart. Women with chronic hypertension should have baseline renal studies performed before conceiving. Hypertension places a woman at increased risk of superimposed pre-eclampsia during pregnancy, even if it is well controlled. Presently, there are many types of medications that control hypertension. The adverse effects of any medication should be investigated to assess whether there are any adverse effects on the fetus. As a general guideline, methyldopa and labetalol are considered safe to take during pregnancy. Angiotensin-converting enzyme inhibitors and angiotensin II receptor antagonists are contraindicated during pregnancy.

Celiac Disease

Celiac disease is an immune-mediated condition affecting the gastrointestinal tract. The symptomatology of the disease is brought on by the ingestion of gluten, which is present in wheat, barley, and rye. This causes a chronic inflammatory process resulting in atrophy of the intestinal villi, which then causes malabsorption. Celiac disease affects 1% of the population and has a genetic component. It is more prevalent in those with other autoimmune disorders including type 1 diabetes and thyroiditis. Classic symptoms include constipation, diarrhea, abdominal pain, anorexia, and vomiting. However, other cases of celiac disease do not have any of the gastrointestinal manifestations. A presenting symptom of celiac disease can be iron deficiency anemia. It also has been associated with infertility and recurrent miscarriages. In

TABLE 4.2

The 2017 American Diabetes Association Threshold Glucose Values for a 2-Hour Glucose Tolerance Test and HgbA1C Values

Test	Normal	Borderline	Diabetes
HgbA1C	≤5.6%	5.7%–6.4%	≥6.5%
Fasting blood glucose[a]	<100 mg/dL	100–125 mg/dL	≥126 mg/dL
2-hour blood glucose after a OGTT[b]	<140 mg/dL	140–199 mg/dL	≥200 mg/dL

[a] Fasting is defined as no caloric intake for at least 8 hours.

[b] The Oral Glucose Tolerance Test (OGTT) involves a fasting blood glucose level, ingesting of 75 g of anhydrous glucose dissolved in water, and then another blood glucose level 2 hours later.

a recent publication by Kumar et al. the prevalence of celiac disease in a group of patients with unexplained infertility was 5.65% compared to 1.30% in the control group [36].

The recommended screening for celiac disease includes the IgA antihuman tissue transglutaminase and IgA endomysial antibody immunofluorescence. If these tests are positive, then an endoscopy with biopsy of the duodenum should be performed. If the biopsies confirm atrophy of the villi, then the diagnosis is confirmed. The recommended treatment is elimination of all gluten from the diet.

Advanced Maternal Age

Current technology has increased the ability for women well over the age of 40 years to achieve a pregnancy with egg donation. However, older women are at increased risk for complications during pregnancy as compared to their younger counterparts. With advancing age, every woman is at increased risk of developing diabetes mellitus, chronic hypertension, and coronary artery disease, which can complicate a pregnancy. Therefore, it is prudent that every woman over the age of 40 undergo a medical evaluation before undergoing treatment to assess her medical fitness for a pregnancy.

Medication Use

All medications that a woman is taking should be investigated for potential detrimental effects on a pregnancy. The Food and Drug Administration (FDA) has placed medications into several categories based on animal and human studies that have investigated the harmful effects during pregnancy (Table 4.3).

It is clear that if a pregnant woman is taking a category X medication, it should be discontinued. However, if a medication falls into one of the other categories, continuation of the medication during pregnancy may be considered if benefits outweigh the risks. Consultation with a specialist is important and the decision to continue the medication is dependent on several factors. If the medical condition is not life-threatening or of significant importance, then serious consideration should be given to discontinuing the medication. In other situations, not treating the medical condition may put the mother or fetus at risk. In this situation, the clinician must try to select a medication that is effective in treating the condition and yet minimizes the risk to the fetus. For any medical therapy, if the benefits of treating the medical condition clearly outweigh the risks to the fetus, then the medication should be continued.

TABLE 4.3

FDA Drug Categories for Fetal Toxicity

Category	Description
A	Adequate, well-controlled studies in pregnant women have not shown an increased risk of fetal abnormalities.
B	Animal studies have revealed no evidence of harm to the fetus; however, there are no adequate and well-controlled studies in pregnant women. **or** Animal studies have shown an adverse effect, but adequate and well-controlled studies in pregnant women have failed to demonstrate a risk to the fetus.
C	Animal studies have shown an adverse effect and there are no adequate and well-controlled studies in pregnant women. **or** No animal studies have been conducted and there are no adequate and well-controlled studies in pregnant women.
D	Studies, adequate well-controlled or observational, in pregnant women have demonstrated a risk to the fetus. However, the benefits of therapy may outweigh the potential risk.
X	Studies, adequate well-controlled or observational, in animals or pregnant women have demonstrated positive evidence of fetal abnormalities. The use of the product is contraindicated in women who are or may become pregnant.

In 2014, the FDA established a new standard that will replace the current pregnancy letter category reporting. As of June 2015, new drugs have separate sections in the labeling for pregnancy, lactation, and female/male reproductive potential. Labeling of previously approved drugs will be phased in gradually.

Reproductive History

A reproductive history is an important part of preconceptional care and the details of previous pregnancies should be obtained. If a woman has had a previous pregnancy with complications, she could be at increased risk for the recurrence of these complications with a future pregnancy. Therefore, any pregnancy with an abnormal outcome should be investigated before attempting pregnancy. The correction of an underlying problem may improve the outcome of a future pregnancy. Some of the more common issues concerning the reproductive history are discussed below.

Recurrent Miscarriages

If a couple has experienced two or more miscarriages, then an evaluation is indicated. A survey of lifestyle issues and environmental factors may give insight into the pregnancy losses. The workup includes serum karyotypes on both the female and male partner to rule out chromosomal anomalies. A balanced translocation can be present in up to 2%–5% of couples. A menstrual history is important to determine whether ovulatory dysfunction may be a contributing factor. The female partner should have an assessment of TSH level, lupus anticoagulant, and anticardiolipin and anti–β-2-glycoprotein antibodies. An assessment of the uterine cavity should also be performed to rule out an anatomical reason for the pregnancy losses such as uterine fibroids and Müllerian defects. An examination of the uterine cavity can be accomplished by a hysterosalpingogram, a sonohysterogram, or a hysteroscopy.

Previous Stillborn or Infant Born with Congenital Anomalies

In most cases, when a previous pregnancy has resulted in a stillbirth or a baby with birth defects, testing has been performed on the fetus and the couple has undergone counseling. However, if there is uncertainty about the depth or scope of the workup, then the couple should be referred to a high-risk obstetrician for a consultation to determine the risk with a future pregnancy.

History of Premature Labor

The causes of premature labor are varied and can be secondary to premature rupture of the membranes, an abnormal uterine cavity (secondary to uterine fibroids, a Müllerian defect, and in utero DES exposure), chorioamnionitis, or an incompetent cervix. A history of premature labor places a woman at increased risk of a similar occurrence with a future pregnancy. A pregnancy complicated with premature labor and a malpresentation increases the likelihood of an underlying Müllerian anomaly, which has an incidence of 2%–3% in the general population. A vaginal ultrasound and a hysterosalpingogram will help to determine whether there has been any anomalous development of the cavity. Painless dilatation before the delivery suggests the diagnosis of incompetent cervix. These women should be counseled on the benefits of a cervical cerclage with a future pregnancy. Finally, a multiple pregnancy should be avoided in women with a previous history of premature labor.

Gestational Diabetes

A woman who has been diagnosed with gestational diabetes during a pregnancy is at increased risk of recurrence during a future pregnancy. In addition, these women are at increased risk of developing adult onset diabetes during their lifetime (approximately 2%–4% chance per year). For this reason, women with a history of gestational diabetes should be screened for glucose intolerance with an HgbA1C, fasting blood glucose, or a 2-hour glucose tolerance test. If diabetes is diagnosed, then referral to a medical endocrinologist or a high-risk obstetrician would be in order before attempting pregnancy. Adequate control of diabetes before conception decreases the chance of congenital anomalies and complications during the pregnancy.

Severe Pre-Eclampsia

Pre-eclampsia complicates 6%–8% of all pregnancies. In most cases, pre-eclampsia occurs during the first pregnancy and does not recur. However, severe pre-eclampsia with onset during the second trimester may recur in 10%–15% of future pregnancies. It may be increased to a greater degree if there are any underlying risk factors including diabetes, renal dysfunction, chronic hypertension, or a thrombophilia. Women with a history of severe pre-eclampsia may benefit from a referral to a high-risk obstetrician for counseling.

Occupational History

There has been increased awareness about the impact of environmental toxic exposures on general and reproductive health. Toxic exposures at the workplace can put some individuals at considerable risk. The Occupational Safety and Health Administration (OSHA), a federal agency of the Department of Labor, was established in 1970 and has monitored safety in the workplace. One of the three categories of hazardous substances monitored by the OSHA is reproductive toxins. Reproductive toxins are categorized as mutagens, teratogens, fertility toxins, and toxins transferred at lactation. It has been estimated that 17% of working women are exposed to known teratogens in the workplace [37]. The following is a discussion of some occupational risks that may pose a risk to reproduction.

Exposure to Anesthetic Gases

It is well documented that women who are exposed to anesthetic gases (i.e., operating room personnel and dental hygienists) are at increased risk for infertility, spontaneous abortion, and congenital anomalies [37–40]. Of interest is that paternal exposure may also be of consequence. Women who were impregnated by men who were exposed to anesthetic gases were found to be at greater risk of having a pregnancy complicated by a spontaneous abortion and congenital anomalies [38].

Exposure to Beauty Salon Chemicals

Beauty salon workers work in a complex environment and are exposed to many chemicals in hair dyes, permanent solutions, and bleaches. Furthermore, nail sculpturing also involves exposure to volatile chemicals that can be inhaled. A previous study concluded that beauty salon workers have an increased risk of miscarriage and infertility [41]. The risk was influenced by the number of hours worked per week, the use of formaldehyde disinfectants, and the practice of using gloves during hair treatments and whether nail sculpturing was done in the salon.

Organic Solvents

All women should be asked about exposure to organic solvents. Organic solvents include aliphatic and aromatic hydrocarbons, phenols, trichloroethylene, xylene, vinyl chloride, and acetone. Women at greatest risk for exposure to these chemicals are those who work in the health care profession and the clothing and textile industries. However, women in other professions may be unknowingly exposed to these agents as well. In a previous prospective study, women who were exposed to organic solvents during the first trimester were followed throughout the pregnancy [42]. When compared to a control group, there was no statistical difference in the rate of a spontaneous abortion and minor malformations. However, the group exposed to organic solvents had a statistically higher incidence of major malformations when compared to controls (12% vs. 1%, $p < 0.001$).

RECOMMENDATION

As part of preconceptional care, it is important to assess whether either the male or female partner is exposed to any toxin in the workplace, which may prove detrimental. All employers must provide material safety data sheets (MSDS) of all chemicals that are present in the workplace. Any potential risk is dependent on the specific toxin, length of time of exposure, and degree of exposure. If there is concern about an exposure, a consultation with a specialist in occupational medicine will help to clarify the risk.

Exposure to Spermatotoxins

From a fertility standpoint, males are more susceptible to toxins since sperm production is an ongoing process. The first report of an occupationally related spermatotoxin appeared in the mid-1970s [43]. It showed that men who worked at factories that produced DBCP (a pesticide) had an increased incidence of infertility—the severity being dependent on the dose and length of exposure. Since this report was released, other spermatotoxins have been discovered, including kepone, ethylene glycol ethers, carbon disulfide, naphthyl methylcarbamate, ethylene dibromide, organic solvents, and lead.

Genetic Counseling and Screening

As our knowledge in the field of genetics grows, increased responsibility will rest with those who counsel and prepare couples for pregnancy. A genetic history should be part of every evaluation of the infertile couple. There is no consensus as to the scope and breadth of the genetic history. Ideally, every couple contemplating pregnancy would be evaluated by a geneticist or genetic counselor to determine their genetic risks. This obviously is not practical but a thorough assessment of genetic risk and counseling is indicated.

It is important that any practitioner who is providing genetic counseling has an understanding of the disease process, its inheritance, and the limitations of the screening tests that are currently available. In addition, it is of utmost importance that the clinician stays abreast of new clinical developments and screening tests that become available. In some cases, referral to a genetic counselor is indicated. Recommendations for genetic counseling and position statements concerning testing have been published by the American College of Obstetrics and Gynecology (ACOG) (www.acog.com) and the American College of Medical Genetics (ACMG) (www.acmg.net).

Ancestral Backgrounds

An important aspect of the genetic history is an exploration of the ancestral backgrounds of both partners. Historically, individuals of a specific ethnic population are more likely to reproduce with others from the same population. This gives an opportunity for the propagation and higher prevalence rate of certain genetic disorders within these populations. Autosomal recessive diseases are most common. In this inheritance pattern, carriers are asymptomatic for the disease and both partners must be carriers to be at risk (one in four chance) of having a child that could be affected by the disease. Some of the commonly inherited conditions and indicated testing are discussed below. Many of these diseases can result in early death or significant morbidity. If an individual does not have an at-risk ancestral background but does have a family history of the disease, he or she should undergo screening (Table 4.4). It is also important that any individual who is identified to be a carrier of a genetic disease should be instructed to tell his or her siblings so that they too can undergo screening.

Presently, the clinician has two approaches when doing carrier screening. The first approach is to do targeted screening focused on the specific ancestry in question. ACOG and ACMG have summarized their recommendations in a joint publication [44]. One problem with this approach is that up to 30% of individuals are unclear of the ancestry. The second approach is to do the expanded carrier

TABLE 4.4

Genetic Testing Based on Ancestral Backgrounds

Ancestral Group	Disease	Screening Test
Caucasian, Native American	Cystic fibrosis[a]	DNA testing
French Canadian, Cajun	Tay–Sachs	Hexosaminidase enzyme activity and DNA testing
Jewish	**ACOG Recommendations**	
	• Canavan disease	DNA testing
	• Cystic fibrosis[a]	
	• Familial dysautonomia	
	• Tay–Sachs	Hexosaminidase enzyme activity and DNA testing
	ACMG Recommendations	
	• All of the above tests plus	
	• Niemann-Pick Type A	DNA testing
	• Bloom syndrome	
	• Fanconi Anemia Group C	
	• Mucolipidosis IV	
	• Gaucher disease	
African, Asian, Cambodia, Caribbean, Central America, India, Indonesia, Laos, Malaysia, Mediterranean, Middle Eastern, Pakistan, Thailand, Turkey, Vietnam	Hemoglobinopathies	CBC, Hgb electrophoresis

[a] It is impractical to screen for all cystic fibrosis mutations since more than 1000 mutations have been identified. Therefore, the clinician must realize the limitations of the screening and counsel couples accordingly. For instance, the detection rate of cystic fibrosis carriers in the Caucasian, Native American, and Jewish populations is 90%, 94%, and 97%, respectively.

screening panel, which is commercially available and is done through genotyping/sequencing. The expanded panel screens for 100 or more diseases, many of which are rare. There are concerns about the expanded panel results. Screening for hemoglobinopathies is best done with a hemoglobin electrophoresis. The panel includes Tay–Sachs DNA testing, which may not be positive in non-Jewish carriers. Therefore, the Tay–Sachs enzyme test is the best screen. There is also the issue of cost. In many cases, both partners end up being tested since 40%–50% of those tested initially will be a carrier of some disorder. Another consideration with carrier screening is that despite a negative screen, there is always a residual risk that the individual may still be a carrier with a mutation that is not detected by the testing—patients need to be counseled accordingly. This is especially important when one partner is a carrier of a condition and the other is not.

Screening for Chromosomal Anomalies

In some situations, a chromosomal analysis may be indicated. The following are some indications in which a karyotype of the male and female partners may be indicated.

Recurrent Miscarriages

Couples with two or more miscarriages have a 2%–5% chance of having a balanced translocation [45,46]. This chromosomal abnormality may explain the repeated miscarriages. While this chromosomal abnormality may put a couple at risk for a miscarriage, the majority of gametes that are produced in affected individuals are chromosomally normal. If a viable pregnancy is established when one of the partners has a balanced translocation, there is concern that the fetus may have a chromosomal imbalance that would increase the risk of congenital anomalies. In these cases, the couple may consider genetic testing with chorionic villus sampling or a genetic amniocentesis.

History of Down Syndrome

If a first-degree relative was diagnosed with Down syndrome, then it should be ascertained whether that affected individual underwent chromosomal testing. Approximately 90% of cases of Down syndrome are trisomy 21, which is a sporadic event. The remaining 10% are the result of a translocation. Of these, half are inherited and the other half occur *de novo*. Therefore, if there is uncertainty about the etiology or the result of the chromosomal analysis of the affected individual with Down syndrome, then a karyotype should be offered.

History of Stillbirth and Congenital Anomalies

In situations when a couple gives birth to a stillborn infant or an infant with a congenital anomaly, the chromosomal makeup of the fetus is usually tested. If this testing was not done or was inconclusive, then chromosomal testing of the couple should be offered.

Severe Male Factor Infertility

In males with azoospermia or severe oligospermia (<5 million sperm/cc) there is a 5%–15% chance of chromosomal anomalies and 3%–15% of microdeletions in the Y chromosome [47–49].

Fragile X Screening

Mental retardation can be caused by many factors including environmental, social, genetic, and unknown factors. The most commonly inherited type of mental retardation is Fragile X syndrome, which affects 1 in 1200 males and 1 in 2500 females. Fragile X syndrome is the result of expansion of the trinucleotide (CGG) repeat section on the long arm of the X chromosome. The degree of mental retardation can be borderline to severe and is related to the number of repeats within the mutation allele. Fragile X is associated with specific findings including a long thin face with prominent jaws, autistic features, and speech and language difficulties. Fragile X syndrome has an atypical inheritance. From one-third to one-half of females who carry the full mutation have Fragile X syndrome. If a woman is a carrier of a premutation, then she will not be affected by Fragile X syndrome but she is at increased risk of premature ovarian failure (before the age of 40). The premutation is identified in 2% and 14% of women with isolated and familial premature ovarian failure, respectively [50]. Fragile X screening should be considered for couples with a family history of unexplained mental retardation, autism, or premature ovarian failure.

Maternal Age Counseling

Advanced maternal age is associated with an increased incidence of post-fertilization chromosomal abnormalities in the embryo. This explains why increased maternal age is associated with an increased incidence of infertility, pregnancy loss, and fetal chromosomal abnormalities. While most pregnancies complicated by a chromosomal anomaly result in a miscarriage, others will progress to term, resulting in a delivery. The incidence of fetal chromosomal abnormalities in relation to maternal age is shown in Table 4.5. Once pregnancy is achieved, the risk of a fetal chromosomal abnormality can be further evaluated.

TABLE 4.5

Chromosomal Abnormalities in Live-Born Infants and Maternal Age

Maternal Age (Years)	Risk for Down Syndrome	Total Risk for Chromosomal Anomalies[a]
20	1/1667	1/526
21	1/1667	1/526
22	1/1429	1/500
23	1/1429	1/500
24	1/1250	1/476
25	1/1250	1/476
26	1/1176	1/476
27	1/1111	1/455
28	1/1053	1/435
29	1/1000	1/417
30	1/952	1/385
31	1/909	1/385
32	1/769	1/322
33	1/602	1/286
34	1/485	1/238
35	1/378	1/192
36	1/289	1/156
37	1/224	1/127
38	1/173	1/102
39	1/136	1/83
40	1/106	1/66
41	1/82	1/53
42	1/63	1/42
43	1/49	1/33
44	1/38	1/26
45	1/30	1/21
46	1/23	1/16
47	1/18	1/13
48	1/14	1/10
49	1/11	1/8

Source: Modified from Hook DB, Cross PK, Schreinemachers DM. Chromosomal abnormality rates at amniocentesis and in live-born infants. *J Am Med Assoc* 1983;249:2034–8; and Hook EB. Rates of chromosomal abnormalities at different maternal ages. *Obstet Gynecol* 1981;58:282–5.

[a] The other chromosomal anomalies that are increased with maternal age in addition to 47,+21 (Down's syndrome) are 47,+18; and 47,+13; 47,XYY (Klinefelter's syndrome); 47,XYY and 47,XXX. The incidence of 47,XXX for women between the ages of 20 and 32 years is not available.

Paternal Age Counseling

There is evidence that advanced paternal age can also pose a risk to the fetus. The increased incidence is not based on chromosomal abnormalities, but in the transmission of new genetic mutations. In contrast to oogenesis, spermatogenesis is an ongoing process that continues throughout a man's life beginning at puberty. The increased frequency of divisions within the spermatocytes increases the chance of errors that can result in a new mutation. These new mutations can result in the passage of an autosomal dominant disorder to an offspring or an X-linked recessive disorder to a grandson, which is called the "grandfather effect." The incidence of the inheritance of an autosomal dominant condition is 1 in

5000–10,000 deliveries. While the paternal age effect on the occurrence of any specific autosomal dominant condition may be low, the combined effect on all autosomal dominant conditions can be significant.
While advanced paternal age increases the risk of these new mutations, testing for all of these autosomal
dominant and X-linked disorders is not possible. Further, there is no consensus as to the definition of
advanced paternal age. It has been estimated that one-third of new autosomal dominant mutations are
the result of advanced paternal age (>40). It seems prudent to suggest that men complete their families
by age 40. Even though there is no easy way to screen for all of these genetic conditions in utero, at the
very least, couples should be made aware of the potential risk and given the opportunity to meet with a
genetic counselor.

Conclusion

Any couple who is interested in pregnancy should have a thorough evaluation to identify factors that
may put the patient at risk for a complicated pregnancy. Depending on the situation, further workup or
counseling may be indicated before the couple attempts pregnancy.

REFERENCES

1. Center for Disease Control (www.cdc.gov/tobacco).
2. The Practice Committee of the American Society for Reproductive Medicine. Smoking and infertility. *Fertil Steril* 2012;90:S254–9.
3. Zenzes MT. Smoking and reproduction: Gene damage to human gametes and embryos. *Hum Reprod Update* 2000;6:122–31.
4. Yang Q, Sherman SL, Hassold TJ et al. Risk factor for trisomy 21: Maternal cigarette smoking and oral contraceptive use in a population-based case-control study. *Genet Med* 1999;1:80–8.
5. Center for Disease Control (www.cdc.gov/ncbddd/fasd/alcohol-use.html).
6. Eggert J, Holger T, Engfeldt P. Effects of alcohol consumption on female fertility during an 18-year period. *Fertil Steril* 2004;81:379–83.
7. Center for Disease Control (www.cdc.gov/nchs/data/hestat/obesity_adult_13_14/obesity_adult_13_14 .htm).
8. Stothard KJ, Tennant PW, Bell R et al. Maternal overweight and obesity and the risk of congenital anomalies: A systematic review and meta-analysis. *JAMA* 2009;301:636–50.
9. Gunatilake RP, Perlow JH. Obesity and pregnancy: Clinical management of the obese gravida. *Am J Obstet Gynecol* 2011:204:106–19.
10. Endler GC, Mariona FG, Sokol RJ et al. Anesthesia-related maternal mortality in Michigan, 1972–1984. *Am J Obstet Gynecol* 1988;159:187–93.
11. http://www.nhlbi.nih.gov/files/docs/guidelines/prctgd_c.pdf
12. The American College of Obstetricians and Gynecologists. Practice Bulletin; Obesity in pregnancy. Number 315, 2015.
13. Bolumar F, Olsen J, Rebagliato M, Bisanti L. Caffeine intake and delayed conception: A European multicenter study on infertility and subfecundity. European Study Group on Infertility Subfecundity. *Am J Epidemiol* 1997;15:324–34.
14. The American College of Obstetricians and Gynecologists. Committee Opinion; Moderate caffeine consumption during pregnancy. Number 462, 2015.
15. Mulinare J, Cordero JF, Erickson JD, Berry RT. Periconceptional use of multivitamins and the occurrence of NTDs. *J Am Med Assoc* 1988;260:3141–5.
16. Bower C, Stanley FJ. Dietary folate as a risk factor for NTDs: Evidence from a case control study in Western Australia. *Med J Aust* 1989;150:613–9.
17. Miles JL, Rhoads GG, Simpson JL et al. The absence of a relationship between the periconceptional use of vitamins and NTDs. *N Engl J Med* 1989;321:430–5.
18. Hall JG, Solehdin F. Folate and its various ramifications. *Adv Pediatr* 1998;45:1–35.
19. McDonald SD, Ferguson S, Tam L et al. The prevention of congenital anomalies with periconceptional folic acid supplementation. *J Obstet Gynaecol Can* 2003;25:115–121.

20. Williams J, Mai CT, Mulinare J et al. Updated estimates of neural tube defects prevented by mandatory folic acid fortification—United States, 1995–2011. *MMWR* January 16, 2015;64(01):1–5.

21. Shaw GM, Velie EM, Schaffer D. Risk of neural tube defect-affected pregnancies among obese women. *J Am Med Assoc* 1996;275:1093–6.

22. MRC Vitamin Study Research Group. Prevention of NTDs: Results of the Medical Research Council Vitamin Study. *Lancet* 1991;338:131.

23. Smithells RW, Nevin NC, Sellers MJ et al. Further experience of vitamin supplementation for the prevention of NTD recurrences. *Lancet* 1983;1:1027.

24. Vergel RG, Sanchez LR, Heredero BL et al. Primary prevention of NTDs with folic acid supplementation: Cuban experience. *Prenat Diagn* 1990;10:149.

25. Rothman KJ, Moore LL, Singer MR et al. Teratogenicity of high vitamin A intake. *N Engl J Med* 1995;333:1369–73.

26. Lammer EJ, Hayes AM, Schunior A, Holmes LB. Unusually high risk for adverse outcomes of pregnancy following fetal isotretinoin exposure. *Am J Hum Genet* 1988;43:A58.

27. Marcus DM, Snodgrass WR. Do no harm: Avoidance of herbal medicines during pregnancy. *Obstet Gynecol* 2005;105:1119–22.

28. Ondrizek RR, Chan PJ, Patton WC, King A. An alternative medicine study of herbal effects on the penetration of zona-free hamster oocytes and the integrity of sperm deoxyribonucleic acid. *Fertil Steril* 1999;71:517–22.

29. Morreale de Escobar G, Obregon MJ, Escobar del Rey F. Is neuropsychological development related to maternal hypothyroidism or to maternal hypothyroxinemia? *J Clin Endocrinol Metab* 2000;85:3975–87.

30. Haddow JE, Palomaki GE, Allan WC et al. Maternal thyroid deficiency during pregnancy and subsequent neuropsychological development of the child. *N Engl J Med* 1999;342:549–55.

31. Alexander EK, Marqusee E, Lawrence J et al. Timing and magnitude of increases in levothyroxine requirements during pregnancy in women with hypothyroidism. *N Engl J Med* 2004;351:241–9.

32. Bayer SR, Turksoy RN, Emmi AM, Reindollar RH. Rubella susceptibility of an infertile population. *Fertil Steril* 1991;56:145–6.

33. Reid KC, Grizzard TA, Poland GA. Adult immunizations: Recommendations for practice. *Mayo Clin* 1999;74:377–84.

34. Rodrigues J, Niederman MS. Pneumonia complicating pregnancy. *Clin Chest Med* 1992;13:679–91.

35. The Practice Committee of the American Society for Reproductive Medicine. Recommendations for reducing the risk of viral transmission during fertility treatment with the use of autologous gametes: A committee opinion. *Fertel Steril* 2013;99:340–6.

36. Kumar A, Meena M, Begum N et al. Latent celiac disease in reproductive performance of women. *Fertil Steril* 2011;95:922–7.

37. Makuc D, Lalich N. Employment characteristics of mothers during pregnancy. Health United States and Prevention Profile 1983. National Center for Health Statistics, DHSS Publication No. (PHS) 841232. Washington, DC: US Government Printing Office, December 1983:25–32.

38. Cohen EN, Bellville JW, Brown BW Jr. Anesthesia, pregnancy and miscarriage: A study of operating room nurses and anesthetists. *Anesthesiology* 1971;35:343–7.

39. Rowland AS, Baird DD, Weinberg CR et al. Reduced fertility among women employed as dental assistants exposed to high levels of nitrous oxide. *N Engl J Med* 1992;327:993–7.

40. Guirguis SS, Pelmear PL, Roy ML, Wong L. Health effects associated with exposure to anesthetic gases in Ontario hospital personnel. *Br J Int Med* 1990;47:490–7.

41. John EM, Savitz DA, Shy DM. Spontaneous abortions among cosmetologists. *Epidemiology* 1994;5:147–55.

42. Khattak S, K-Moghtader G, McMartin K et al. Pregnancy outcome following gestational exposure to organic solvents: A prospective controlled study. *J Am Med Assoc* 1999;281:1106–9.

43. Whorton D, Krauss RM, Marshall S et al. Infertility in male pesticide workers. *Lancet* 1977;2:1259–61.

44. Edwards JG, Feldman G, Goldberg J et al. Expanded carrier screening in reproductive medicine—Points to consider. *Obstet Gynecol* 2015;125:653.

45. Plouffe L, White EW, Tho ST et al. Etiological factors of recurrent abortion and subsequent reproductive performance of couples: Have we made any progress in the past 10 years? *Am J Obstet Gynecol* 1992;167:313.

46. Harger JH, Archer DF, Marchese SG et al. Etiology of recurrent pregnancy losses and outcome of subsequent pregnancies. *Obstet Gynecol* 1983;62:574.
47. DeBraekeler M, Dao TN. Cytogenetic studies in male infertility: A review. *Hum Reprod* 1991;6:245–50.
48. Pryor JL, Kent-First M, Muallem A et al. Microdeletions in the Y chromosome of infertile men. *N Engl J Med* 1997;336:534–9.
49. Kent First MG, Kol S, Muallem A et al. The incidence and possible relevance of Y-linked microdeletions in babies born after intracytoplasmic sperm injection and their infertile fathers. *Mol Hum Reprod* 1996;2:943–50.
50. Sherman SL. Premature ovarian failure in the fragile X syndrome. *Am J Genet* 2000;97:189–94.

5

Clinical Algorithms

Michael M. Alper and Nina Resetkova

This chapter contains clinical algorithms that will aid the physician in the day-to-day management of the infertile couple. Each infertile couple presents with a different set of circumstances, and the scope of the testing and recommended treatment will vary accordingly.

The clinical algorithms are general guidelines regarding patient care, and other circumstances, including patient choice, may dictate a course of management other than that presented.

The following clinical algorithms are presented:

1. Infertility evaluation (Figure 5.1)
2. Unexplained infertility (Figure 5.2)
3. Reduced ovarian reserve (Figure 5.3)
4. Ovulatory dysfunction (Figure 5.4)
5. Uterine factor (Figure 5.5)
6. Tubal/peritoneal factor (Figure 5.6)
7. Male factor (Figure 5.7)

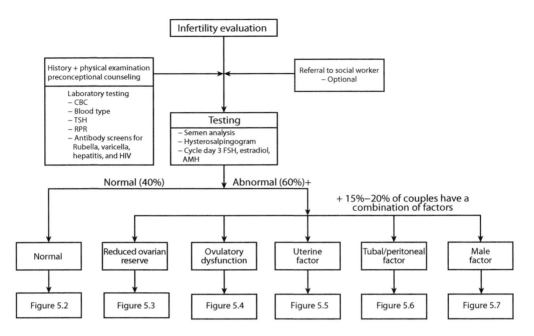

FIGURE 5.1   AMH, anti-mullerian hormone; CBC, complete blood count; FSH, follicle-stimulating hormone; HIV, human immunodeficiency virus; RPR, rapid plasma regain; TSH, thyroid-stimulating hormone.

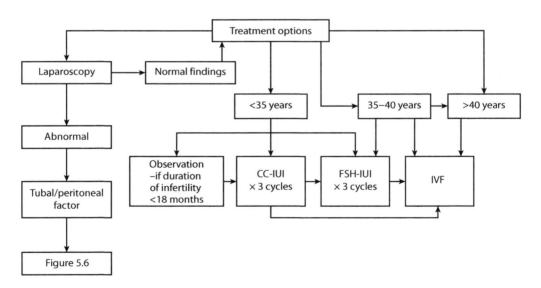

FIGURE 5.2   Unexplained infertility. CC, clomiphene citrate; FSH, follicle-stimulating hormone; IUI, intrauterine inseminations; IVF, in vitro fertilization.

DIAGNOSIS

The diagnosis of reduced ovarian reserve is supported by any of the following:

1. Cycle day 3 FSH > 10 mIU/mL or estradiol > 70 pg/mL
2. Abnormal clomiphene challenge test
   To perform:
   - Cycle day 3 FSH, estradiol levels
   - Clomiphene citrate 100 mg cycle days 5–9
   - Cycle day 10 FSH level

   If any of the FSH levels are >10 mIU/mL or the estradiol is >70 pg/mL, the test is considered abnormal.
3. AMH level < 1.0 mL
4. Documented poor response to aggressive ovulation induction

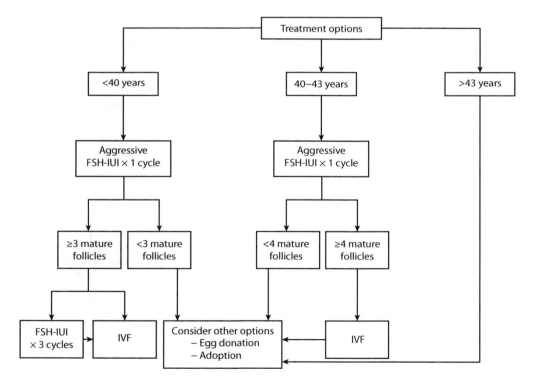

FIGURE 5.3 Reduced ovarian reserve. FSH, follicle-stimulating hormone; IUI, intrauterine inseminations; IVF, in vitro fertilization.

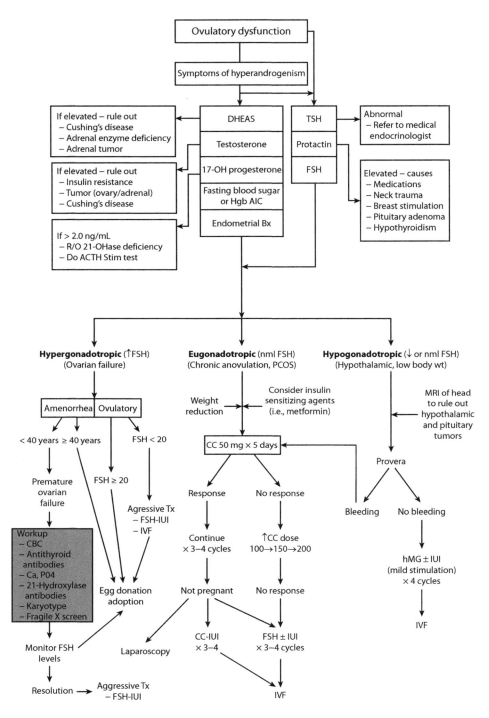

FIGURE 5.4 Ovulatory dysfunction. ACTH, adrenocorticotropic hormone; CBC, complete blood count; CC, clomiphene citrate; DHEAS, dehydroepiandrostenedione; FSH, follicle-stimulating hormone; hMG, human menopausal gonadotropins; IUI, intrauterine inseminations; IVF, in vitro fertilization; MRI, magnetic resonance imaging; PCOS, polycystic ovarian syndrome; TSH, thyroid-stimulating hormone.

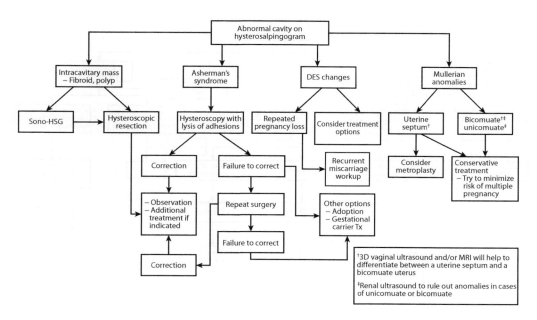

FIGURE 5.5 Uterine factor. DES, diethylstilbestrol; MRI, magnetic resonance imaging; Sono-HSG, sonohysterogram.

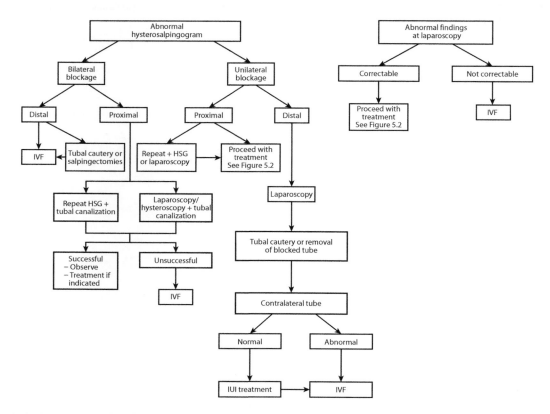

FIGURE 5.6 Tubal/peritoneal factor. HSG, hysterosalpingogram; IVF, in vitro fertilization; IUI, intrauterine inseminations.

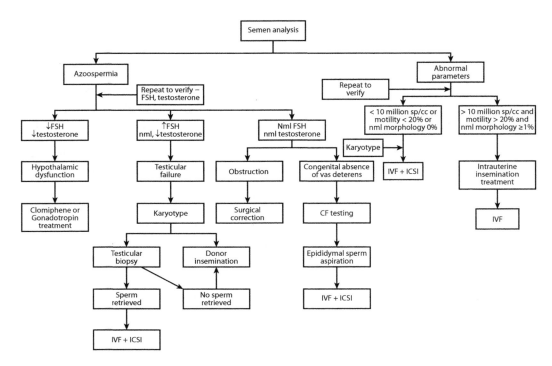

FIGURE 5.7 Male factor. CF, cystic fibrosis; FSH, follicle-stimulating hormone; ICSI, intracytoplasmic sperm injection; IVF, in vitro fertilization.

6

Treatment Options: I. Ovulation Induction

Selwyn P. Oskowitz and Alan S. Penzias

Approximately 20% of infertile patients present with underlying ovulatory dysfunction as a major contributing factor to their infertility. Compared to other etiologies, ovulatory problems are often the easiest to correct in most cases. However, before any treatment is started, it is important to delineate the underlying cause of the ovulatory dysfunction (refer to Chapter 5). The causes of ovulatory dysfunction are varied and can be categorized into *hypergonadotropic* (ovarian failure), *eugonadotropic* (chronic anovulation), and *hypogonadotropic* (hypothalamic, weight-related) states. Women who have ovarian failure or are perimenopausal generally do not respond favorably to medical treatment. There are many different medications, both oral and injectable, that can be used as part of ovarian stimulation. The choice of medication depends on the clinical presentation and the goal of the specified treatment. This chapter will review the current approach to ovulation induction.

Clomiphene Citrate

Clomiphene citrate (CC) was first introduced in 1961 and is the most commonly prescribed medication for the infertile woman. It can be prescribed for different reasons, but its primary indication is for the correction of ovulatory dysfunction. When compared to other ovulation induction agents, CC is inexpensive, is easy to administer, and does not require close monitoring that is required with injectable ovulation induction agents. Historically, CC was the first-line treatment for those patients with polycystic ovary syndrome (PCOS). Those patients with hypothalamic dysfunction who fail to have withdrawal bleeding after a progesterone challenge will not respond well to CC in most cases.

Pharmacology

CC is a triphenylethylene derivative that is related to tamoxifen and diethylstilbestrol. CC exists in two isomeric forms, zuclomiphene and enclomiphene citrate. The pharmacological effect of this medication is from the zuclomiphene citrate isomer. Commercial preparations of CC contain equal amounts of these two isomers. CC is an estrogen antagonist and binds for an extended period to intranuclear estrogen receptors, which decreases the replenishment of these receptors. The hypothalamus responds to the *psuedo-hypoestrogenic* state by increasing GnRH pulse frequency, which, in turn, increases the secretion of FSH and LH from the anterior pituitary. CC has a half-life of 5 days and can be detected in the blood and stool up to 6–8 weeks after administration. Despite the long half-life of CC, there are no reported increase in congenital anomalies that can be attributed to the use of this medication.

Side Effects

Since CC is a synthetic hormonal agent, side effects are common and are not dose related. Many of the side effects that result are related to the pseudo-hypoestrogenic state that is created. The more common side effects and their incidence are as follows:

DEFINITION OF TERMS

Ovulation induction is the term for the stimulation of ovulation in the anovulatory patient. The aim is to stimulate the growth of a single follicle with the release of its egg.

Superovulation (SO) is the term for stimulating the growth of multiple follicles with the release of multiple eggs. SO is an integral part of intrauterine insemination and in vitro fertilization (IVF) treatments.

- Irritability, mood changes (20%)
- Vasomotor symptoms (10%)
- Abdominal discomfort (6%)
- Breast discomfort (2%)
- Nausea/vomiting (2%)
- Visual symptoms (1%)
- Headaches (1%)

The use of ovulation induction agents, especially CC, may result in more pain associated with ovulation. Prolonged administration of CC through its anti-estrogenic action can diminish cervical mucus production and thin the endometrial lining, which could lower the chance of pregnancy.

Dosage and Administration

CC is available in 50-mg tablets. The recommended initial dose of CC for treatment of anovulatory infertility is 50 mg daily for 5 days after either a spontaneous or progesterone-induced menstrual period. Many practitioners begin CC in anovulatory women following confirmation of a negative pregnancy test without inducing menses. After the treatment is started, if ovulation is confirmed and the menstrual cycle is less than 32 days in length, then the current dose should be continued for three cycles. Couples should be instructed to use an ovulation predictor kit or time intercourse around the predicted periovulatory period. If the induced cycles are greater than 32 days or there is no indication of ovulation by LH kit, the dosage of the CC should be increased to 100 mg for 5 days. If this dose is inadequate, then the dose should be increased to 150 mg. If pregnancy is not achieved after three ovulatory cycles, then other factors should be ruled out. If no other factors are identified, then intrauterine inseminations can be added to the CC treatment since CC may have an adverse effect on cervical mucus in 15% of cases. Although higher doses up to 250 mg/day may be attempted, the majority of pregnancies occur at dosages of 150 mg daily or less. If the patient with chronic anovulation does not respond to a dose of 150 mg daily, then our approach is to proceed on with injectable gonadotropins.

Outcome

Proceeding in the stepwise fashion as described above, the ovulatory rates on the 50-mg, 100-mg, and 150-mg dosage regimens are 50%, 22%, and 12%, respectively [1]. However, despite 80% of anovulatory patients ovulating with CC treatment, only 40%–50% of women will achieve pregnancy [2].

- *Pregnancy rate*: 10% per ovulatory cycle.
- *Multiple pregnancy rate*: 8%–10%—most are twins, but there is a 1% chance of triplets.

Management of CC Failures

Lack of Ovulation

Serial increases in CC dose without a new period, if no sign of follicle growth 14 days after the last CC dose [3]

- Metformin—pretreatment with 1500–2000 mg qd for 4–6 weeks before another course of CC [4]
- Dexamathasone—0.5 mg PO qd, for cases where dehydroepiandrostenedione (DHEAS) is higher than 430 µg/dL

Ovulation but No Pregnancy

- Add a surrogate LH surge with an injection of hCG (10,000 units) or recombinant hCG (250 µg) subcutaneously when the lead follicle is 18–25 mm in diameter.
- Improving cervical mucus with estradiol 2 mg daily from CD 9 to ovulation.
- Combined approach of estradiol from day 12 followed by progesterone starting 3 days after the LH surge detected by ovulation predictor kit [5].
- Add intrauterine inseminations.

Unexplained Infertility

In clinical practice, CC is commonly prescribed for the woman with unexplained infertility. Theoretically, it seems that CC would improve fecundity by increasing the number of eggs that are released at the time of ovulation and CC may correct subtle ovulatory dysfunction. However, previous studies including a recently published Cochrane review of seven trials fail to show that CC improves fertility over doing nothing at all [6–8]. Nevertheless, some couples and clinicians feel that this is a reasonable initial treatment to pursue. As with any therapy, most pregnancies are achieved within the first few months of treatment. Therefore, the duration of treatment should be limited to three to four cycles at which time the treatment plan should be reassessed.

Recommended dosage: CC 100 mg administered between cycle days 3 and 7. Limit duration of treatment to 3–4 months. Instruct couples to use an ovulation predictor kit or have intercourse every other day between cycle days 10 and 18.

Pregnancy rate: 6% per cycle.

Letrozole

Letrozole is an aromatase inhibitor that is a supplemental treatment for hormonally responsive breast cancer. There has been interest in the utility of this medication as a fertility drug but it is not approved by the Food and Drug Administration (FDA) for this indication. The use of letrozole in the infertile population was the topic of a previous review [9]. By inhibiting the aromatase enzyme, letrozole causes a drop in estrogen levels, which results in release of FSH by the pituitary gland. Unlike CC, letrozole does not have detrimental effects on the cervical mucus and endometrial lining. Letrozole is available in 2.5-mg tablets and is taken once a day beginning in the early follicular phase. The standard dose is 2.5 mg/day increasing up to 7.5 mg/day for 5 days. The incidence of side effects with letrozole is similar to those noticed from CC including hot flashes, nausea, dizziness, and headaches. The risk of a multiple pregnancy is from 5% to 10%, most of which are twins, and high-order multiple pregnancies are rare. Ovarian hyperstimulation syndrome (OHSS) is theoretically possible.

NOTE: There was an initial report concluding that there was an increased rate of fetal anomalies with letrozole [10]. However, larger studies have not shown any increased risk to the offspring [11,12]. Despite this reassurance, patients should be counseled that this medication is not FDA approved for ovulation induction purposes.

Other Medications That Can Be Used with CC

In some women with ovulatory dysfunction, other medications may be considered, which can be administered by themselves or in addition to CC.

Oral Hypoglycemic Agents

It is now believed that insulin resistance plays a central role in the pathogenesis of PCOS. Insulin resistance is a condition in which the action of insulin is hampered either by a defective insulin receptor or by a post-receptor defect. With insulin resistance, higher circulating levels of insulin are necessary to maintain normal glucose homeostasis. Hyperinsulinism can explain many of the associated findings of PCOS. Insulin increases ovarian and adrenal androgen production, decreases the production of sex hormone binding globulin, and stimulates the pituitary secretion of LH. All of this leads to an androgenic *milieu* that interferes with the normal follicular development and ovulation. Insulin resistance is a metabolic disorder and ovulatory dysfunction is only one of its manifestations. Other medical issues associated with insulin resistance include type 2 diabetes, hypertension, dyslipidemia, centripetal obesity, and an increased risk of cardiovascular disease.

Those with adult-onset diabetes mellitus have been treated effectively with oral hypoglycemic agents, such as metformin, which improves the actions of insulin in several ways. It increases the uptake of glucose into fat and muscle cells. In addition, it decreases intestinal absorption of glucose and reduces hepatic gluconeogenesis. There are published data that have confirmed that metformin improves the insulin resistance in patients with PCOS, which results in a correction of the ovulatory dysfunction [4,13,14]. This was a significant breakthrough in the treatment of PCOS. Many women with PCOS respond poorly to CC and have to be treated with injectable gonadotropins to induce ovulation, which is associated with a higher multiple pregnancy rate and greater chance of OHSS. In a previous meta-analysis, it was concluded that metformin alone improved the rate of ovulation [15,16]. The ovulation rates were different between the metformin and placebo groups, 46% versus 26%. Also, the rate of ovulation in those who took metformin plus CC or CC alone was 76% versus 42%, respectively. While metformin may be effective by itself, it may take up to 6 months to appreciate ovulatory cycles [14,16]. After these studies were published, it was felt by many infertility specialists that metformin treatment should be the initial treatment for PCOS patients. However, many of the initial studies included a small number of patients. A well-designed study published by Legro et al. provided the data that helped to define the role of metformin treatment in PCOS [17]. This multicenter blinded study involved 626 infertile women with PCOS who were randomly assigned to one of three arms: CC plus placebo (CC), metformin plus placebo (MET), and metformin plus CC (MET/CC). Patients were then followed for 6 months after the treatment was begun. The live birth rate was 22.5% in the CC group, 7.2% in the MET group, and 26.8% in the MET/CC group. The difference in pregnancy rates was statistically significant between CC and MET groups and between MET/CC and MET groups but not for CC versus MET/CC (Figure 6.1). The conclusion from this study is that initial treatment with CC for the PCOS patient is warranted. However, metformin does have a role in the treatment of the PCOS patient, which is discussed below.

Evaluation

Renal studies (creatinine, BUN) and liver function tests (SGOT, SGPT) should also be obtained. One potential risk of metformin treatment is lactic acidosis. The incidence of this side effect is increased in those patients with renal or hepatic dysfunction.

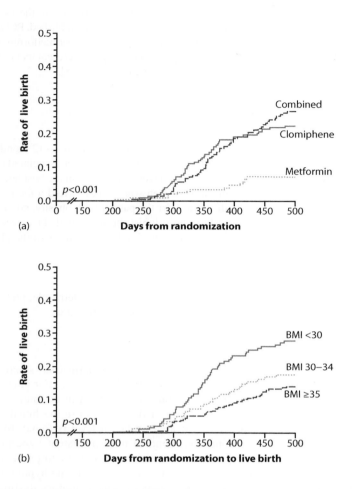

FIGURE 6.1   Kaplan–Meier curves for live birth rates according to study group (a) and BMI (b). Clomiphene is a superior treatment for infertility. BMI affects prognosis for all treatment groups. (Reprinted with permission from Legro RS, Barnhart HX, Schlaff WD et al. Clomiphene, metformin, or both for infertility in the polycystic ovarian syndrome. *N Engl J Med* 2007;356(6):551–66. Copyright 2007 Massachusetts Medical Society. All rights reserved.)

Recommended Dosage

Metformin is available in standard and extended release (XR) formulations. Initiation of metformin should be done in a gradual fashion to decrease the incidence of side effects. One tablet (500 mg) should be taken daily for 1 week, then twice a day for 1 week, and then 3–4 times a day (1500–2000 mg/day). The medication should be taken with meals. There are benefits in the XR formulation—for some, it is better tolerated and the total dose can be taken at once on a daily basis.

Side Effects

Gastrointestinal symptoms, including nausea, vomiting, diarrhea, bloating, and flatulence, occur in 30% of patients who take metformin. These side effects are usually temporary, but in some patients, the side effects do not abate. In these cases, decreasing the dose may reduce the side effects, and at some time in the future, a higher dose may be tried again. Lactic acidosis is a serious metabolic disorder that may be increased in those with renal and/or hepatic dysfunction. There have been reports of metformin-induced lactic acidosis after the administration of intravenous iodine contrast agents, which can result in transient nephrotoxicity. Therefore, metformin should be withheld 24 hours before and 48 hours after the performance of the x-ray procedure. Metformin is a schedule B drug but should be discontinued when pregnancy is established. PCOS patients are at increased risk of miscarriage and there has been some controversy as to whether metformin decreases the chance of a first-trimester loss if taken throughout the early part of pregnancy. In a recent meta-analysis, it was concluded that metformin does not decrease the chance of a first-trimester loss [18].

Clinical Application

Long-Term Treatment

In some cases, long-term treatment with metformin can be considered for up to 6–12 months. This is an especially attractive treatment for those women with obesity and possibly other associated consequences of insulin resistance (i.e., hypertension, glucose intolerance) who may not be in the best health for a pregnancy. Metformin should also be considered in those women who want to avoid a multiple pregnancy that is associated with ovarian stimulation medications. For the patient with obesity, good nutrition and an exercise program should be stressed. A referral to a nutritionist should strongly be considered. Weight loss will increase the effectiveness of metformin. The patient should follow up with the physician periodically every 6–8 weeks to monitor for treatment efficacy.

Short-Term Treatment

For those patients who have failed to respond to moderate doses of CC or letrozole, pretreatment with metformin (4–8 weeks) before moving on to another cycle may prove efficacious.

Dopaminergic Agents

Hyperprolactinemia is a cause of ovulatory dysfunction. A serum prolactin assay should be obtained on any woman who presents with irregular or absent menstrual periods and/or galactorrhea. It is important that the prolactin level is assessed on a blood sample drawn in the morning during the follicular phase of the menstrual cycle. At other times of the day, and in the luteal phase, physiological elevations of prolactin can occur. If an elevated prolactin level is found, the assessment should be repeated for verification. If a woman is found to have persistent hyperprolactinemia, then a cause should be determined. Hyperprolactinemia can be secondary to previous breast surgery, neck trauma, medication use, renal insufficiency, a pituitary tumor, and hypothyroidism. Any woman with unexplained hyperprolactinemia when associated with ovulatory dysfunction should have a magnetic resonance imaging of the brain to rule out a pituitary tumor. Several dopaminergic agents are available to correct the hyperprolactinemia (e.g., bromocriptine, cabergoline). Most times, these agents are effective by themselves in correcting the ovulatory dysfunction. In a previous review reporting on 22 clinical trials, it was noted that 80% of women with hyperprolactinemia had restoration of their menstrual function after treatment with bromocriptine [19]. On average, menstrual function returned 5.7 weeks after treatment was started. If the patient fails to develop normal ovulatory cycles despite the establishment of a normal prolactin level, then the clinician may consider adding CC or another ovulation induction agent to the treatment regimen. Many patients will resume ovulatory cycles with slightly elevated prolactin levels.

How do we explain the woman who has normal menstrual cycles in the presence of hyperprolactinemia? In addition to the biologically active monomeric prolactin, other larger prolactin species (termed macroprolactins) are present in the bloodstream. These macroprolactins are inactive and are of no clinical significance but are measured in the conventional prolactin assay. A macroprolactin level can be measured to determine the true circulating levels of bioactive monomeric prolactin. For this reason, routine screening of women with normal cycles and no complaints of galactorrhea should be discouraged.

Available Agents and Doses

1. *Bromocriptine* is available in 2.5-mg tablets. Start with half a tablet (1.25 mg) at bedtime for 1 week then increase up to one tablet (2.5 mg). Repeat the prolactin level in 4 weeks. If the prolactin level is still elevated, the dose can be increased in an incremental fashion.
2. *Cabergoline* is available in 0.5-mg tablets. Start with one tablet (0.5 mg) twice a week. Repeat the prolactin level in 4 weeks. If the prolactin level is still elevated, the dose can be increased by 0.25 mg twice weekly up to a total dose of 1 mg twice a week.

Side Effects

The more common side effects include gastrointestinal upset, fatigue, dizziness, and nasal stuffiness. For those with persistent gastrointestinal side effects, vaginal administration of the medication may be considered.

Dexamethasone

Dexamethasone can be considered for the anovulatory woman who fails to respond to increasing doses of CC or is noted to have an elevated DHEAS level. An elevated DHEAS level may suggest an attenuated adrenal enzyme deficiency. Other causes include an adrenal tumor and Cushing's syndrome, which must be considered but are, nonetheless, rare. If associated with an elevated 17-OH-progesterone level, a 21-hydroxylase deficiency must be ruled out. The administration of dexamethasone will decrease the adrenal androgen contribution to the pool of androgens. In some cases, this will be enough to improve the response to CC. Dexamethasone can be administered at night at a dose of 0.5 mg. One month after starting the dexamethasone, a morning cortisol level should be checked. A cortisol level less than 2 µg/dL suggests significant depression of cortisol synthesis by the adrenal gland, which could interfere with a stress response by the adrenal gland. In this circumstance, the dose or frequency of administration should be decreased. The use of dexamethasone should be avoided during pregnancy.

Dexamethasone can be considered in clomiphene failures in the absence of elevated androgen levels. In a previous prospective study, 223 CC-resistant patients were randomized to receive CC 200 mg days 5–9 + dexamethasone (DEX) 2.0 mg days 5–14 and the other group was given CC 200 mg days 5–9 + a placebo [20]. In the CC–Dex group, 88% ovulated compared to only 20% in the CC–placebo group.

Dexamethasone Treatment Options

- 0.5 mg qd—Check morning serum cortisol plasma level 3–4 weeks after treatment started and if it is <2.0 µg/dL, reduce the dose.
- 2.0 mg cycle days 5–14 during CC cycle.

Gonadotropins

Gonadotropins are injectable medications that are effective in correcting ovulatory dysfunction. A list of current agents that are available appears in Chapter 8. The agent used depends on the clinical presentation. One must exercise caution when administering these agents to correct ovulatory dysfunction (as compared to their use in the context of superovulation) to minimize the risk of multiple pregnancy.

Hypothalamic Dysfunction

Since these patients are deficient in FSH and LH, both of these hormones need to be replaced. Therefore, human menopausal gonadotropins is the drug of choice. It is important that low doses (75 IU) be administered initially and one is cautious in raising the dose.

1. hMG 75 IU × 5–7 days then check E2 and US
   a. If E2 < 50, increase by 37.5 IU × 3 days then repeat the E2/US. Increase HMG by no more than ½ amp every 3–4 days.
   b. If E2 > 50, continue the same dose and repeat monitoring for 2–3 days.
2. Administer hCG when lead follicle is ≥16 mm.

CAUTION: These patients are at significant risk of a multiple pregnancy—the goal of the stimulation is 1–2 follicles. If more than 2 follicles are ≥16 mm or if several secondary follicles are present >12 mm, consideration should be given to canceling the cycle or converting to IVF.

OHSS can be a risk related to gonadotropin use. In addition to the aforementioned mature follicles, careful study of the ultrasound results is needed to assess the number of small follicles 10–14 mm.

Polycystic Ovarian Disease

These patients are deficient in FSH and may have elevated circulating levels of LH. Therefore, only FSH-containing medications are needed to correct the ovulatory dysfunction.

1. FSH 37.5 to 75 IU × 5 days then check E2 and ultrasound.
   a. If E2 < 50, increase by 37.5 IU × 3 days then repeat the E2/US. Increase HMG by no more than ½ amp every 3–4 days.
   b. If E2 > 50, continue the same dose and repeat monitoring for 2–3 days.
2. Administer hCG when lead follicle is ≥16 mm.

CAUTION: These patients are at risk of a multiple pregnancy and OHSS—the goal of the stimulation is 1–2 follicles. However, the success rate in the PCO population is lower than those patients with hypothalamic dysfunction. If more than 3–4 follicles ≥16 mm develop on ultrasound examination or if several secondary follicle >12 mm are present, then consideration should be given to canceling the cycle or converting to IVF.

REFERENCES

1. Gysler M, March CM, Mishell DR, Bailey EJ. A decade's experience with an individualized clomiphene treatment regimen including its effect on the post-coital test. *Fertil Steril* 1982;37:161.
2. Practice Committee of the American Society of Reproductive Medicine. Use of clomiphene citrate in infertile women: A committee opinion. *Fertil Steril* 2013;100(2):341–8.
3. Hurst B, Hickman M, Matthews R et al. A novel Clomiphene "stair-step" protocol reduces time to ovulation in women with polycystic ovary syndrome. *Am J Obstet Gynecol* 2009;510, 200.
4. Nestler JE, Jakubowicz DJ, Evans WS, Pasquali R. Effects of metformin on spontaneous and clomiphene-induced ovulation in the polycystic ovary syndrome. *N Engl J Med* 1998;338:1876–80.
5. Elkind-Hirsch KE, Phillips K, Bello SM et al. Sequential hormonal supplementation with vaginal estradiol and progesterone gel corrects the effect of clomiphene on the endometrium of oligo-ovulatory women. *Hum Reprod* 2002;17:295–8.
6. Hughes E, Brown J, Collins JJ, Vandekerckhove P. Clomiphene citrate for unexplained subfertility in women. *Cochrane Database Syst Rev* 2010; Jan 20(1):CD 00005.

7. Hughes EG. The effectiveness of ovulation induction and intrauterine insemination in the treatment of persistent infertility: A meta-analysis. *Hum Reprod* 1997;12:1865–72.

8. Fujii S, Fukui A, Fukushi Y et al. The effects of clomiphene citrate on normally ovulatory women. *Fertil Steril* 1997;68:997–9.

9. Requena A, Herrero J, Landeras J et al. Use of letrozole in assisted reproduction: A systematic review and meta-analysis. *Hum Reprod Update* 2008;14:571–82.

10. Biljan MM, Hemmings R, Brassard N. The outcome of 150 babies following the treatment with letrozole or letrozole and gonadotropins. *Fertil Steril* 2005;84(suppl. 1);S95.

11. Tulandi T, Martin J, Al-Fadhli R et al. Congenital malformations among 9111 newborns conceived after infertility treatment with letrozole or clomiphene citrate. *Fertil Steril* 2006;85(6):1761–5.

12. Forman S, Gill R, Moretti M et al. Fetal safety of letrozole and clomiphene citrate for ovulation induction. *J Obstet Gynaecol Can* 2007;29, 668–71.

13. Velazquez EM, Acosta A, Mendoza SG. Menstrual cyclicity after metformin therapy in polycystic ovary syndrome. *Obstet Gynecol* 1997;90:392–5.

14. Velazquez EM, Mendoza SG, Hamer et al. Metformin therapy in polycystic ovary syndrome reduces hyperinsulinemia, insulin resistance, hyperandrogenemia, and systolic blood pressure, while facilitating normal menses and pregnancy. *Metabolism* 1994;43:647–54.

15. Lord JM, Flight IHK, Norman RJ. Metformin in polycystic ovary syndrome: Systematic review and meta-analysis. *BMJ* 2003;327:951–7.

16. Ibanez L, Valls C, Ferrer A et al. Sensitization to insulin induces ovulation in nonobese adolescents with anovulatory hyperandrogenism. *J Clin Endocrinol Metab* 2001;863:595–8.

17. Legros RS, Barnhart HX, Schlaff WD et al. Clomiphene, metformin, or both for infertility in polycystic ovary syndrome. *N Engl J Med* 2007;356:551–66.

18. Paolmba S, Falbo A, Orio F, Zullo F. Effect of preconceptional metformin on abortion risk in polycystic ovary syndrome: A systematic review and meta-analysis of randomized controlled trials. *Fertil Steril* 2009;92:1646–58.

19. Cuellar FG. Bromocriptine mesylate (Parlodel) in the management of amenorrhea/galactorrhea associate with hyperprolactinemia. *Obstet Gynecol* 1980;55:278.

20. Parsanezhad ME, Alborzi S, Motazedian S, Gholamhossein O. Use of dexamethasone and clomiphene citrate in the treatment of clomiphene-resistant patients with polycystic ovary syndrome and normal dehydroepiandrosterone sulfate levels: A prospective, double-blind, place-controlled trial. *Fertil Steril* 2002;78:1001–4.

7

Treatment Options: II. Intrauterine Insemination

Sonia Elguero and Marsha Forman

Intrauterine insemination (IUI) is a common fertility treatment that involves concentrating motile sperm and placing it high within the uterine cavity. It is utilized in a variety of clinical situations including cervical factor, mild male factor, severe vaginismus, and ejaculatory dysfunction; however, the most common indication is unexplained infertility. It is also the best approach to therapeutic donor sperm insemination (TDI). Prerequisites for performing IUI include ovulation, patency of at least one fallopian tube, and adequate number of motile sperm for insemination. A natural cycle approach may be considered in some instances. In most cases of unexplained or male factor infertility, the use of fertility medications to increase the development of multiple follicles has been shown to increase the chance of success. In addition, the success rate with ovulation induction plus IUI is higher than that with ovulation induction alone. How does an IUI increase the chance of pregnancy? The explanation remains obscure, but may be the result of several factors. The sperm washing procedure may eliminate toxins or bacteria in the seminal plasma and has been shown to induce the acrosome reaction causing activation of the sperm. Performance of the IUI may bypass an impediment in the cervical mucus. In contrast to intercourse, the IUI results in a higher number of motile sperm that find their way into the uterine cavity. Finally, the IUI may overcome faulty coital technique on the part of the couple. Despite all of these theoretical benefits of IUI, the overall success of IUI treatment is low in comparison to in vitro fertilization (IVF). Nevertheless, for many infertility patients, IUI is their first introduction to treatment. This chapter will provide an overview of the treatment.

Approaches to IUI Treatment

Natural Cycle

A natural or non-medicated approach is most often used with TDI, but in the context of infertility, this approach is associated with a low success rate. A natural cycle IUI may be suitable in a couple with coital factor infertility such as ejaculatory dysfunction or vaginismus. It may be the desire of the couple who wants to completely avoid medications or a multiple pregnancy. When considering this treatment approach, it is essential that the patient is ovulatory.

Monitoring

The patient is instructed to start testing her urine with an ovulation predictor kit 3–4 days before the anticipated time of ovulation. For the woman who has cycles that are 28–30 days in length, she is instructed to start testing her urine on day 11. When the ovulation predictor test turns positive, she is instructed to come in the following day for the insemination.

Clomiphene Citrate

Clomiphene citrate (CC) can be the initial medicated approach for younger women under the age of 35. For women over the age of 35, a more aggressive ovulation induction (e.g., gonadotropins) is the preferred approach. CC is the most widely prescribed fertility medication. For a detailed description of this medication, please refer to Chapter 6. CC is administered at a dose of 100 mg for 5 days between cycle days 3 and 7. Alternatively, it can be administered between cycle days 5 and 9.

Femara (Letrozole)

Letrozole is another option for ovulation induction. In women with polycystic ovary syndrome and an elevated body mass index greater than 30, it has been shown to be more effective in inducing ovulation with higher live birth rates as compared to CC [1]. In the setting of unexplained infertility, letrozole and CC have been shown to have similar live birth rates [2]. The starting dose is typically 2.5 mg/day and can be increased up to 7.5 mg/day. At higher doses, it can be associated with thin endometrium, similar to CC. For women with unexplained infertility, letrozole can result in lower rates of multiple gestation. It is currently used off label as it is not approved by the US Food and Drug Administration for ovulation induction. It can be potentially teratogenic if used during early pregnancy and patients should be counseled about off-label use before prescribing.

Monitoring

The patient is instructed to use an ovulation predictor kit beginning on cycle day 11. When the test turns positive, a single insemination treatment is done the following day. In our experience, approximately 90% of patients will detect the LH surge between cycle days 11 and 15. An alternative is to perform vaginal ultrasound examinations beginning cycle day 12 and to administer human chorionic gonadotropin (hCG) (10,000 IU, or 250 µg of Ovidrel) when the follicle reaches 18 mm and the insemination is scheduled 36 hours later. There is no difference in the success rate with CC-IUI when ultrasound monitoring and hCG trigger versus monitoring the LH surge with urine testing [3]. However, the advantage of doing an ultrasound exam is that it provides valuable information about the ovarian response. If just a single follicle develops, then there should be consideration to substituting FSH injections for the CC. The average success rate after CC-IUI treatment is 8%–10% per cycle, and the multiple pregnancy rate is 10% (9% twins; 1% triplets). An important factor that affects treatment success is the maternal age. The Boston IVF experience with CC-IUI of more than 4000 cycles was reported by Dovey et al. [4], and the results are reported in Table 7.1.

TABLE 7.1

Boston IVF CC-IUI Success Rates

Age	Pregnancies Achieved		Pregnancies Achieved after 3 Cycles of Treatment
	Per Cycle	**Per Patient**	
<35	11.5%	24.2%	89.5%
35–37	9.2%	18.5%	91%
38–40	7.3%	15.1%	95%
41–42	4.3%	7.4%	67%
>42	1.0%	1.8%	100%

Source: Data taken from Dovey S, Sneeringer RM, Penzias AS. Clomiphene citrate and intrauterine inseminations: Analysis of more than 4100 cycles. *Fertil Steril* 2008;90:2281–6.

Note: A pregnancy was defined as ultrasound confirmation of an intrauterine sac.

Gonadotropins

The use of FSH injections for ovulation induction as part of IUI treatment increases the success rate. For older women or women with a diminished ovarian reserve, this may be a more suitable option compared to CC or letrozole. For a detailed discussion on these medications, the reader is referred to Chapter 8. The injections of FSH are started on day 3 and continued until mature follicles have developed. The initial dose will be dependent on many factors including previous response and age. In general, the first cycle of treatment requires more caution with the starting dose (75–150 U) since it is unknown how the patient will respond to the medication. This is of less concern for the older patient over the age of 40 who most likely has some reduced ovarian reserve, and the starting dose may be increased to 150–225 U. The goal of the treatment may vary as well. For a younger woman, the goal is to obtain two to four mature follicles that are 16 mm or larger. If more than five mature follicles are present or there are multiple follicles between 12 and 16 mm, then there is an increased risk of a multiple pregnancy. These cycles should be either canceled or converted to an IVF treatment cycle. For the woman over the age of 40, the chance of a multiple pregnancy is reduced and the goal of the stimulation is to obtain four to six mature follicles.

Monitoring

The assessment of serum estradiol levels and a vaginal ultrasound exam are recommended 4–5 days after starting injections. If the estradiol level is >400 pg/mL, then the dose is reduced by 75 U. The goal is to have the estradiol level increase by 50%–100% every 2–3 days. The vaginal ultrasound will determine the number and size of the follicles. A mature follicle is between 16 and 20 mm in diameter. The final goal of the treatment is to have a peak estradiol level between 500 and 2000 pg/mL at the time of the hCG administration. A single insemination is performed 36 hours after hCG administration.

Success Rate

As with any fertility treatment, several factors influence success. One important factor is the semen quality. Pregnancy rates are higher when the total motile sperm count is >2 million, post-wash motility is >40%, and/or normal sperm morphology is >4% [5]. However, interpretation of sperm morphology can vary from laboratory to laboratory. Age is an important determinant of treatment success [6,7]. Duran et al. reported on more than 1000 cycles and reported the live birth rate in the different age groups (see Table 7.2).

In comparison to CC-IUI, success rates after FSH-IUI tend to be higher, but one must also take into consideration the increased multiple pregnancy rate of 15%–20%, which includes a higher incidence of high-order multiple pregnancies.

TABLE 7.2

FSH-IUI Success Rates

Age	Number of Cycles	Live-Birth Rate, % (95% CI)
<25	15	26.7 (4.3, 49.4)
25–29	219	14.2 (9.6, 18.8)
30–35	556	12.5 (9.8, 15.2)
36–39	221	9.5 (5.6, 13.4)
≥40	106	8.5 (3.2, 13.8)

Source: Data taken from Duran HE, Morshedi M, Kruger T, Oehninger S. Intrauterine insemination: A systematic review on determinants of success. *Hum Reprod Update* 2002;8:373–84.

Preparation of the Semen Sample

A semen sample is produced on the day of the IUI. It is best to collect the sample in a sterile specimen container supplied by the laboratory since it has been tested for sperm survivability. Several plastics are harmful to sperm and may reduce the vitality of the sample. It is preferred that semen is collected via masturbation; however, collection condoms can be purchased online from fertility specialty stores. Drug store condoms should never be used since they are developed to kill sperm with or without spermicide. Lubricants should not be used to produce the sample. Semen samples can be produced on site or at home and then transported to the laboratory. It is best if the sample collected outside of the office can be delivered within 60 minutes after production. The sample should be kept at body temperature from the time of collection until it is received by the laboratory staff. Exposure to temperatures other than body temperature for an extended time between collection and processing may be responsible for poor motility of the specimen. For security reasons, we only accept sperm samples from the male patient/intended parent and not another party (including the wife). His identification is confirmed by examination of his government-issued picture ID. Our sperm washing procedure is as follows.

Once the sample is received by the laboratory staff, it will be assessed for concentration and motility. The semen sample is then washed and prepared for insemination. Washing can be performed in a complex or simple fashion. Washing of the sample removes prostaglandins and bacteria found in the seminal plasma. A simple wash will concentrate the sperm, both motile and immotile, into the pellet for insemination. A complex wash uses a density gradient to filter the seminal fluid, resulting in an elevated post-washed motility. Washing also concentrates the sperm into a reduced volume for insemination.

Process all specimens using sterile technique and practicing universal precautions. Examination gloves should be worn at all times, and facial protection should be used if the sample is not processed under a hood. Check the laboratory requisition for any special instructions.

1. The semen sample is produced by masturbation into the provided sterile specimen cup.
2. Allow semen sample to liquefy for 20–60 minutes.
3. Measure volume with a 10-ml pipette.
4. Divide the sample into two test tubes labeled "pellet" with the patient's name.
   a. Simple method: Add an equal volume of sperm wash to each of the tubes and mix well.
   b. Complex method: Layer semen in a 2:1 ratio over 80% gradient.
5. Remove any coagulates that may pellet to bottom of tubes.
6. Centrifuge for 10 minutes at 1200 rpm (300 g).
7. Remove supernatant and place in the tube labeled "super."
8. Resuspend the pellets in a total of 2 mL fresh sperm wash; the two pellet tubes should be combined at this step. The wash medium should not exceed 2 mL.
9. Centrifuge (second time) for 5 minutes at 1200 rpm (300 g).
10. Remove supernatant.
11. Resuspend the pellet in a total of 0.5 mL sperm wash.
12. Mix thoroughly and count the sample.
13. Place washed sample on the 37°C warmer until ready to use.

Performing the IUI

Depending on the state, nurses or physicians can perform the IUIs. If there is any difficulty with the insemination, a physician is called to complete the procedure. Before the insemination, the patient's name is verified and she confirms that her name is on the tube containing the washed sperm sample. To perform the IUI treatments, a speculum examination is performed and the cervix is visualized. The cervix is wiped with a large cotton tip applicator. The washed sperm sample is loaded into a catheter, which is inserted through the cervical canal and into the uterine cavity. Immediately after the IUI, the patient is discharged and normal activity can be resumed. A pregnancy test is scheduled 14 days later. Patients should be reassured that mild cramping or discomfort can occur along with increased wetness. Luteal phase support can be considered with IUI cycles particularly in patients utilizing gonadotropins.

Single versus Double Inseminations

The decision to do one versus two inseminations has been the subject of ongoing debate. In a meta-analysis, Polyzos et al. reported on 68 randomized controlled studies including 829 women [8]. The pregnancy rate in double versus single insemination groups was 13.6% versus 14.4%, respectively. These findings have been supported by other investigators [9,10]. The odds ratio was 1.33 (95% CI 0.99, 1.73). However, two of the studies included used CC as a stimulatory agent. Both of these studies using CC confirmed a benefit of a second insemination. The explanation as to why a second insemination is needed with CC remains uncertain. When the CC studies were excluded, the results did not confirm that the additional IUI improved the success. The data published to date prevent any conclusive evidence that a second insemination is necessary. From a theoretical standpoint, a second insemination may not be necessary if one considers that sperm generally maintain their viability for 48–72 hours and the oocyte has a 12- to 24-hour window to be fertilized.

Cost Analysis

As couples weigh their treatment options, the financial aspect no doubt is a part of the decision-making process. It is clear that IVF is the most successful option, but for many couples, the treatment may be too costly. There are only 15 states with mandated insurance coverage for infertility treatment, and the degree of coverage can vary from state to state. Massachusetts has the best insurance coverage and allows the couple to choose the treatment they want—many go directly to IVF while others will try a few insemination cycles first. In New York, some have coverage for insemination treatments but not for IVF. The vast majority of infertile couples in the United States do not have insurance coverage for treatment. So what is the most cost-effective approach for couples to take? Boston IVF participated in a study that helps to put this into better perspective. The FASTT (fast track and standard treatment trial) involved more than 500 couples with unexplained infertility [11]. The couples were randomized to one of two arms: the first arm included three cycles of CC-IUI followed by three cycles of FSH-IUI and then up to six cycles of IVF; the second "accelerated" arm involved three cycles of CC-IUI and then directly moving to IVF. The conclusions from the study were as follows:

- An increased pregnancy rate was noted in the accelerated group.
- Median time to pregnancy was quicker in the accelerated group 8 versus 11 months.
- Per-pregnancy rates for CC-IUI, FSH-IUI, and IVF were 7.6%, 9.8%, and 30.7%, respectively.
- Average charges per delivery were $9800 lower for the accelerated arm.
- FSH-IUI treatment had no added value.

Thus, the most cost-effective approach for the couple with unexplained infertility is CC-IUI × 3 cycles and then move on to IVF.

Commentary

Intrauterine insemination is the oldest infertility treatment and still has a place in the treatment paradigm, but its utility may be fading. Over the years, IVF success rates have continued to increase and this has resulted in the transfer of fewer embryos, thus decreasing the chance of a multiple pregnancy. The complications and risks associated with a multiple pregnancy are well documented. By following

ASRM/ACOG guidelines and reducing the number of embryos transferred, we have essentially eliminated high-order multiple pregnancies and there is now focus on decreasing the twin pregnancy rate, which makes up 20%–25% of IVF pregnancies. Preimplantation genetic screening (PGS) is beginning to take hold and is now offered at most IVF programs. If PGS becomes a standard part of the IVF treatment cycle, then all patients will have the transfer of a single euploid blastocyst. Realizing the strides we have made in the IVF patient population, we now have to take a closer look at the multiple pregnancies associated with the conservative treatments. There seems to be a disconnect—for those undergoing IVF, we are trying to do everything to avoid a multiple pregnancy, but for those undergoing medicated IUI treatment, we are somewhat complacent and accepting of the chance of a multiple pregnancy. To this end, we should try to phase out FSH-IUI treatment. And at some point in the future, we may want to bypass even other more conservative treatment options that utilize CC and letrozole.

REFERENCES

1. Legro RS et al. Letrozole versus clomiphene for infertility in the polycystic ovarian syndrome. NICHD Reproductive Medicine Network. *N Engl J Med* 2014;371:119–29.
2. Diamond MP, Legro RS, Coutifaris C et al. Letrozole, gonadotrophin or clomiphene for unexplained infertility. NICHD Reproductive Medicine Network. *N Engl J Med* 2015;373:1230–40.
3. Lewis V, Queenan J, Hoeger K et al. Clomiphene citrate monitoring for intrauterine insemination timing: A randomized trial. *Fertil Steril* 2006;85:401–6.
4. Dovey S, Sneeringer RM, Penzias AS. Clomiphene citrate and intrauterine inseminations: Analysis of more than 4100 cycles. *Fertil Steril* 2008;90:2281–6.
5. Haebe J, Martin J, Tekepety F et al. Success of intrauterine insemination in women aged 40–42 years. *Fertil Steril* 2002;78:29–33.
6. Harris ID, Missmer SA, Hornstein MD. Poor success of gonadotropin-induced controlled ovarian hyperstimulation and intrauterine insemination for older women. *Fertil Steril* 2010;94:144–8.
7. Duran HE, Morshedi M, Kruger T, Oehninger S. Intrauterine insemination: A systematic review on determinants of success. *Hum Reprod Update* 2002;8:373–84.
8. Polyzos NP, Tzioras S, Mauri D, Tatsioni A. Double versus single intrauterine insemination for unexplained infertility: A meta-analysis of randomized trials. *Fertil Steril* 2010;94:1261–6.
9. Osuna C, Matorras, R, Pijoan JL, Rodriguez-Escudero FJ. One versus two inseminations per cycle in intrauterine insemination with sperm from patients' husbands: A systematic review of the literature. *Fertil Steril* 2004;82:17–24.
10. Bagin T, Haydardedeoglu B, Kilicdag EV et al. Singe versus double intrauterine insemination in multifollicular ovarian hyperstimulation cycles: A randomized trial. *Hum Reprod* 2010;25:1684–90.
11. Reindollar RH, Regan MM, Neumann PJ et al. A randomized clinical trial to evaluate optimal treatment for unexplained infertility: The fast track and standard treatment (FASTT) trial. *Fertil Steril* 2010; 94:888–910.

8

Treatment Options: III. In Vitro Fertilization

Michael M. Alper

In vitro fertilization (IVF) is one of the most significant advances in the field of reproductive medicine. The first IVF baby, Louise Brown, was born in England in 1978. This was the result of a decade of research by Dr. Robert Edwards who was ultimately awarded the Nobel Prize in Medicine in 2010 for his work. Since the first IVF success, more than 400 IVF units have been established in the United States alone. More than 5 million babies have been born as a result of this technology, and now 1%–2% of all babies born in the United States are conceived with IVF. Initially, IVF was developed for women with tubal disease but now it is the treatment of choice for many other causes of infertility that are refractory to more conservative treatment. Since its introduction, all of the steps of IVF treatment have been improved, resulting in continuously rising success rates over the last 20 years (Figure 8.1). IVF is the most successful infertility treatment that can be offered. IVF has also provided a platform for the development of other treatments including egg donation, gestational surrogacy, and preimplantation diagnosis and screening. This chapter will provide a basic overview of the IVF treatment.

The following four steps of IVF will be reviewed:

1. Ovarian hyperstimulation
2. Oocyte retrieval
3. Oocyte insemination
4. Embryo transfer

Ovarian Hyperstimulation

IVF treatment initially utilized non-medicated or natural cycles. The timing of the egg retrieval was based on the initiation of the endogenous luteinizing hormone (LH) surge as detected from multiple blood tests throughout the day. Overall, the natural cycle and those cycles that used mild stimulation with clomiphene citrate were extremely inefficient since few follicles developed. One of the first modifications that increased IVF success rates significantly was the use of gonadotropins to stimulate the growth of multiple ovarian follicles. The term *gonadotropins* refers to medications that contain follicle-stimulating hormone (FSH) and LH. This was a definite improvement, but premature ovulation complicated approximately 30% of cycles, making timing of the egg retrieval a challenge, and many of these cycles were canceled. The next breakthrough occurred in the late 1980s when the gonadotropin-releasing hormone (GnRH) agonist was introduced. The addition of the GnRH agonist virtually eliminated any chance of a premature LH surge and resulted in more control of the cycle. Later in the 1990s, the GnRH antagonists were developed and provided another approach to suppressing a premature LH surge. The ovarian hyperstimulation step is extremely important since the success rate is directly related to the number of oocytes that are retrieved, which, in turn, affects the number

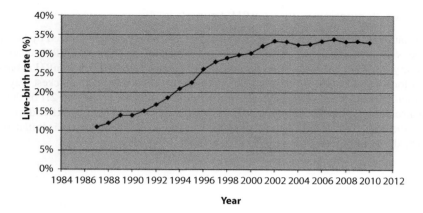

FIGURE 8.1 IVF treatment success rates have continued to increase over time. The live-birth rate (per oocyte retrieval for all women treated during the calendar year) increased 3.0-fold between 1987 and 2003. The increase in the success rates has been paralleled by an increased number of ART procedures that have been performed in the United States.

of embryos that are available for transfer. Over the years, there has been a change using gonadotropins obtained from urine of postmenopausal women to those preparations created by recombinant DNA technology. The newer gonadotropins are more purified, allowing subcutaneous injection. The medications used for ovarian hyperstimulation are listed in Table 8.1. The ovulation induction protocols that are used today are described below.

TABLE 8.1

Fertility Medications

Gonadotropin—Gonadotropins are injectable medications used for ovarian hyperstimulation for intrauterine insemination and IVF treatment. Two types of gonadotropins can be administered and are discussed below:

1. FSH (Gonal-F®, Follistim®)—These medications contain only FSH and are administered by subcutaneous injection. These are the most commonly prescribed medications for ovulation induction.
2. Human menopausal gonadotropins (Menopur)—This medication contains equal amounts of FSH and LH, and are administered on a daily basis by subcutaneous injections.

GnRH agonist (Lupron)—This is a synthetic hormone that is administered by subcutaneous injection. The administration of a GnRH agonist initially causes release of FSH and LH from the pituitary gland. However, with continued administration, there is down-regulation of the GnRH receptors, which minimizes release of FSH and LH by pituitary gonadotrophs and prevents an LH surge. GnRH agonists are administered with gonadotropins in women undergoing IVF treatment. The main benefit is that pretreatment with a GnRH agonist prevents an LH surge.

GnRH antagonists (Ganirelix®, Cetrotide®)—GnRH antagonists reversibly bind to GnRH receptors and prevent release of FSH and LH. The major benefit of the use of GnRH antagonists in conjunction with FSH is the suppression of the LH surge. In contrast to GnRH agonists, the GnRH antagonists have an immediate action in prevention of an LH surge and require fewer injections during the treatment cycle.

Human chorionic gonadotropin (Profasi®, Pregnyl®, Ovidrel®, Novarel®)—This medication contains naturally occurring pregnancy hormone, hCG, which functions similarly to LH. Since LH is not available in the United States as a separate medication, we use hCG as its surrogate. LH (with low levels throughout the follicular maturation stage) is an important hormone that works alongside FSH to help mature the eggs. However, the final maturation of the egg to undergo meiosis is triggered with an LH surge in the natural cycle or by the administration of hCG during IVF. The IVF cycle egg retrieval (or IUI if an IUI cycle) is typically done 36 hours after the administration of hCG just before ovulation would otherwise occur.

Progesterone supplements—Progesterone supplements are used in women undergoing IVF treatment to help prepare the endometrium for implantation and support a pregnancy. Progesterone can be administered by intramuscular injection, vaginally and orally. In general, oral progesterone (Prometrium®) is not as effective owing to hepatic metabolism to inert metabolites. Vaginal progesterone has the advantage of having a direct effect on the endometrium and ease of use. The two approved vaginal products in the United States are Crinone® (usually given once daily after the egg retrieval) and Endometrin (given two to three times daily).

Pituitary Down-Regulation with a GnRH Agonist

Traditionally, pituitary down-regulation has been the most common protocol utilized by IVF programs. Daily injections of a GnRH agonist results in "down-regulation" of pituitary GnRH receptors, which reduces pituitary FSH and LH release and prevents an LH surge. Generally, the GnRH agonist must be administered for a period of 10–15 days before down-regulation occurs. The quickest way to achieve down-regulation is to start the GnRH agonist in the mid-luteal phase (cycle day 21) of the preceding cycle. It can also be started in the early follicular phase with the onset of menses. After down-regulation has occurred, the dose of the GnRH agonist is reduced and the ovulation induction is initiated with FSH injections. The dose of FSH required may vary from 150 to 450 U/day.

Microdose Lupron

This protocol is used for women who are poor responders or who have evidence of reduced ovarian reserve. This protocol typically involves the administration of oral contraceptives for a period of 3 weeks. Theoretically, the administration of the oral contraceptives suppresses gonadotropin release and puts the ovaries to rest. After the 3-week course of the oral contraceptives has been completed, small doses of a GnRHa and an FSH are administered twice daily. When Lupron is administered in this fashion, it acts as a stimulatory agent because it induces the release of FSH and LH, and after continued administration, there is inhibition of the LH surge (down-regulation).

Pituitary Suppression with a GnRH Antagonist

GnRH antagonists result in the immediate suppression of FSH and LH release from the pituitary gland, as opposed to agonists that take several days to suppress the pituitary. The use of GnRH antagonist protocols is becoming more popular. The advantages include fewer injections, avoidance of the ovarian suppression that can occur after administration of a GnRHa, and a lower chance of ovarian hyperstimulation syndrome (OHSS). For this protocol, gonadotropins are started on cycle day 2. When the lead follicle reaches a diameter of 14 mm and/or the serum estradiol level is >500 pg/mL, the daily administration of the GnRH antagonists is started (alongside the gonadotropins). The administration of the antagonist initially results in a decrease in the serum estradiol level in part because the antagonist reduces both endogenous FSH and LH secretion. Some have advocated the addition of LH activity when the antagonists are started to offset the reduction in endogenous LH—this can be in the form of human menopausal gonadotropins or low-dose human chorionic gonadotropin (hCG) (10 IU/day).

Monitoring

During the ovarian stimulation, the woman's response is monitored with serum estradiol levels and vaginal ultrasound examinations. The estradiol level is used to determine the dose of gonadotropins and whether under- or overstimulation occurs. However, some studies have concluded that serum estradiol monitoring is not always necessary and the response to treatment can be followed with ultrasound monitoring alone. The goal of the ovarian hyperstimulation is to develop at least three mature follicles that are 17 mm in diameter or larger. Once this is achieved, FSH and other medications are discontinued, and a single injection of hCG is given to mature the eggs to allow fertilization. The hCG administration will also cause ovulation, but this does not occur until 40 hours or later after the injection. Therefore, it is standard that the hCG injection is administered 36 hours before the scheduled egg retrieval such that this will allow adequate maturation of the eggs and yet there would be little risk of ovulation. When the GnRH antagonist protocol is being used and there is concern about OHSS, a GnRH agonist can be used (in place of hCG) to induce an endogenous LH surge for final oocyte maturation.

Oocyte Retrieval

The egg retrieval is performed under vaginal ultrasound guidance. First, the vagina is cleansed with normal saline. Betadine is not used since it may be toxic to the eggs. The vaginal ultrasound probe is then placed in the vagina and the ovarian follicles are located. A 17-gauge needle is directed through the back wall of the vagina and into the ovarian follicles (Figure 8.2). The fluid is aspirated and then examined by an embryologist to identify the microscopic egg (Figure 8.3). All follicles within both ovaries are aspirated. Once the eggs are retrieved, they are placed in culture plates with nutrient media and then placed in the incubator. The procedure is performed under light anesthesia and generally takes less than 10–15 minutes to complete. Prophylactic antibiotics are routinely administered. The overall complication rate is <1%.

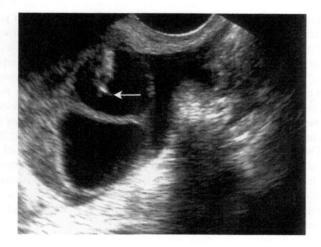

FIGURE 8.2 Vaginal ultrasound–guided egg retrieval. This is an ultrasound image taken at the time of egg retrieval. During the procedure, the ovary is positioned on the other side of the vaginal wall. A needle has been inserted through the vaginal wall, and the tip of the needle is positioned in the center of the follicle (arrow). After proper placement of the needle, the fluid from the follicle is aspirated.

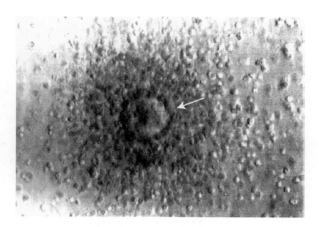

FIGURE 8.3 An oocyte. This picture is of an oocyte obtained at the time of egg retrieval. The oocyte (arrow) is surrounded by a group of granulosa cells called the cumulus oophorus. During normal fertilization, the acrosome of the sperm releases enzymes that disperse the cumulus cells, therefore allowing the sperm to penetrate and fertilize the oocyte.

Oocyte Insemination

Standard Insemination

On the day of egg retrieval, the sperm concentration and motility are assessed. If the sperm sample is adequate, then a sperm prep is done to isolate the most motile sperm. A total of 50,000 motile sperm are placed with the eggs in a culture dish, which is then placed in the incubator.

Intracytoplasmic Sperm Injection

Intracytoplasmic sperm injection (ICSI) is used in cases of male factor or in cases when a prior standard IVF resulted in <30% of eggs fertilized. It was first introduced more than 20 years ago by Palermo which revolutionized the field of IVF, and it was then realized that all you need is only one viable sperm to fertilize the egg. ICSI involves the injection of a single sperm directly into the oocyte (Figure 8.4). In the United States, ICSI is used in more than half of all IVF cycles. Fertilization rates after this procedure are between 60% and 70% (comparable to the rates achieved with a standard insemination when the semen parameters are normal). Males with severe oligospermia (count <5 million sperm/cc) should have a karyotype performed since they are at greater risk for having a chromosomal abnormality. Couples should be counseled that there is an increased risk of sex chromosomal anomalies in infants born after the ICSI procedure when it is performed in cases of severe oligospermia. The rate of sex chromosomal aneuploidy in infants conceived naturally is 0.2% and is 0.8% after the ICSI procedure. These chromosomal abnormalities are likely not the result of the ICSI procedure itself but are attributed to the low level of mosaicism present in the spermatogonia. Couples may opt for a prenatal genetic testing during the pregnancy to detect potential chromosomal problems. Studies have confirmed that many cases of male factor infertility are caused by microdeletions on the Y chromosome. Couples should be counseled that this genetic testing is available, and if a defect is found, then it could be transmitted to a male offspring.

The morning after insemination, the eggs are examined to determine whether fertilization has occurred. A fertilized egg is shown in Figure 8.5. Note that the two pronuclei (one from the sperm and the other from the egg) should be present within the egg. Within a few hours, the nuclei unite and the embryo will start to divide.

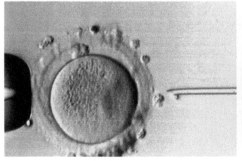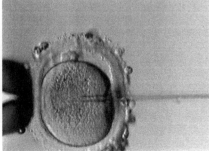

FIGURE 8.4   The ICSI procedure is performed with very fine instruments under a microscope. After the granulosa cells have been stripped away from the oocyte with enzymes, the oocyte is held in place by a holding pipette. The other pipette, which is much smaller and sharper, is used to pick up a single sperm. The smaller pipette is then brought into proper position (left panel) and then inserted through the zona pellucida and into the cytoplasm of the oocyte where the sperm is injected (right panel). ICSI, intracytoplasmic sperm injection.

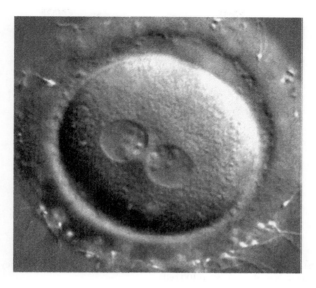

FIGURE 8.5   A fertilized egg. Note the two pronuclei (one from the sperm and one from the egg) present within the egg.

Embryo Transfer

The embryo transfer can be performed either day 3 (cleavage stage embryo) or day 5 (blastocyst stage) after the egg retrieval. In the United States, most transfers occur on day 5 when the embryo is at the blastocyst state. On day 3, good quality embryos are generally between 6 and 8 cells (Figure 8.6). Single-medium culture systems allow the embryo to develop from day 3 to day 5 without the need to change the culture system (Figure 8.7). The advantage of waiting until day 5 is that it provides additional time to select the better-quality embryos since only 50%–60% of embryos have the ability to develop into blastocysts and therefore fewer embryos are available for transfer and freezing. Published evidence supports a higher implantation potential for a blastocyst embryo compared to a cleavage stage embryo. However, there are theoretical risks with blastocyst culture. The blastocyst culture environment may not be optimal for all embryos, so theoretically an embryo may do better in

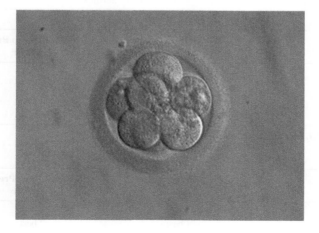

FIGURE 8.6   An eight-cell embryo. This state of development is achieved at approximately 48 hours after fertilization has been confirmed. Note the outer membrane called the zona pellucida that surrounds the embryo.

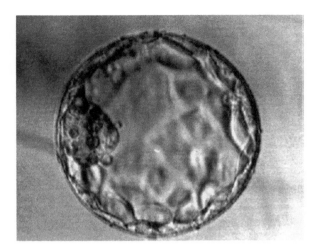

FIGURE 8.7 A blastocyst. Approximately 30% to 50% of embryos will develop to the blastocyst state 5 to 6 days after the egg retrieval. The blastocyst is made up of 50 to 100 cells.

the uterus versus the incubator. Another disadvantage is that there is a higher chance of monozygotic twinning (MZT) with a day 5 versus a day 3 transfer.

The recommended number of embryos to transfer is determined by the woman's age and the timing of the embryo transfer (Table 8.2). We perform the embryo transfer under abdominal ultrasound guidance. A full bladder creates a window so that the uterus can be easily visualized. An echogenic catheter can be easily seen as it courses through the cervical canal and up into the cavity (Figure 8.8). The catheter is positioned 1–2 cm from the top of the cavity where the embryos are placed. Extra embryos that are of sufficient quality can be frozen and stored for future use. A serum pregnancy test is performed 11 days later (after cleavage stage embryo transfer) or 9 days after a blastocyst transfer.

TABLE 8.2

Boston IVF Recommended Embryo Transfer Guidelines

	Day 3 Embryo Transfer Guidelines	
Age	If HG Embryo Present, Transfer	If No HG Embryo Present, Transfer
<35	1 best	2 best
35–37	1 best	2 best
38–40	2 best	3 best
>40	5 best	5 best

Note: HG, High-grade embryo defined as ≥6 cell Grade B.

	Day 5 Blastocyst Transfer Guidelines	
Age	If HG Blast Present, Transfer	If No HG Blast Present, Transfer
<35	1 best	2 best
35–37	1 best	2 best
38–40	2 best	3 best
>40	3 best	3 best

Note: HG, High-grade blastocyst is at least a 2BB or better (Gardner classification).

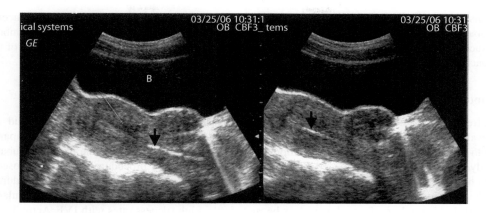

FIGURE 8.8 Ultrasound-guided embryo transfer. In the left panel, the filled bladder (B) allows adequate visualization of the uterine cavity. The tip of the catheter (arrow) has been advanced to the lower aspect of the uterine cavity. In the right panel, the catheter has been advanced to approximately 1.5 cm from the top of the cavity where the embryos are placed. A small anterior serosal fibroid can be seen slightly impinging on the bladder.

Luteal Phase Support

Progesterone, a hormone produced by the ovary after ovulation, matures the lining of the uterus for implantation. Studies have shown that women who are undergoing IVF treatment need supplemental progesterone. For this reason, it is standard to administer progesterone after the egg retrieval. Natural progesterone is available and can be administered vaginally (Crinone®, Endometrin®, and Prometrium®) or by intramuscular injection. If pregnancy occurs, the progesterone is continued for a period of time. We will generally continue the progesterone supplementation until fetal viability is confirmed. Studies have supported that there is no increased risk of birth defects or health risks to women who take natural progesterone supplements during pregnancy. In lieu of progesterone, hCG injections (1500 U every 3 days × 3 doses beginning the day after the oocyte retrieval) can be administered in the luteal phase. However, hCG is rarely used to supplement the luteal phase owing to the higher incidence of OHSS.

IVF-Related Procedures

Frozen Embryo Transfer

Embryos that are cryopreserved during an IVF cycle can be replaced after a spontaneous ovulation (natural cycle) or the creation of an "artificial" endometrium with estrogen and progesterone. Embryos are frozen using vitrification technology; approximately 90% of vitrified embryos will survive the freeze/thaw process. If the embryo survives, the chances of implantation are virtually the same as a fresh embryo transfer. In fact, several reports have suggested that transferring embryos in a frozen embryo transfer (FET) may actually be associated with a higher pregnancy rate than fresh transfers, suggesting that the endometrium during a stimulated fresh IVF cycle may not be optimal for implantation. The main advantage of a frozen embryo transfer as compared to a medicated IVF cycle is that there is no need for the surgical egg retrieval, no anesthesia, and no gonadotropins, which makes FET far less involved and less expensive. It is reassuring that there is no increased risk of congenital anomalies in infants born after the transfer of cryopreserved embryos.

Natural Cycle IVF

For couples who want to minimize the risk of a multiple pregnancy or would like to avoid the risks of the ovulation induction drugs, a natural cycle IVF approach can be considered. The woman undergoes monitoring with blood work and ultrasound examinations beginning on cycle day 10. The hCG is administered when a mature follicle is identified. If an LH surge occurs, then the cycle must be canceled. The goal of the natural cycle approach is the retrieval of one egg and the replacement of one embryo. The success rate is much lower (<10%) than conventional IVF, which is a major disadvantage of this approach.

Gamete Intrafallopian Transfer

This treatment involves the first two steps of IVF treatment: ovarian hyperstimulation and egg retrieval. In contrast to IVF, the gamete intrafallopian transfer (GIFT) procedure involves a laparoscopy to place eggs and sperm into the fallopian tube, allowing the tube to be the natural incubator. Usually, four to six eggs are replaced. The disadvantage of the GIFT procedure is that a laparoscopy has to be performed under general anesthesia. A prerequisite to performing the GIFT procedure is that the woman must have at least one normal fallopian tube. This procedure was quite popular in the 1980s but is rarely performed nowadays because of the high success rates with IVF. Actually less than 1% of assisted reproductive technology (ART) procedures are GIFT. Indications for resorting to GIFT include altered cervical anatomy that prevents a successful uterine transfer, or if religious reasons preclude IVF.

Tubal Embryo Transfer

This treatment involves the first three steps of IVF: ovarian hyperstimulation, egg retrieval, and fertilization of the eggs in the laboratory. In contrast to IVF, the tubal embryo transfer (TET) procedure involves the laparoscopic placement of the embryos in the fallopian tube(s), allowing the tube to be the natural incubator. The disadvantage of the TET procedure is that two separate procedures requiring anesthesia are performed, including the egg retrieval and a laparoscopy. This procedure is rarely performed but might be considered when there is altered cervical anatomy preventing a transcervical embryo transfer.

Egg Donation

Egg donation can be considered for a woman who is a poor responder to the ovulation induction medications, has evidence of reduced ovarian reserve, or is a carrier of a genetic condition.

The source of the donor eggs can be a fresh cycle or frozen eggs from a donor egg bank. The recipient is treated with hormones including estrogen and progesterone, which create an endometrium that will allow implantation of the embryos. Before this treatment is begun, all parties involved should undergo medical, psychological, and legal counseling. This option is discussed in detail in the next chapter.

Gestational Surrogacy

Some women cannot carry a pregnancy but can produce eggs and embryos from IVF. Indications for gestational carrier treatment are when the woman has no uterus (e.g., prior hysterectomy), has a congenitally deformed uterus, has a uterus that is unable to support a pregnancy, or has a medical condition that precludes her from safely carrying a pregnancy. All the steps of IVF treatment are performed except that the embryos are transferred into a gestational carrier. Before this treatment is begun, all parties involved must undergo medical, psychological, and legal counseling.

Embryo Donation

When a couple decides that they do not want any more children or they want to stop treatment, they must decide what to do with their frozen embryos. Because of religious or moral beliefs, some couples find it unacceptable to discard the embryos. One option is to donate the embryos to another couple. Agencies around the country can assist matching recipient couples to donated embryos. Medical, psychological, and legal counseling are important components of the treatment.

Epididymal/Testicular Sperm Aspiration

In some cases of azoospermia, sperm are being produced but do not find their way to the ejaculate. This may be the result of an obstruction (e.g., previous vasectomy, infection), congenital absence of the vas deferens, or cases of severely impaired sperm production. In these cases, aspiration of epididymal sperm or testicular sperm by a urologist may be considered. In years past, the only way to aspirate epididymal sperm was via the microscopic epididymal sperm aspiration (MESA) procedure. This procedure is performed in the operating room under general anesthesia. More recently, the percutaneous epididymal sperm aspiration procedure has become more popular. It can be accomplished under local anesthesia in the office with a much shorter recuperation than the MESA procedure. If epididymal sperm aspiration does not produce viable sperm, then the urologist can resort to testicular sperm extraction. In all cases of sperm aspiration, the motility of the sample is quite poor; thus, the ICSI procedure must be performed. To accomplish this procedure, there must be coordination with the urologist and the IVF team. The sperm aspiration can be performed on the day of the oocyte recovery or before the IVF cycle and the samples are frozen.

Laboratory Procedures

Assisted Hatching

Assisted hatching is a procedure in which the zona pellucida, the outer membrane surrounding the embryo, is thinned by either the application of a dilute acidic solution or more recently with microscopic laser, mechanical disruption. It has been theorized that some implantation failures may be the result from failure of the embryo to hatch out from the confines of the zona pellucida. However, published studies are inconclusive about the benefit of this procedure. Therefore, it should not be used universally but might be considered in patients who have undergone several IVF cycles that have been unsuccessful or in older women.

Preimplantation Genetic Diagnosis and Preimplantation Genetic Screening

In the past, when a couple was at risk of having a child with a genetic condition, the only options for genetic diagnosis were a chorionic villous sampling or a genetic amniocentesis. These choices are not optimal since terminating a pregnancy can be quite stressful and, for many couples, is not considered an option. Preimplantation genetic diagnosis (PGD) provides couples with another option. The refinement of micromanipulation techniques has provided the ability to perform genetic diagnosis from a few cells that are removed from the embryo before transfer. The first successful case of PGD was performed in 1990 for a couple who were at risk of having a child with cystic fibrosis. Since that time, centers worldwide have developed the expertise to perform PGD. It can be performed for autosomal recessive and dominant conditions. PGD is an emerging technology, and as more and more genetic probes become available, there will be an increased demand for this procedure.

Preimplantation genetic screening (PGS) is becoming a popular adjunct to IVF treatment. In contrast to PGD, which detects specific mutations that can cause a specific disease in a child, PGS is used to detect whether an embryo has the normal 23 pairs of chromosomes. Many embryos have an extra or missing chromosome (called aneuploidy), which prevents them from implanting or causes a miscarriage. Embryos with the normal chromosome complement (called euploidy) have a higher chance of implanting (additional 15%–20%) compared to untested embryos. PGS is typically done on blastocyst embryos. A few cells are biopsied before cryopreservation. The cells are sent to the laboratory and the DNA amplified and the chromosome status is determined. This takes several days, so no fresh transfer is done. Only euploid embryos are transferred subsequently.

Cost was a major limiting factor to PGS usage in the past, but because of new technologies (NexGen sequencing), the cost has been reduced. A significant issue with PGS is "mosaicism," which refers to the fact that some embryos have some abnormal cells that are eventually marginalized in nature and a normal baby results. If these abnormal cells were biopsied, then the embryo would have been erroneously discarded. The incidence of mosaicism is not known but could range between 3% and 15%.

Oocyte Freezing

Oocyte freezing is another emerging technology. The oocyte, in contrast to the embryo, is quite sensitive to the cryopreservation process. This is related to the high water content in the egg, which predisposes it to ice crystal damage. Recently, breakthroughs have been made in the technique, resulting in improved survival at the time of thawing. Techniques involving vitrification (fast-freezing) that have revolutionized the success with egg freezing have been developed. It is anticipated that egg freezing will become a common method to preserve fertility in women not prepared to have a family and, for the first time in human history, the biological clock can be stopped. The indications for oocyte freezing are manifold. It gives opportunity to women undergoing cancer treatment to preserve fertility. It also would benefit the younger woman who doesn't anticipate motherhood in the near future and wants to preserve her fertility. Finally, couples undergoing IVF could freeze extra eggs instead of embryos. Once the couple decides that their family is complete, it is much easier emotionally to discard frozen eggs instead of frozen embryos.

Success Rates

IVF success rates continue to improve and the reasons are manifold, including improved ovulation induction medications, refined laboratory techniques, less traumatic embryo transfer catheters, and the introduction of ancillary procedures such as ICSI. The success rate for any individual patient after IVF is influenced by countless factors including the number of embryos transferred, cycle number, ovarian reserve, age, and diagnosis. Center-specific data are difficult to compare owing to the variation in patient selection and philosophy regarding treatment.

Maternal Age

One of the most important factors that influence a couple's fertility is the woman's age. Generally, younger women have a greater quantity and quality of eggs that, once fertilized, are more likely to implant in the uterus and result in a pregnancy. Furthermore, the chance of a miscarriage is lower in younger women. The decreased fertility associated with advancing age is a gradual process that seems to begin around age 35 and then accelerates after the age of 40. One reason for the decreased fertility associated with aging is that there is a higher rate of aneuploidy. Women over the age of 40 should be counseled about the decreased chances of pregnancy even with aggressive treatment, such as IVF (Figure 8.9). IVF using one's own eggs should be discouraged in women who are 44 years and older because of the dismal chance of a successful outcome. These women should be counseled and encouraged to pursue other more fruitful options such as egg donation and adoption.

Diagnosis

Women with ovulatory problems, except those with reduced ovarian reserve, tend to have higher pregnancy rates with the various treatments. Women with tubal factor infertility or severe male factor infertility seem to fair poorly with conservative interventions (i.e., ovulation induction with or without intrauterine inseminations). While the cause of the infertility may affect success rates of the conservative treatments, there is virtually little difference between the success rates for the different diagnostic categories with IVF treatment (Figure 8.10).

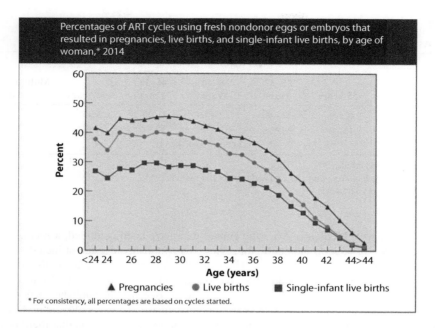

FIGURE 8.9 Pregnancy and live-birth rates for ART cycles using fresh (non-donor) embryos by age of the woman. (Obtained from published data from the Centers for Disease Control, 2014 Assisted Reproductive Technology Success Rates.)

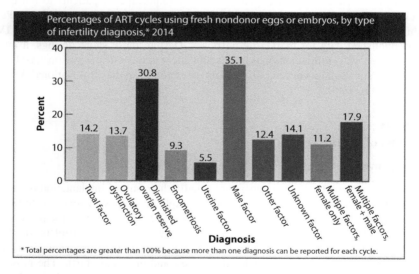

FIGURE 8.10 Live-birth rates after IVF by primary diagnosis. (Obtained from published data from the CDC, 2014 Assisted Reproductive Technology Success Rates.)

Fertility Clinic Success Rate and Certification Act of 1992

Since the passage of the Fertility Clinic Success Rate and Certification Act of 1992, it is mandatory that all IVF centers in the United States submit their annual success rates to a federal registry. In the past, this was a joint venture of the United States Centers for Disease Control and Prevention (CDC) and the Society of the Assisted Reproductive Technologies (SART), a subsidiary of the American

TABLE 8.3

Society of Assisted Reproductive Technology (SART) 2014 Report

	Live-Birth Rates by Age Group (%)					Multiple Pregnancy Rate
Treatment	<35 Years	35–37 Years	38–40 Years	41–42 Years	>42 Years	
IVF (±ICSI)[a]	42.6%	34.0%	22.4%	11.9%	3.9%	26.9%[b]
Frozen embryo transfer[c]	42.7%	39.6%	33.7%	27.3%	19.6%	
Egg donation[c]	Fresh 53.6%; Frozen 38.5%					

[a] Live-birth rates per cycle initiated.
[b] Multiple pregnancy rate includes twins (23.7%) and triplets and more (1.5%).
[c] Live-birth rates per embryo transfer.

Society for Reproductive Medicine. After the annual data have been compiled, a finalized report is published and made available to the public for review. The published document includes a summary of national and clinic-specific success rates. The main impetus behind this law is that the reporting of clinic success rates would help the infertile couple select the "best" IVF clinic for their treatment. Unfortunately, there are several shortcomings to this process. Because the published data are based on live-birth rates, the most recent data that have been published are 2–3 years old and may not reflect a clinic's current success rate. Another pitfall to the interpretation of the data is that there is no way to decipher the inclusion and exclusion criteria that any individual center used in selecting patients for treatment. Therefore, as these criteria are highly variable for each program, center-by-center comparison of success rates is not valid. Some highly experienced IVF programs attract more difficult cases, which causes their statistics to be lower. Therefore, it is important for patients to not use the CDC statistics to choose an IVF program. What is more important is to determine an individual's chance of success within a particular program. An unfortunate outcome to the process is that some IVF centers have used the published data for marketing purposes. Despite these shortcomings, a major benefit of the data collection is to follow national trends and success rates of the various ART procedures. The CDC ART statistics can be viewed online. Data extracted from the 2014 National ART Summary report are presented in Table 8.3.

Complications of Treatment

Multiple Pregnancy

Most multiple pregnancies after IVF treatment are usually the result of implantation of more than one embryo (fraternal twins). Therefore, the chance of a multiple pregnancy increases with the number of embryos that are transferred. In the most recently published CDC/SART report, the percentage of pregnancies delivered that were twins was approximately 10%–15%, and that for triplets was 1%. Multiple pregnancies are associated with an increased risk of most complications of pregnancy including miscarriage, toxemia, congenital anomalies, gestational diabetes, and premature birth. The most concerning risk of a multiple pregnancy is prematurity. Babies born from triplet pregnancies have a 20% chance of a major handicap, a 17-fold increase in cerebral palsy, and a 20-fold increase in death during the first year after birth (as compared to a singleton pregnancy) [1]. MZT is a multiple pregnancy that results from the splitting of a single embryo, which will lead to a set of identical twins. The incidence of MZT is increased in pregnancies conceived after IVF. MZT pregnancies are more complicated because of the risks of twin-to-twin transfusion and cord accidents. A multiple pregnancy may also pose increased emotional and financial hardship for a couple. If a multiple pregnancy develops, the couple may consider a multi-fetal reduction procedure. This procedure, which is performed in the first trimester of pregnancy, reduces the number of fetuses to a lower and safer number. Although the success rate is 90%–95%, a miscarriage may result from the procedure.

During the early 1990s, there was a progressive increase in the number of triplet pregnancies. Since 1997, there has been a reduction in the number of high-order multiple pregnancies. In the 1990s, there was a concerted effort from the American College of Obstetricians and Gynecologists and the American Society for Reproductive Medicine to develop guidelines to help reduce the number of embryos transferred [2,3]. In addition, the continued progress in the field has produced higher implantation rates, which also has provided a further impetus to reduce the number of embryos transferred without affecting pregnancy rates [4]. With the continued improvement in outcomes, transferring a single embryo is now the preferred approach for most patients.

Birth Defects

The possibility that IVF could increase the risk of birth defects has been a great concern for patients and clinicians. This is of particular interest since >1% of all children are now conceived after IVF. Although many studies have looked at malformations in IVF children, most have had limitations in sample size and there has been a lack of a standard definition of a minor versus a major congenital malformation. However, the majority of studies point to a slightly increased risk of congenital malformations. A previous meta-analysis including seven studies compared the rate of birth defects between those conceived after ART (IVF and ICSI) with those naturally conceived [5]. The pooled odds ratio was 1.40 (95% CI 1.28–1.53) and confirmed an increased risk of major birth defects in the babies conceived by ART. In a recent case-control study, the researchers confirmed a higher incidence in singleton IVF pregnancies of septal heart defects, cleft lip/palate, esophageal atresia, and anorectal atresia [6].

The explanation for the increased risk of malformations is unclear but may be the result of some aspect of the treatment itself or genetic factors in the couple who are undergoing the treatment. A major deficiency of most studies is that they do not include babies born to infertile women who were not treated by IVF—this is unfortunate since it is well known that congenital malformation are more common in the infertile population. ICSI does not appear to increase the rate of malformations in comparison to the standard insemination technique [7,8]. The transfer of previously cryopreserved embryos does not convey a higher rate of malformations in comparison to the transfer of fresh embryos [9,10]. It is probable that infertile women who are treated or not treated may be at risk for children with congenital malformations.

It is unclear whether there is an increased risk after IVF itself but, if so, the overall risk is still low when one considers the baseline major malformation rate, which is 3% in the United States. This information needs to be conveyed to our patients and should be part of the informed consent process. We counsel our couples that the incidence of birth defects in naturally conceived pregnancies is 2%–3% and may be increased to 3%–4% in babies born after IVF treatment.

Ovarian Hyperstimulation Syndrome

OHSS can be a complication after the use of any ovulation induction agent but is more common after the use of injectable medications. It is a clinical situation whereby multiple follicles develop in the ovaries after hCG administration. The symptoms that occur depend on the number and sizes of the follicles that are present. Patients at risk for OHSS are those with PCOS and high estradiol levels and those with many smaller follicles (<12 mm) at the time of the hCG trigger. However, most patients who develop OHSS don't have any risk factors and are difficult to predict. The timing of the development of symptoms is generally 7–10 days after the hCG administration. More than half of cases of OHSS are brought on by the rising β-hCG levels during the early stages of pregnancy. Approximately 20%–30% of IVF patients develop mild OHSS, and their symptoms include mild lower abdominal discomfort and distention. The symptoms are self-limited and resolve in a week. Approximately 1%–2% of women who undergo IVF develop symptoms compatible with severe OHSS. The abdominal pain and distention are more significant and can be accompanied by the development of shortness of breath, nausea, vomiting, and decreased urine output. With severe OHSS, there is the accumulation of ascitic fluid, which, via the lymphatics, can traverse into the pleural spaces. With the accumulation of ascites, there can be contraction of intravascular volume with resultant hemoconcentration that can lead to thrombotic events resulting in stroke, kidney damage, and possibly death.

Management

All patients should be educated on the symptoms of OHSS. Any patient who develops symptoms of OHSS must be evaluated. If the symptoms are mild, then the patient is instructed to take daily weights and maintain oral fluids. The patient is called on a daily basis to be assessed. If she increases her weight by 2 lb or more, has worsening pain, or develops shortness of breath, she is brought in for an evaluation. A physical exam is performed along with vital signs. The presence of tachycardia can be a sign of contraction of the intravascular volume, which can occur with acute ascites. On the lung exam, reduced breath sounds at the bases can be a sign of a pleural effusion. A gentle abdominal exam will provide an idea as to the severity of the ascites. A pelvic exam is not performed since the ovarian cysts are prone to rupture. A vaginal and abdominal ultrasound exam will delineate the extent of the ascites. Laboratory studies, including a CBC, PT/PTT, and electrolytes, are obtained. The result of the CBC is most important and will give an idea of the degree of the hemoconcentration. If the hematrocrit is >48%, then prophylactic anticoagulation is administered (Lovenox 40 mg qd) until the syndrome resolves.

Traditionally, the treatment for severe OHSS was hospitalization with fluid restriction and careful fluid management. Albumin was intravenously administered to mobilize the fluids. Our present management is to perform a vaginal ultrasound–guided paracentesis to remove the ascites [11]. We have found that this approach speeds up the recovery and resolution of the process. We have removed up to 3 L of fluid without any problem. This has essentially eliminated the need for hospitalization [12].

Ovarian Cancer

In the general population, every woman has a 1-in-70 chance of developing ovarian cancer during her lifetime. Known risk factors for ovarian cancer include infertility, nulliparity, and genetics. Alternatively, birth control pill use and pregnancy reduce a woman's lifetime risk of developing ovarian cancer. It has been theorized that the number of ovulations that occur during a woman's lifetime increases the chance of cancer formation. Hence, there is concern that the use of fertility medications could heighten the risk. This topic has been studied extensively. The Danish cohort of 50,000 infertile patients is the largest study to date that helped to shed light on the topic. The investigators in the initial study reported a higher incidence of breast and ovarian cancer in the infertile population [13]. In a follow-up study of the cohort, the investigators sought out to determine the impact of fertility medications on the risk of ovarian cancer [14]. They concluded that the incidence of ovarian cancer was not increased in those infertile women who took fertility medications. These findings were supported by a review by Brinton et al. [15]. Therefore, while it is a fact that infertile women are at greater risk of developing ovarian cancer, this risk is not heightened with the use of fertility medications.

Conclusions

There is no question that IVF is safe and the most successful treatment for the infertile couple. The emergence of genetic testing with PGS has allowed the selection of the embryos that have the best chance of establishing a viable pregnancy. As this technology continues to emerge, it will become a standard part of the IVF cycle, thus allowing the transfer of a single euploid embryo. At some point in the future, the infertility treatment paradigm will shift, conservative treatments will be bypassed, and all infertile couples will go directly to IVF treatment. The issue with IVF relates to the cost of the technology which hopefully will become more affordable in the future.

REFERENCES

1. American College of Obstetricians and Gynecologists. Clinical Management Guideline for Obstetricians and Gynecologists. Multiple gestation: Complicated twin, triplet and high order multifetal pregnancy. Number 56, October 2004.
2. American Society for Reproductive Medicine. Guidelines on number of embryos transferred. A Practice Committee Report-A Committee Opinion. (Revised). American Society for Reproductive Medicine, 1999.
3. American College of Obstetricians and Gynecologists. Nonselective embryo reduction: Ethical guidance for the obstetrician-gynecologist ACOG Committee Opinion 215. Washington: American College of Obstetricians and Gynecologists, 1999.
4. Tepleton A, Morris JK. Reducing the risk of multiple births by transfer of two embryos after in vitro fertilization. *N Engl J Med* 1998;339(9):573–7.
5. Hansen M, Bower C, Milne E et al. Assisted reproductive technologies and the risk of birth defects—A systematic review. *Hum Reprod* 2005;20:328–38.
6. Reefhuis J, Honein MA, Schieve LA et al. Assisted reproductive technology and major structural birth defects in the United States. *Hum Reprod* 2009;24:360–6.
7. Bonduelle M, Liebaers I, Deketalaere V et al. Neonatal data on a cohort of 2889 infants born after ICSI (1991–1999) and of 2995 infants born after IVF (1983–1999). *Hum Reprod* 2002;17:671–94.
8. Palermo GD, Colombero LT, Schattman GI et al. Evolution of pregnancies and initial follow-up of newborns delivered after intracytoplasmic sperm injection. *JAMA* 1996;276:1893–7.
9. Wennerholm UB, Albertsson-Wikland K, Bergh C et al. Postnatal growth and health in children born after cryopreservation as embryos. *Lancet* 1998;351:1085–90.
10. Wada I, Macnamee MC, Wick K et al. Birth characteristics and perinatal outcome of babies conceived from cryopreserved embryos. *Hum Reprod* 1994;9:543–6.
11. Alper MM, Smith L Sills ES. Ovarian hyperstimulation syndrome: Current views on pathophysiology, risk factors, prevention, and management. *J Exp Clin Assist Reprod* 2009 Jun;10;6:3.
12. Smith LP, Hacker MR, Alper MM. Patients with severe ovarian hyperstimulation syndrome can be managed safely with aggressive outpatient transvaginal paracentesis. *Fertil Steril* 2009;92(6):1953–9.
13. Jensen A, Sharif H, Olsen J, Kjaer SK. Risk of breast cancer and gynecologic cancers in a large population of nearly 50,000 infertile Danish women. *Am J Epidemiol* 2009;168:49–57.
14. Jensen A, Sharif H, Frederiksen K, Kjaer SK. Use of fertility drugs and risk of ovarian cancer: Danish population based cohort study. *BMJ* 2009;338:1–8.
15. Brinton LA, Moghissi KS, Scoccia B et al. Ovulation induction and cancer risk. *Fertil Steril* 2005;83:261–74.

9

Treatment Options: IV. Third-Party Reproduction

Brian M. Berger

Over the past 30 years, the use of assisted reproductive technologies has changed the choices available for older women. These choices include donor egg in vitro fertilization (DE IVF), which is now a standard treatment offered by most IVF centers. Women who would benefit from DE IVF include those with premature ovarian failure, those with ovarian failure attributed to either chemotherapy or radiation, and women with gonadal dysgenesis. A second and much larger group includes women with diminished ovarian function and age-related infertility. Other candidates include women who have previously failed multiple IVF attempts and women carrying transmittable genetic abnormalities that could affect their offspring.

Increasing Number of DE IVF Cycles

There are many reasons for the increase in the number of women who are candidates for egg donation such as those with diminished ovarian function. Surveys have shown that many women choose to delay childbearing and rear their children only after establishing a stable relationship and financial security. There are also increasing numbers of late and second marriages and more women now wish to finish their education and establish a career before trying to start a family [1]. So many women find themselves in their 40s looking at their options. For most in this age group, the IVF success rate using their own eggs is low and egg donation is the best option for a successful pregnancy. In 2014, more than 400 IVF programs reported on the use of donor oocytes to the American Society for Reproductive Medicine (ASRM)/Society for Assisted Reproductive Technology Registry. Donor eggs (fresh and frozen) were used in approximately 10% of all assisted reproductive technology (ART) cycles performed. The live birth rate using fresh and frozen donor eggs was 53.6% and 38.5%, respectively [2,3].

Ethics of DE IVF

Several publications have addressed the important ethical considerations and social issues related to egg donation in postmenopausal women. Generally, there are three main objections related to this treatment: (i) the physical risk to the older woman during pregnancy [4], (ii) the rights of the children born to older women [5], and (iii) the use of scarce health care resources that might deprive younger patients of treatment. Other issues that have been raised against treating older patients include the views of donors about using their oocytes for treating older women, and the psychological effect of giving birth beyond the age of 50, which is unknown at present [4]. Those who are in favor of treating older patients argue that, by careful selection of patients, the risk of complications is reduced to a minimum and most older women wanting children are quite willing to accept the small risk of complications. There is also argument about the definition of what constitutes advanced maternal age, especially given the fact that the life expectancy of both men and women has increased considerably [6].

TABLE 9.1

Five Steps to Completing a Donor Egg Cycle

Responsible Party	Steps
IVF center	Completion of the recipient eligibility screening process
Recipient/IVF center	Determination of insurance eligibility/financial clearance
Recipient	Selection or identification of a potential donor
IVF center	Screening of the potential donor
IVF center	Cycle coordination

Steps to Completing a Cycle of DE IVF

The process of completing a DE IVF cycle has five distinct steps (see Table 9.1). The patients are instructed to first set up an appointment with their physician to discuss the medical aspects of DE IVF. Spouses or partners must accompany the recipient to this appointment.

The Donor Egg Team

At Boston IVF, we have a designated DE Team that is responsible for working with all recipients. The team helps to ensure that the recipient and her partner (if applicable) and the egg donor have been properly screened and helps to coordinate the treatment cycle. First, the recipients are instructed to attend an Egg Recipient Seminar with the program coordinator. At this seminar, comprehensive information about egg donation is given and all questions regarding the process are answered. We also have the patients meet with the financial coordinator. They will learn about what their insurance policy may cover and the eligibility testing, which may be required, and learn about the out-of-pocket expenses. The cost of a donor egg cycle has continued to increase over the years, and the charges including the IVF cycle, payment to the donor and agency, and costs of screening the egg donor can total up to $30,000–$40,000. The cost can be reduced if the couple uses a known egg donor.

FDA Regulations and Egg Donation

In 2004, the Food and Drug Administration (FDA) published the final rules to strengthen regulation of human tissue and expanded the regulations to include human cells, tissues, and cellular and tissue-based products [7]. The regulations apply to reproductive tissues such as eggs, embryos, and semen. The FDA began requiring various establishments to register with the agency and list the products manufactured. These establishments include those that recover, process, store, label, package, or distribute the products, or those that screen or test donors. More than 350 reproductive establishments, including semen banks and fertility clinics, registered with the FDA. Reproductive establishments including IVF centers were required to comply with donor eligibility requirements, which became effective on May 25, 2005. These requirements establish screening and testing criteria for donors of human cells, tissues, and cellular and tissue-based products to help prevent the transmission of communicable diseases. People who are donating to their own sexual partners are not required to be screened or tested.

For egg donors, the collection of a donor specimen for testing must occur up to 30 days before recovery of the oocytes or egg retrieval [8] (see Table 9.2). For sperm donors (fresh specimen), the center may collect the donor specimen up to 7 days before or after the sperm is donated [8] (see Table 9.3).

Required testing must be performed by an FDA-certified laboratory. Centers must also use an appropriate FDA-licensed, -approved, or -cleared donor screening test if available. A donor whose specimen tests reactive on a non-Treponemal screening test for syphilis and negative on a specific Treponemal confirmatory

TABLE 9.2

FDA-Required Testing for Communicable Disease
Agents or Diseases for Oocyte Donors

- Human immunodeficiency virus (HIV), types 1 and 2
- Hepatitis B virus (HBV)
- Hepatitis C virus (HCV)
- *Treponema pallidum* (syphilis)
- *Chlamydia trachomatis*
- *Neisseria gonorrhoeae*

Source: Food and Drug Administration, HHS, *Fed Regist*, 69(101), 29785–834, 2004 May 25.

TABLE 9.3

FDA-Required Testing for Communicable Disease
Agents or Diseases for Sperm Donors

- Human immunodeficiency virus (HIV), types 1 and 2
- Hepatitis B virus (HBV)
- Hepatitis C virus (HCV)
- *Treponema pallidum* (syphilis)
- *Chlamydia trachomatis*
- *Neisseria gonorrhoeae*
- Human T-lymphotropic virus, types 1 and 2
- Cytomegalovirus

Source: Food and Drug Administration, HHS, *Fed Regist*, 69(101), 29785–834, 2004 May 25.

test may nevertheless be considered eligible, as long as all other required testing and screening are negative. A donor whose specimen tests reactive on a Treponemal confirmatory test is not eligible.

The Egg Recipient Evaluation

All recipients are tested according to FDA regulations as described above. In addition, the recipients will have a uterine cavity evaluation via a hysterosalpingogram, sonohysterogram, or hysteroscopy. Routine prenatal blood work will be done and the partner will have a semen analysis. All recipients are required to schedule an appointment with a social worker. Once again, the spouse/partner must attend this appointment. This consultation allows them to explore the psychological issues involved in egg donation. If recipients are working with an egg donor who is known by or related to them (known donor or KD), we require that they meet once with a social worker as a couple, the donor and her spouse (if applicable) meet with the social worker once as a couple, and then all four meet again for a joint consultation. After the testing is completed, the intended parents will schedule an appointment with their physician who will review the results of the recipient evaluation and write orders for the treatment cycle.

To prevent miscommunication and confusion, we only allow the screening of one potential egg donor at a time. Recipients are also told that they are financially responsible for services rendered to the donor, even if she is not accepted as a donor after her medical screening.

Anonymous Egg Donation

Boston IVF allows anonymous donors to be recruited by approved egg donor agencies only. We will not permit recipients to recruit their own donors through the Internet or through any other means. This

TABLE 9.4

Features to Seek in a Donor Egg Agency

Qualities	Importance
Medical expertise	An agency that offers a staff member with medical training is invaluable. Medical expertise is important to make decisions about which donors the agency will accept and make available to recipients.
Legal counsel for both the donor and recipient	Legal consultation for both the donor and the recipient protects the interests of both parties by establishing a mutually acceptable legal contract. An agency should facilitate this process and should provide this service as a part of the agency package.
Short-term medical insurance policy for the egg donor	Should an egg donor experience any adverse medical event related to the egg retrieval or the medications, the recipient is financially responsible for her medical care and treatment. A good agency should offer a short-term insurance policy for purchase that covers any potential problems related to the procedure and the medications.
Professional, courteous staff	A staff that is professional and courteous will treat egg donors and recipients with respect and ensure that the needs of each are met in an efficient manner. Professional demeanor usually reflects a company that is organized and efficient.

policy is necessary to ensure that anonymity is preserved and that the necessary legal contracts are properly in place. Recipients are given tremendous guidance in selecting an appropriate egg donor (see Table 9.4). Egg donors should be healthy, between the ages of 21 and 35 [9,10], and free of infectious diseases. All egg donors, whether anonymous or known, must be screened to ensure that their motivation appears reasonable and voluntary [11]. Egg donation presents a number of unique medical, legal, and emotional issues, which need to be carefully considered.

Known Egg Donors

Known egg donors include sisters, relatives, or friends. Known egg donors must be medically and psychologically screened as rigorously as anonymous donors. Cross-generation egg donation in which a daughter donates to her mother or a mother donates to her daughter is not permitted at Boston IVF.

Legal Contracts

We require legal consultation and establishment of a legal contract with the donor, anonymous or known. The recipient couple is generally responsible for legal fees incurred by the donor, although many donor egg agencies include this fee in their administrative fees.

Initiating the Treatment Cycle

When recipients have selected a potential donor, the agency (or recipient if using a known donor) calls the Egg Donation Program Coordinator who will send them application and history forms, register the donor at Boston IVF, and schedule the donor's appointments. The donor should bring her completed forms and any previous medical records with her to her appointments. If using an agency, it is important for recipients to find out all of the costs of the agency before selecting an agency or paying a fee. Agency fees typically include the egg donor's compensation, a short-term medical insurance policy for the egg donor, and legal fees. In addition, if they select a donor who lives out of state, we require that she travels to Boston IVF twice: once for her screening appointments, and once again for the monitoring and egg retrieval. At the time of the egg retrieval, she usually stays locally for 1 week.

Screening Donors

Boston IVF screens potential egg donors thoroughly according to FDA regulations. An eight-page phone screen is first performed and a decision is made on whether or not to schedule a screening appointment. The Boston IVF physician, social worker, and the DE Program Coordinator work as a team to determine whether a donor candidate is appropriate. We perform an expanded genetic carrier screening that tests for more than 100 recessive diseases. If a donor completes her screening and is approved by the medical director, the DE Program Coordinator is responsible for synchronizing the recipient's cycle with the egg donor's cycle.

Cycle Coordination

Donors

Implantation and Success in DE IVF

The process of implantation remains poorly understood, but two factors are clearly required: endometrial receptivity and synchronization of embryo and endometrial development. In the natural cycle, these factors are induced by the simultaneous development of the follicle and the surrounding hormonal events surrounding ovulation. In the DE IVF treatment, these events are, by definition, separated and need to be controlled and synchronized by a sequence of ovarian down-regulation and endometrial preparation. Because of these factors, controlled timing of follicle growth, egg maturation, and ovulation in the donor, and adequate stimulation of the endometrium with an estrogen–progesterone sequence in the recipient need to be performed.

Donor Ovulation Induction Protocol

All donors are initially started on oral contraceptives (OCP). The OCP is started with the donor's menses and continues for 16 to 35 days. OCP pretreatment in high responders has been shown to improve the success of the treatment and also reduce the risk of ovarian hyperstimulation syndrome [12]. The OCP is stopped on a Monday and the donor is instructed to call with the first day of her withdraw bleed. Gonadotropin stimulation is then started the following Saturday. This regimen assures that the egg retrieval will most often occur in the middle of the week [13].

For several years, we have used a regimen consisting of FSH/low-dose human chorionic gonadotropin (hCG) and a gonadotropin-releasing hormone (GnRH) antagonist (see Table 9.5). This protocol allows us a maximum flexibility in treatment and has also allowed us to almost eliminate the incidence of ovarian hyperstimulation (<0.2%) [14]. We perform frequent estradiol measurement in the beginning of the cycle in order to adjust the stimulation and also to ensure that the donor is responding adequately (see Table 9.6). We have also successfully utilized a protocol in which early adjustments in FSH dose are implemented based on the estradiol measurement on day 3 and day 5 [15]. We have found that modification of the initial and subsequent FSH dose yields similar clinical outcomes in oocyte donors with a significantly lower basal antral follicle count (BAFC). In donors with a high BAFC (>30), this management strategy also minimizes the risk of ovarian hyperstimulation syndrome (1/249) [16]. All donors are triggered with Lupron 80 mg unless they have contraindications such as hypothalamic amenorrhea (in which case, an hCG trigger is used). A confirmatory progesterone (P4) and luteinizing hormone (LH) are performed the day after ovulation to document efficacy.

Recipients

Down-Regulation of Recipients

Before the uterine preparation treatment, down-regulation of the cycle is usually performed owing to studies that have clearly indicated that adequate down-regulation of the menstrual cycle beforehand is

TABLE 9.5

Donor Ovulation Induction Protocol

Medication Regimen:

- OCP start date:_____
- OCP stop date **Monday**[a]:_____
- Start FSH/low-dose hCG on **Saturday**[b]:_____
- FSH dose 225 units/low-dose hCG 10 units QD × 2 days or
- FSH dose_____units/_____ low-dose hCG × 2 days

Antagonist

With lead follicle ≥ 14 mm:

- Cetrotide 0.25 mg sc QD_____
- Ganirelix 0.25 mg sc QD_____

[a] Stop OCPs on Monday, start FSH/low-dose hCG on Saturday.
[b] If menses on Tues/Wed, begin FSH/low-dose hCG on Friday.

TABLE 9.6

Monitoring Protocol for Donors

- E2 only on stimulation day 3 and day 5
- Ultrasound only after stimulation day 5
- On stimulation day 3 if E2 > 150, decrease by 75 IU
- On stimulation day 3 if E2 < 75, increase by 75 IU
- On stimulation day 5 if E2 > 500, decrease by 75 IU
- On stimulation day 5 if E2 < 150, increase by 75 IU

beneficial. Borini et al. [17] studied the effect of long-term down-regulation on pregnancy and implantation rates in 122 cyclic patients who received donor oocytes. Recipients who were either menopausal or cyclic but had long-term down-regulation had significantly higher pregnancy and implantation rates. Apart from the improved pregnancy and implantation rates after long-term down-regulation, these data not only demonstrate an important role of the endometrium in implantation but also suggest that a period of amenorrhea improves the pregnancy rate.

In cyclic patients with natural menstrual cycles, suppression of the cycle is accomplished with a GnRH agonist analog (Lupron®). Lupron® has the added advantage that it can be used for several months at a time without causing any permanent changes to the reproductive system or detrimental effect on the success of the cycle. This ensures a degree of flexibility that allows egg donation to function successfully.

Estrogen Replacement for Recipients

Lutjen et al. [18] first reported egg donation to a recipient with premature ovarian failure in 1984. They used a steroid replacement regimen for the recipient consisting of estrogen valerate (Progynova®; Schering, Sydney, Australia) and progesterone suppositories (Utrogestan®; Piette, Brussels, Belgium). Since then, many different regimens of estrogen and progesterone replacement have been tried successfully, differing in both the method of administration and timing.

There are many reports dealing with the recommended type and dosage of estrogen and progesterone supplementation in artificial endometrial preparation before the transfer of embryos. We know from oocyte donation programs that a maximum flexibility is necessary to synchronize the recipient until oocytes are available. The aim is an open so-called "window of implantation" with a highly receptive-appearing endometrium at the time of embryo transfer—this period lasts a maximum of 48 h. At the end of endometrial preparation should be an overlapping between the "window of transfer," during which a transfer is planned.

Many studies have examined the effects of different estrogen replacement regimens. Most have shown that the length of estrogen administration could be varied and delayed. In fact, successful implantation was observed in an extreme situation even after 100 days of unopposed estradiol valerate administration [19]. Ovulatory patients in this study received a GnRH analog simultaneously. Breakthrough bleeding increasingly appeared according to the duration of estrogen replacement. These clinical observations provide evidence that the concept of "prolonged follicular phase" estrogen replacement for ovum donation can be maintained, at least as long as 15 weeks. Because of the high incidence of breakthrough bleeding after 9 weeks (>44%), the authors recommended stopping estrogen replacement after this time. Yaron et al. [20] extended uterine preparation with estradiol as long as 5 weeks without significantly decreased pregnancy rates.

It was suggested that shorter and lower dosage protocols of estradiol priming of the endometrium could result in higher abortion rates. This indicates an optimal endometrial proliferation, which is necessary to enable optimal development of progesterone receptors and subsequent transformation into an endometrium receptive to the transferred embryo [21]. Neither endometrial thickness nor serum estradiol was able to predict optimal receptivity and therefore outcome in oocyte donation.

At Boston IVF, we continue estrogen replacement (both oral and transdermal) until 10 weeks estimated gestational age.

Progesterone Replacement for Recipients

Much controversy surrounds the issue of progesterone replacement in DE IVF cycles. Unfortunately, prospective studies comparing different types and durations of progesterone supplementation before transfer of DE IVF embryos with regard to treatment outcome have not yet been performed. With regard to timing of progesterone, several retrospective studies have shed light on the implantation window. In one study, 4–5 days of progesterone administration were optimal for embryo transfer comparing results after transfers between day 2 and day 7 of progesterone administration. Rosenwaks [22] reported best results after transfers on days 3–5 of progesterone supplementation.

Prapas et al. [23] performed an interesting retrospective study on the association between the "window of embryo transfer" and the duration of progesterone therapy. They transferred day 2 embryos (4- to 6-cell) after 2, 3, 4, 5, and 6 days after initiation of endometrial exposure to progesterone. Their results indicate that the window of implantation depends on the duration of progesterone treatment. It begins ~48 h after starting progesterone administration and lasts for ~4 days. Highest pregnancy rates were achieved after 5 days (48.3%), with lower rates after 4 days (40%), 6 days (20.4%), and 3 days (12%). No pregnancies were observed after 2 days of progesterone administration.

- Progesterone is also a critical factor in the late follicular phase of fresh IVF cycles. There is much debate on the question of whether a subtle, late follicular phase, pre-hCG rise of progesterone above a certain threshold (1.5 ng/mL) has an impact on the outcome of treatment in IVF cycles [24]. Our guideline at Boston IVF is to cancel cycles when the P4 measurement rises above a threshold of more than 1.5 ng/mL.

- We use both vaginal and intramuscular progesterone replacement regimens, and a retrospective study we performed did not see a significant difference in success rates [25]. Another retrospective analysis also showed similar rates in patients doing frozen embryo transfers and receiving either vaginal gel versus intramuscular progesterone [26]. However, more recent prospective data (unpublished) have shown a potential difference when intramuscular progesterone is used either alone or in conjunction with vaginal progesterone, versus vaginal progesterone alone. Because of this, if patients are willing to try intramuscular progesterone, we recommend giving intramuscular progesterone 50 mg every 3 days along with twice daily vaginal gel. The medications and forms of administration are listed in Table 9.7. As with the estrogen replacement, we continue progesterone replacement until 10–12 weeks estimated gestational age.

Recipient Monitoring

In most cases, recipients are monitored only once with an ultrasound to measure the endometrial thickness. This typically occurs on days 5–7 of the donor's stimulation cycle. This allows us to adjust the medications in the event that the lining is not adequate (≥7 mm) [27].

TABLE 9.7

Administration of Medications

Class of Medication	Typical Form
Oral contraceptives	Oral tablet
Low-dose hCG	Subcutaneous injection
Cetrotide/Ganirelix	Subcutaneous injection
Lupron	Subcutaneous injection
Lupron Trigger	Subcutaneous injection
Estrogen	Oral tablet; skin patch
Progesterone	Vaginal gel, vaginal suppository, or intramuscular injection

Gestational Carrier IVF

In 1985, Utian et al. [28] described the first successful pregnancy using a gestational carrier. The patient had undergone a hysterectomy. She had her eggs removed and then fertilized with her husband's sperm. The embryos were then transferred into the gestational carrier. There are two groups of patients that are candidates for gestational carrier IVF (GC-IVF): women without a functioning uterus or those whose pregnancy would severely exacerbate a medical condition. It is important to note that IVF with a gestational carrier differs from traditional surrogacy. In a traditional surrogacy arrangement, the surrogate mother provides the oocyte *and* the uterus to foster a pregnancy. With a gestational carrier IVF cycle, the gestational carrier is not the genetic mother because she does not provide the oocyte. At Boston IVF, we do not participate in traditional surrogacy treatment.

Prescreening and Counseling

At our center, the minimum age of gestational carriers is 21 years, with an upper limit of 40 at the initiation of the IVF cycle. All gestational carriers must have carried at least one child and preferably have completed their families. As with egg donor and recipients, both genetic mothers (intended patents or IPs) and gestational carriers undergo prenatal screening as recommended by the guidelines of the ASRM. Before ovarian stimulation, issues discussed with the IPs, the gestational carrier, and her partner include selective reduction for multiple gestations in excess of twins, chorionic villus sampling, amniocentesis, risks of the procedure, and mode of delivery. All of the IPs, the gestational carriers, and their partners undergo psychological and legal counseling, including appropriate legal contracts. Unlike DE IVF, there are no agencies and therefore legal contracts must be done with an attorney specializing in reproductive law. It is important that the IPs and the gestational carrier have separate representation.

Cycle Synchronization and Ovulation Induction

Cycle synchronization between the IP and the gestational carrier can be achieved with oral contraceptives and down-regulation with leuprolide acetate. The ovulation induction protocol for the IP can be individualized. Estrogen replacement for the carrier (both oral and transdermal) and progesterone replacement are continued until 10 weeks estimated gestational age.

FDA Regulations

Both of the IPs are regarded as "gamete donors" according to FDA regulations [7]. The intended mother must therefore be screened for the same tests as an oocyte donor up to 30 days before the egg retrieval (Table 9.2), and the intended father must be screened for the required tests (Table 9.3) within 7 days before or after the egg retrieval.

Embryo Donation

In the current practice of ART, more embryos are created than can be transferred during the cycle. Embryos that meet criteria for cryopreservation are stored for future use by the patients. When the genetic parents decide that their family is complete and embryos are still available, they are faced with a dilemma: donating their embryos to research, thawing them and rendering them nonviable, or donating them to a couple who is unable to conceive. A survey sent to all 430 ART facilities in the United States in 2002 estimated that a total of 396,526 embryos had been placed in storage in the United States [29]. In 2011, this number is estimated to have increased to well over 500,000 embryos.

In 2009, the ethics committee of the ASRM issued a report strongly objecting to the term embryo "adoption" as inaccurate and misleading [30]. Their point is that donating an embryo to another person is a medical procedure, subject to the rules and regulations for medical procedures, not subject to the legal and social work regulations associated with adoption of an actual human being. On the other hand, despite ASRM's insistence that donation of embryos is strictly a medical procedure, there are embryo donation programs on the Internet that will arrange "open" embryo adoptions, allowing the donor and recipient to actually share the future child like in traditional open adoptions of existing children. Some embryo adoption agencies will allow the donor to choose the recipient of their embryos. As with donor oocyte, donor sperm, and gestational carrier procedures, in the United States, the FDA oversees the process through comprehensive regulations that apply to all donated human tissues, reproductive and non-reproductive alike.

In 2016, the ASRM reissued guidelines for ART practices that offer embryo donation [31]. The guidelines stated that the practice should be knowledgeable in the storage, thawing, and transfer of frozen embryos and that the practice may charge a professional fee to the potential recipients for embryo thawing, the embryo transfer procedure, cycle coordination and documentation, and infectious disease screening and testing of both recipients and donors. However, the selling of embryos per se is ethically unacceptable. Embryos should be quarantined for a minimum of 6 months before the potential donors are screened and tested or retested, with documentation of negative results. Last, physicians and employees of an infertility practice should be excluded from participating in embryo donation as either donors or recipients within that practice.

For embryos derived from gametes obtained from an anonymous donor or donors, the donor or donors must have met all FDA screening and testing requirements and must have been determined eligible for anonymous donation. If donor sperm were used, the sperm donor must have met all current FDA requirements for donation, the sperm sample used to fertilize the oocytes must have met the minimum 6-month quarantine requirement for donor sperm, and the female partner must have met all screening and testing requirements for oocyte donors within the 30 days preceding oocyte retrieval. If donor oocytes were used, the oocyte donor must have met all current FDA requirements for donation within the 30 days preceding the oocyte retrieval, and the male partner must have met all screening and testing requirements, including the minimum 6-month quarantine for donor sperm. Embryos derived from the gametes of a sexually intimate couple and created for use by that couple are exempt from the requirements for donor screening and testing before creation of the embryos.

Per the ASRM guidelines: The decision to proceed with embryo donation is complex, and patients may benefit from psychological counseling to aid in this decision. Psychological consultation with a qualified mental health professional should be offered to all couples participating in the donor-embryo process. The physician should require psychological consultation for couples in whom there appear to be factors that warrant further evaluation [28].

Sperm Donation

Sperm donation is the most common type of gamete donation. The guidelines for sperm donation have been published by the ASRM [27].

There are several indications for sperm donation, including male factor infertility, when the male partner is a carrier of a genetic condition or has a transmissible disease that can not be eradicated, and for the woman who does not have a male partner. Before the outbreak of HIV, it was common that fresh donor sperm samples were used, but now exclusively frozen sperm samples are obtained from licensed sperm banks. The frozen sperm samples are quarantined for a period of 6 months and only released after the donor has tested negative for syphilis, hepatitis, and HIV. More commonly, the sperm donation is done anonymously but on occasion the choice is a known donor. For a couple, the male partner may desire to use a relative such as a brother or less commonly his father for the sperm donor since this will allow him to have a genetic tie to the offspring. For the single woman, she may choose an identified sperm donor as well. It is standard that any couple or woman pursuing sperm donation meet with a social worker for counseling. In cases of known sperm donation, all parties will meet with the social worker over several sessions before moving forward. In cases of known sperm donation, it is also of extreme importance that legal counseling be obtained to specify who controls the sperm samples, the parental rights and obligations of the recipient woman or couple, and the lack of parental rights and obligations of the sperm donor. This legal counseling should result in the development of a contract that protects all parties involved.

Egg Banking

Since the introduction of an efficient method of oocyte vitrification by Kuwayama in 2005, there has been a growing body of clinical evidence demonstrating the potential of this procedure with applications in donor oocyte programs and, in particular, for donor egg banking [32]. This procedure has been demonstrated to be safe, and more than 900 oocyte cryopreservation babies were born with no apparent increase in congenital anomalies [33]. Forman et al. confirmed that oocyte vitrification does not increase the risk of embryonic aneuploidy or diminish the implantation potential of blastocysts created after intracytoplasmic sperm injection [34]. Furthermore, a prospective randomized sibling–oocyte study comparing embryo development in fresh versus vitrified oocytes in patients undergoing cycles with their own oocytes found no statistical differences between fertilization rates or embryo development/quality in the two groups [35]. There has been much debate in the reproductive endocrinology community regarding the current status and clinical applicability of oocyte cryopreservation. Whereas sperm and embryo freezing has been used with good pregnancy success rates for a long enough time to gain widespread acceptance, oocyte freezing previously suffered from being labeled "experimental." This changed in January 2013, when the ASRM announced that oocyte cryopreservation was no longer experimental [36]. Improved methods for oocyte preservation and demand for donor oocytes have led to the emergence of a new phenomenon in the United States and worldwide commercial egg banks and networks, entities able to provide cryopreserved oocytes to intended recipients of egg donation. With the establishment of more egg banks, their impact on overall egg donation cycles is likely to increase. As egg bank donor egg IVF becomes a growing segment of the donor egg IVF market, it is crucial to intensify research on oocyte cryopreservation techniques and provide ethical and legal guidance for this promising new treatment option.

Evaluation

Prescreen evaluation for patients using donor sperm

1. Uterine evaluation—hysterosalpingogram.
2. Cycle day 3 FSH, E2, TSH.
3. Prenatal blood work and indicated genetic testing based on ancestral background.
4. Cytomegalovirus (CMV) IgG and IgM titers—if the woman is found to be CMV negative, then she should choose a CMV negative donor. CMV is a herpes virus and there is concern that a CMV-positive donor may excrete active virus in the semen.
5. Cervical cultures.

6. Male partner (of recipient couple) should be screened for RPR, hepatitis B antigen, hepatitis C antibody, and HIV.

7. Consultation with social worker.

REFERENCES

1. Bloom DE, Trussell J. What are the determinants of delayed childbearing and permanent childlessness in the United States? *Demography* 1984;21(4):591–611.
2. Centers for Disease Control (CDC) 2014 Assisted Reproductive Technology (ART) Report.
3. Society for Reproductive Technology. 2014 National Report, https://www.sartcorsonline.com/.
4. Joseph KS, Allen AC, Dodds L et al. The perinatal effects of delayed childbearing. *Obstet Gynecol* 2005;105(6):1410–8.
5. Benagiano G. Pregnancy after the menopause: A challenge to nature? *Hum Reprod* 1993;8(9):1344–5.
6. Olshansky SJ, Passaro DJ, Hershow RC et al. A potential decline in life expectancy in the United States in the 21st century. *N Engl J Med* 2005;352(11):1138–45.
7. Food and Drug Administration, HHS. Eligibility determination for donors of human cells, tissues, and cellular and tissue-based products. Final Rule. *Fed Regist* 2004 May 25;69(101):29785–834.
8. Food and Drug Administration, HHS. Human cells, tissues, and cellular and tissue-based products; donor screening and testing, and related labeling. Interim final rule; opportunity for public comment. *Fed Regist* 2005 May 25;70(100):29949–52.
9. Shulman A, Frenkel Y, Dor J et al. The best donor. *Hum Reprod* 1999;14(10):2493–6.
10. Cohen MA, Lindheim SR, Sauer MV. Donor age is paramount to success in oocyte donation. *Hum Reprod* 1999;14(11):2755–8.
11. Ethics Committee of the American Society for Reproductive Medicine. Financial incentives in recruitment of oocyte donors. *Fertil Steril* 2004 Sep;82 Suppl 1:S240–4.
12. Damario MA, Barmat L, Liu HC et al. Dual suppression with oral contraceptives and gonadotrophin releasing-hormone agonists improves in-vitro fertilization outcome in high responder patients. *Hum Reprod* 1997;12(11):2359–65.
13. Barmat LI, Chantilis SJ, Hurst BS, Dickey RP. A randomized prospective trial comparing gonadotropin-releasing hormone (GnRH) antagonist/recombinant follicle-stimulating hormone (rFSH) versus GnRH-agonist/rFSH in women pretreated with oral contraceptives before in vitro fertilization. *Fertil Steril* 2005;83(2):321–30.
14. Morris RS, Paulson RJ, Sauer MV, Lobo RA. Predictive value of serum oestradiol concentrations and oocyte number in severe ovarian hyperstimulation syndrome. *Hum Reprod* 1995;10(4):811–4.
15. Berger BM, Ezcurra D, Alper MM. A standardized protocol with minimal monitoring for controlled ovarian stimulation of egg donors results in improved pregnancy rates. *Fertil Steril* 2004;82:S121.
16. Berger BM, Ezcurra D. Treatment modification based on basal antral follicle count maintains high pregnancy rates while preventing OHSS in egg donor IVF. *Fertil Steril* 2009;92:S3.
17. Borini A, Violini F, Bianchi L et al. Improvement of pregnancy and implantation rates in cyclic women undergoing oocyte donation after long-term down-regulation. *Hum Reprod* 1995;10(11):3018–21.
18. Lutjen P, Trounson A, Leeton J et al. The establishment and maintenance of pregnancy using in vitro fertilization and embryo donation in a patient with primary ovarian failure. *Nature* 1984;307(5947):174–5.
19. Remohi J, Gutierrez A, Cano F, Ruiz A, Simon C, Pellicer A. Long oestradiol replacement in an oocyte donation programme. *Hum Reprod* 1995;10(6):1387–91.
20. Yaron Y, Amit A, Mani A et al. Uterine preparation with estrogen for oocyte donation: Assessing the effect of treatment duration on pregnancy rates. *Fertil Steril* 1995;63(6):1284–6.
21. Navot D, Scott RT, Droesch K et al. The window of embryo transfer and the efficiency of human conception in vitro. *Fertil Steril* 1991;55(1):114–8.
22. Rosenwaks Z. Donor eggs: Their application in modern reproductive technologies. *Fertil Steril* 1987 Jun;47(6):895–909.
23. Prapas Y, Prapas N, Jones EE et al. The window for embryo transfer in oocyte donation cycles depends on the duration of progesterone therapy. *Hum Reprod* 1998;13(3):720–3.

24. Bosch E, Labarta E, Crespo J et al. Circulating progesterone levels and ongoing pregnancy rates in controlled ovarian stimulation cycles for *in vitro* fertilization: Analysis of over 4000 cycles. *Hum Reprod* 2010;25:2092–100.
25. Berger BM, Phillips JA. Pregnancy outcomes in oocyte donation recipients: Vaginal gel versus intramuscular injection progesterone replacement. *J Assist Reprod Genet* 2012;29:237–42.
26. Shapiro DB, Pappadakis JA, Ellsworth EM et al. Progesterone replacement with vaginal gel versus IM injection: Cycle and pregnancy outcomes in IVF patients receiving vitrified blastocysts. *Hum Reprod* 2014;29:1706–11.
27. Zenke U, Chetkowski RJ. Transfer and uterine factors are the major recipient-related determinants of success with donor eggs. *Fertil Steril* 2004;82(4):850–6.
28. Utian WH, Sheean L, Goldfarb JM, Kiwi R. Successful pregnancy after in vitro fertilization and embryo transfer from an infertile woman to a surrogate. *N Engl J Med* 1985;313(21):1351–2.
29. Hoffman DI, Zellman GL, Fair CC, Mayer JF, Zeitz JG, Gibbons WE, Turner TG. Cryopreserved embryos in the United States and their availability for research. *Fertil Steril* 2003 May;79(5):1063–9.
30. Ethics Committee of the American Society for Reproductive Medicine. American Society for Reproductive Medicine: Defining embryo donation. *Fertil Steril* 2009;92:1818–9.
31. Ethics Committee of the American Society for Reproductive Medicine. Defining embryo donation: An Ethics Committee Opinion. *Fertil Steril* 2016;106:56–8.
32. Kuwayama M, Vajta G, Kato O, Leibo SP. Highly efficient vitrification method for cryopreservation of human oocytes. *Reprod Biomed Online* 2005;11:300–8.
33. Noyes N, Porcu E, Borini A. Over 900 oocyte cryopreservation babies born with no apparent increase in congenital anomalies. *Reprod Biomed Online* 2009;18:769–76.
34. Forman EJ, Li S, Ferry KM et al. Oocyte vitrification does not increase the risk of embryonic aneuploidy or diminish the implantation potential of blastocysts created after intracytoplasmic sperm injection: A novel, paired randomized controlled trial using DNA fingerprinting. *Fertil Steril* 2012;98:644–9.
35. Rienzi L, Romano S, Albricci L et al. Embryo development of fresh "versus" vitrified metaphase II oocytes after ICSI: A prospective randomized sibling-oocyte study. *Human Reprod* 2010;25:66–73.
36. Practice Committees of ASRM, Society for Assisted Reproductive Technology. Mature oocyte cryopreservation: A guideline. *Fertil Steril* 2013;99:37–43.

10

Fertility Care for the LGBT Community

Samuel C. Pang

Introduction

For many years, children have been raised in families where their parents are lesbian, gay, bisexual, or transgender (LGBT; see Table 10.1 for definitions). Studies have found that children of lesbian or gay parents are not different from children of heterosexual parents in terms of their emotional development or relationships with others [1]. Historically, many of these children were conceived and born from heterosexual relationships, after which one parent (or in some cases both parents) "come out" as LGBT. More recently, LGBT people are "coming out" in their youth so that they are less likely to have children from prior heterosexual relationships. Therefore, they are building their families by having children as an LGBT couple. Some choose adoption, but many lesbian couples use donor sperm to conceive. Some use donor sperm from friends, acquaintances, or family members of their partners, but the majority use donor sperm from a commercial sperm bank. For lesbian couples in which one (or both) has infertility, many are able to conceive with assisted reproductive technologies (ART). Historically, gay male couples have built their families through adoption or co-parenting arrangements with lesbian friends, but some have used surrogacy to have children. More recently, transgender people have also been able to use ART to have genetically related children [2].

After the U.S. Supreme Court *Obergefell v. Hodges* decision, which legalized same-sex marriage in the United States, same-sex couples are marrying in increasing numbers [3–5]. Same-sex couples who marry are increasingly seeking to build families, which has resulted in increased demand for ART services [6].

LGBT individuals frequently experience discrimination or disparities in their health care. The Ethics Committees of the American Society for Reproductive Medicine (ASRM) and the American Congress of Obstetricians and Gynecologists (ACOG) have opined that ethical arguments supporting denial of access to fertility services on the basis of marital status, sexual orientation, or gender identity cannot be justified [7–9]. Health care providers need to be informed regarding ART options available to LGBT people so that they may counsel their LGBT patients appropriately.

Psychosocial Counseling

Psychosocial counseling associated with use of ART services is not unique to LGBT patients. All couples who plan to conceive with donor gametes (sperm or eggs) or a surrogate need to have psychoeducational counseling to discuss concerns and feelings that arise when family building involves the assistance of a third party. For the parent who is not contributing genetic material, there is the lack of a genetic connection to the child(ren) conceived with donor gametes. There are also practical issues such as the challenges of choosing the appropriate gamete donor, the differences between known and recruited donors, the option of selecting donors who are open to contact with offspring in the future, and when and how to

TABLE 10.1

Glossary

Sexual orientation:	A person's sexual, physical, romantic, and/or emotional attraction to a particular sex (male or female).
Heterosexuality:	Sexual, physical, romantic, and/or emotional attraction between persons of the opposite sex or gender.
Homosexuality:	Sexual, physical, romantic, and/or emotional attraction between persons of the same sex or gender.
Gay:	Describes a man whose enduring sexual, physical, romantic, and/or emotional attraction is to other men.
Lesbian:	Describes a woman whose enduring sexual, physical, romantic, and/or emotional attraction is to other women.
Bisexual:	An individual who is sexually, physically, romantically, and/or emotionally attracted to both genders, although not necessarily to the same degree.
Gender identity:	A person's internal perception of their gender.
Transgender:	An individual who identifies with a gender different from what society expects based on the sex the individual was assigned at birth. Transgender individuals can be heterosexual, lesbian, gay, or bisexual in their sexual orientation.
Cisgender:	An individual who identifies with the gender that society expects based on the sex the individual was assigned at birth. Cisgender individuals can be heterosexual, lesbian, gay, or bisexual in their sexual orientation.

discuss with the child(ren) conceived with donor gametes the circumstances of their conception. When surrogacy is part of the treatment plan, group counseling involving all parties is mandatory to ensure that everyone is in agreement regarding the expectations of their relationship during and beyond the surrogacy process. For LGBT couples, who frequently experience situations or remarks that are inappropriate or hurtful, it is important to discuss feelings and responses to sociocultural challenges for LGBT families who are marginalized and discriminated against in subtle ways. Counseling with a professional counselor is done before proceeding with treatment.

Donor Sperm

Donors who donate sperm to a commercial sperm bank have all been tested for a standard list of infectious diseases mandated by the Food and Drug Administration (FDA), which has published regulations regarding donation of human tissues [10]. These regulations mandate testing of all donors for these infectious diseases, which may potentially be transmitted in semen, before collecting semen specimens intended for donation. Sperm specimens are frozen and quarantined for a period of 6 months, after which the donor is retested for the same list of infectious diseases. If all the repeat tests for infectious diseases result negative, the quarantined frozen sperm specimens may then be released by the sperm bank for donation. If any test for infectious diseases is positive, the quarantined sperm specimens may not be released for donation and must be discarded.

Sperm donated to a commercial sperm bank have usually been washed with special cell culture media fluids and concentrated into a small volume before cryopreservation. These vials are designated for intrauterine insemination (IUI) and are ready for immediate use upon thaw. If the vial of donor sperm obtained from a commercial sperm bank is labeled "ICI," it is intended for intracervical or intravaginal insemination and needs to be washed with special culture media fluids in the laboratory and concentrated into a small volume before IUI.

Occasionally, some lesbian couples choose to use sperm from a known (or directed) donor, typically a family member of the partner who is not conceiving, or a friend, or an acquaintance. Family building with sperm from a known donor has significant psychosocial and legal ramifications; therefore, psychosocial and legal counseling, as well as legal contracts, are mandatory. The counseling and legal contracts address the questions of who owns the donor sperm specimens and controls their use, parental rights and obligations of the intended parents (IPs), as well as the lack of parental rights and obligations of the donor. If a lesbian couple wishes to use sperm from a known donor, the most efficient process is for the designated donor to bank his sperm at a commercial sperm bank and specifically designate the banked sperm specimens for use by the recipient IPs. There are FDA regulations specifically governing use of sperm from a known/directed donor if the insemination is being performed by a clinician in a medical facility, which are similar to the regulations governing use of sperm from donors recruited by a commercial sperm bank [10]. After initial testing for potentially transmissible infectious diseases, sperm specimens are frozen and quarantined for a period of 6 months, after which the donor is retested for the same list of infectious diseases. If all the repeat tests result negative for these infectious diseases, the frozen sperm specimens may then be released by the sperm bank for use by the recipient IPs. If any test for infectious diseases is positive, the recipient IPs must be counseled regarding the potential risk of infection with the infectious disease, after which they may choose to use the frozen donor sperm specimens for insemination, but would have to sign a waiver acknowledging that they have been counseled regarding the risk of potential infection from use of these donor sperm specimens.

Options for Lesbian Couples

Insemination with Donor Sperm

Donor sperm insemination is the least invasive procedure and is the primary method of conception for lesbians who do not have infertility issues. One option is intravaginal insemination at home, timed with urinary ovulation predictor kits. Alternatively, insemination performed by a clinician in a medical facility is typically IUI, in which donor sperm are placed directly inside the uterus on the day that the woman is determined to be ovulating. IUI serves to deliver the maximum number of sperm to the fallopian tubes where fertilization of the oocyte takes place.

IUI may be done with or without the use of fertility medications. Most lesbians who do not have fertility issues may do donor sperm IUI without the use of fertility medications. However, lesbians who have ovulatory dysfunction may benefit from use of fertility medications such as letrozole, clomiphene, or injectable gonadotropins. There is an increased risk of multiple gestations in pregnancies resulting from use of fertility medications.

IVF with Donor Sperm

Some lesbians are unable to conceive with donor sperm IUI because they have an infertility issue such as endometriosis, pelvic adhesive disease, advanced reproductive age, or unexplained infertility. For these women, they may benefit from treatment with in vitro fertilization (IVF), just like any woman who has infertility.

IVF with Partner's Oocytes

A lesbian who is unsuccessful in conceiving with her own eggs owing to primary ovarian insufficiency (premature ovarian failure), diminished ovarian reserve, advanced reproductive age, or other infertility diagnosis may potentially conceive with IVF using oocytes provided by her partner. This process has been referred to as partner-assisted reproduction.

Reciprocal IVF

Some lesbian couples who have never attempted conception with donor sperm insemination and do not have infertility may choose to have children with IVF using the eggs from one partner, inseminated with donor sperm, and have the resultant embryo(s) transferred into the uterus of the other partner who then gestates the pregnancy and gives birth. This enables both partners in the relationship to be directly and physically involved in having their child(ren), and is an appealing concept for many lesbian couples. After the birth of their first child, they may choose to repeat the reciprocal IVF process, but reverse roles so that the partner who gestated the pregnancy for their first reciprocal IVF cycle then provides her oocytes for their second reciprocal IVF cycle, and the partner who provided oocytes for their first reciprocal IVF cycle then gestates the pregnancy.

Some couples choose to use reciprocal IVF if one of them has no intentions of ever being pregnant, so this is an option for her to have a genetically related child without having to be pregnant. After they have a child successfully with reciprocal IVF, the partner who gestated the pregnancy may then return to conceive her genetically related child with donor sperm insemination so they each have genetically related child(ren).

IVF with Donor Eggs

Some lesbian couples may need to use donor eggs from a third party because of the absence of ovaries or the inability of both women to produce viable oocytes. In this situation, their egg donor may either be a known or directed donor (family member, friend, or acquaintance), or an egg donor recruited by an approved egg donor agency, or frozen donor eggs from a frozen donor egg bank. (See section on Anonymous Egg Donation in Chapter 9.)

IVF with Gestational Surrogacy

In rare situations, some lesbian couples may need to use a gestational surrogate because of the absence of a uterus or the absence of a normally functional uterus in both women, or the presence of other medical impediments to healthy pregnancy. In this situation, embryos may be created with oocytes provided by either of the two women, inseminated with donor sperm, and the resulting embryo(s) are transferred into the uterus of a gestational surrogate. (See section on Gestational Carrier IVF in Chapter 9.)

Options for Gay Male Couples

Historically, gay men who desired genetically related children have had children through co-parenting arrangements with close friends (usually, but not necessarily lesbian friends), or through traditional surrogacy. In traditional surrogacy, sperm of the intended father(s) are inseminated into the surrogate. At birth, the baby conceived in this manner is given up by the traditional surrogate for adoption by the IPs. Traditional surrogacy has significant pitfalls owing to historical cases in which the traditional surrogate changed her mind and decided to keep the baby after birth. These cases have led to litigation in which the IPs have sued for custody of their baby. In these cases, the courts have historically ruled in favor of the traditional surrogate who then retains custody of the baby. Nowadays, traditional surrogacy is rarely, if ever, done.

With the advent of IVF, the option of gestational surrogacy became possible. A gestational surrogate has no genetic relationship with the fetus that she carries. Gay male couples have been using IVF with donor eggs and gestational surrogacy to build their families since the late 1990s. Oocytes donated by an egg donor may be inseminated with sperm provided by one or both of the intended fathers, and the resulting embryo(s) may be transferred into the uterus of the surrogate. In 1998, the Reproductive Science Center of New England (now known as IVF New England, a Boston IVF partner) was the first IVF center in New England, and one of the first IVF programs in the United States and in the world, to treat a gay male couple with donor eggs and gestational surrogacy.

There are significant psychosocial and legal ramifications to having a child through gestational surrogacy, so psychosocial and legal counseling of all parties involved are mandatory, as are legal contracts. Surrogacy is prohibited by law in some states, surrogacy laws vary from state to state, and some states have no laws specifically addressing surrogacy, so it is critical to have legal counseling regarding the implications of the state in which the surrogate delivers the baby.

The roles of egg donor and gestational surrogate may be filled by female relatives or friends, or by women who provide these services through a fee-based agreement facilitated by an agency. (See sections on Anonymous Egg Donation and Gestational Carrier IVF in Chapter 9.)

Egg Donors

Ideally, donors recruited by egg donor agencies are healthy young women who are between the ages of 21 and 29 years, although women who are up to the age of 32 years may be acceptable as recruited egg donors. However, known egg donors (family members or close friends of the IPs) may be women in their mid to late 30s, and may be acceptable as egg donors if they are healthy and have good ovarian reserve.

Donors recruited and matched through an egg donor agency are typically compensated for their time, effort, inconvenience, time off from work, and the pain of undergoing a surgical egg retrieval procedure under anesthesia. They are not considered to be "selling" their eggs and are compensated a fixed amount (that is agreed upon) per donation cycle, regardless of the number of eggs retrieved. They are compensated even if no oocyte is retrieved, assuming that the failure to retrieve oocytes is not a result of reckless noncompliance on the part of the donor. A legal contract is mandatory between the egg donor and the IPs, who must be represented by separate attorneys.

Donor egg cycles are typically coordinated with the woman who is carrying the pregnancy such that fresh embryo(s) is (are) transferred, and any untransferred embryos are cryopreserved for potential future use. More recently, the ability to successfully cryopreserve unfertilized human oocytes has resulted in the development of frozen donor egg banks, which has become an alternative source of donor oocytes for those needing to use donor eggs to conceive. Women who are recruited for frozen donor egg banks are extensively evaluated in the same way that all egg donors are evaluated. These donors are stimulated with gonadotropins and undergo transvaginal oocyte retrieval, after which all the mature oocytes are cryopreserved. Their detailed profile is then posted on the list of available donors on the website of the frozen donor egg bank. IPs who need donor eggs may choose to use frozen donor eggs instead of searching for a donor through an egg donor agency. The live birth success rates from frozen donor egg treatment cycles are comparable to those from fresh donor egg treatment cycles. The frozen donor egg option eliminates the need to search for an appropriate donor through an egg donor agency, waiting for evaluation of the potential donor and, if she is accepted as an appropriate donor, the gonadotropin stimulation of the donor followed by transvaginal oocyte retrieval. It also eliminates the necessity of coordinating and synchronizing the cycles of the egg donor and the woman who is carrying the pregnancy, as frozen donor eggs are ready to be used when thawed. The overall cost of using frozen donor oocytes is also significantly lower than the cost of using donor oocytes from a donor recruited and matched through an egg donor agency, and may result in overall cost savings of approximately $15,000 for a male couple who choose this option. The main advantage of a fresh donor egg treatment cycle is the higher probability of having excess untransferred embryos cryopreserved for potential future use, because frozen donor egg treatment cycles are typically allotted six to eight frozen eggs per treatment cycle, whereas with fresh donor egg treatment cycles, the IPs receive all of the oocytes retrieved from their designated donor.

Gestational Surrogates

Gestational surrogates (or gestational carriers) may be known (a female relative or friend), or may be recruited and matched through a surrogacy agency. Regardless of whether a surrogate is known or recruited through an agency, psychosocial and legal counseling for all parties involved and a legal contract between the surrogate and IPs are mandatory. Legal counseling must be provided by an attorney (or law firm) who specializes in reproductive law.

Once the prospective surrogate has been selected and matched, she undergoes extensive evaluation, including psychological testing, medical testing, and screening for potentially infectious diseases that may inadvertently infect the fetus during pregnancy or childbirth. After comprehensive evaluation, the surrogate's cycle needs to be synchronized with that of the egg donor. Synchronization of the two women's cycles is typically accomplished with a combination of oral contraceptive pills and a gonadotropin-releasing hormone agonist such as leuprolide acetate. On rare occasions, because of unanticipated events, synchronization of the two women's cycles is unachievable, in which case all the embryos created are cryopreserved for frozen embryo transfer (FET) in a subsequent cycle. If frozen donor oocytes are being used, synchronization with the egg donor's cycle is unnecessary. However, in either case, the surrogate's endometrium needs to be programmed with estradiol and progesterone, such that it is at the window of implantation when the embryo is ready for transfer.

Recently, the option to screen embryos for aneuploidy using preimplantation genetic screening (PGS) has become available (see Chapter 12). The current technology for PGS is very accurate, and the cost of doing PGS is very reasonable considering the total cost of having a baby with donor eggs and gestational surrogacy. Many IPs, especially those who are using a donor recruited and matched through an egg donor agency, are opting to do PGS on their embryos, which are then cryopreserved for future FET into their gestational surrogate. The advantage of doing PGS for aneuploidy is the higher probability that transfer of a reportedly euploid embryo is more likely to result in successful implantation [11] and potentially a higher probability of live birth, and a lower risk of spontaneous abortion or pregnancy with a fetus affected with aneuploidy such as Trisomy 21 (Down syndrome). When the IPs have euploid embryos (as determined by PGS), which are cryopreserved and suitable for transfer, their gestational surrogate is then brought in for the FET. This strategy results in more efficient utilization of their gestational surrogate's time and decreases the risk of their gestational surrogate experiencing a spontaneous abortion owing to aneuploidy, or the unfortunate situation of pregnancy with an aneuploid fetus, where the IPs are faced with the dilemma of requesting termination of pregnancy in their gestational surrogate.

Options for Transgender People

The desire to become a parent is compelling for many people, regardless of sexual orientation or gender identity. Transgender individuals who want to have genetically related children need to plan ahead, as some of the hormonal and surgical procedures employed in their transition to their affirmed gender identity may render them incapable of having genetically related children post-transition. Reproductive options for transgender individuals depend on where in the transition process they are, and whether they are ready to have children immediately or in the future.

Fertility Preservation

Most transgender individuals are not ready to have children before or at the time of their transition, so they choose to undergo fertility preservation procedures. While the ability to cryopreserve sperm has been available for decades, effective and reliable cryopreservation of unfertilized human oocytes has only recently become available. There is good evidence that fertilization and pregnancy rates are similar to IVF with fresh oocytes when previously vitrified oocytes from young women are thawed for use in IVF. Although data are limited, no increase in chromosomal abnormalities, birth defects, and developmental deficits have been reported in the offspring born from cryopreserved oocytes when compared to pregnancies from conventional IVF and the general population. Therefore, the ASRM has declared that vitrification of mature oocytes should no longer be considered experimental [12]. Oocyte cryopreservation technology is currently being used for frozen donor egg banks, as well as for the purpose of fertility preservation in young women who have been diagnosed with cancer, or women who are freezing oocytes for delayed childbearing. This same technology is also used for the purpose of fertility preservation in transgender men.

Fertility Preservation for Transgender Men

Transgender men may cryopreserve their oocytes for potential future use. Ideally, this should be done before initiation of testosterone therapy, which suppresses ovulation. However, transgender men who have initiated testosterone therapy may also undergo oocyte cryopreservation if they are willing to discontinue testosterone therapy for a few months in order to undergo oocyte cryopreservation procedures. They may resume testosterone therapy after their oocytes have been successfully cryopreserved. The process for oocyte cryopreservation for transgender men is virtually identical to the process that is used for egg donors who are donating oocytes for a frozen donor egg bank. Controlled ovarian stimulation is achieved with daily gonadotropin injections for an average of 10 to 12 days, after which transvaginal oocyte retrieval is performed under anesthesia. Depending on how many oocytes are desired, more than one oocyte cryopreservation cycle may be done.

Fertility Preservation for Transgender Women

Transgender women may cryopreserve their sperm for potential future use. Ideally, this should be done before initiation of estrogen therapy, which suppresses spermatogenesis. Sperm banking can be done conveniently at any commercial sperm bank. Banking of multiple specimens is recommended.

Reproductive Options for Transgender Individuals Who Are Ready to Have Children

Transgender individuals who have planned ahead and have cryopreserved their gametes (either sperm or eggs) may return to use their cryopreserved gametes to have children when they are ready to do so.

Use of Cryopreserved Oocytes in Transgender Men

When transgender men are ready to use their cryopreserved oocytes to have children, the frozen oocytes may be thawed for IVF. Intracytoplasmic sperm injection (ICSI) is recommended when IVF is being done with previously vitrified oocytes that have been thawed, as the fertilization rate with conventional drop insemination may be very low with previously vitrified oocytes.

Depending on the relationship status of the transgender man, his previously vitrified oocytes may be thawed for insemination with donor sperm or sperm from his cisgender male partner. Depending on his relationship status, the resulting embryo(s) may be transferred into the uterus of his cisgender female partner or a gestational surrogate. If he has not had a hysterectomy, he may choose to gestate the pregnancy himself, in which case the embryo(s) would be transferred into his own uterus.

Use of Cryopreserved Sperm in Transgender Women

When transgender women are ready to use their cryopreserved sperm to have children, their frozen sperm may be thawed for either IUI or IVF, depending on the quantity and quality of the frozen sperm, as well as their partnership status.

If the transgender woman is partnered with a cisgender woman, her frozen sperm may be thawed for either IUI or IVF in her cisgender female partner. If the transgender woman is partnered with a cisgender man or another transgender woman, her frozen sperm may be thawed for IVF with donor oocytes, and the resulting embryo(s) may be transferred into a gestational surrogate.

If the transgender woman is partnered with a transgender man, her frozen sperm may be thawed for IVF with oocytes previously cryopreserved by her partner or with donor oocytes, and the resulting embryo(s) may be transferred into a gestational surrogate, or into the uterus of her partner if he has not had a hysterectomy and chooses to gestate the pregnancy himself.

Reproductive Options for Transgender Individuals Who Have Not Cryopreserved Their Gametes

Transgender individuals who have not cryopreserved their gametes may have the opportunity to have genetically related children if they have not undergone any surgical procedure during the course of their transition that renders them permanently sterile.

Reproductive Options for Transgender Men

Transgender men who transitioned before the availability of oocyte cryopreservation, or who have not previously cryopreserved their oocytes, can have genetically related children if they have not had bilateral oophorectomy and are willing to discontinue testosterone therapy temporarily. Their options for procreation depend on their relationship status and whether they have had a hysterectomy.

A transgender man who is partnered with a cisgender woman may do reciprocal IVF in which he provides oocytes that are inseminated with donor sperm, and the resulting embryo(s) is (are) transferred into the uterus of his partner.

A transgender man who has not had bilateral oophorectomy or hysterectomy may choose to conceive himself with sperm from his cisgender male partner or with donor sperm insemination. Alternatively, he may do IVF with sperm from his cisgender male partner, or sperm from his transgender female partner who previously cryopreserved her sperm, or with donor sperm. The resulting embryos may be transferred into a gestational surrogate, or into his own uterus if he chooses to carry the pregnancy himself, or into the uterus of his transgender male partner who may choose to carry the pregnancy (reciprocal IVF).

Reproductive Options for Transgender Women

Transgender women who transitioned without having previously banked their sperm may or may not be able to have genetically related children, depending on whether they have had bilateral orchiectomy or whether spermatogenesis is still present if they have not had bilateral orchiectomy. In general, estrogen therapy suppresses spermatogenesis to the point of azoospermia, but spermatogenesis may or may not recover if estrogen therapy is discontinued. There are no studies that have been done to document the recovery of spermatogenesis in transgender women who discontinue estrogen therapy, but anecdotally, I have seen a case in which a transgender woman who discontinued estrogen therapy after 5 years had resumption of spermatogenesis, although the sperm count in the ejaculate was extremely low (less than 1 million/mL). Assuming that viable sperm is present in the ejaculate, these may be used in an IVF cycle with ICSI. If the transgender woman is partnered with a cisgender woman, her female partner may undergo an IVF cycle in which the oocytes are inseminated with sperm provided by the transgender woman, and the resulting embryo(s) is (are) transferred into the uterus of her female partner.

If the transgender woman is partnered with a transgender man, her sperm may be used to inseminate donor oocytes or oocytes previously cryopreserved by her partner, and the resulting embryo(s) may be transferred into the uterus of a gestational surrogate to gestate the pregnancy, or into the uterus of her partner if he has not had a hysterectomy and chooses to carry the pregnancy himself. If the transgender woman is partnered with a cisgender man or another transgender woman, sperm from either one or both of them may be used to inseminate donor oocytes, and the resulting embryo(s) may be transferred into the uterus of a gestational surrogate.

Conclusion

The same ART that are used to treat heterosexual couples with infertility have been used very successfully to assist members of the LGBT community who have genetically related children. In addition to being informed about the treatment options that may be offered to LGBT people, it is also very important that medical providers (and their office staff) who treat LGBT people be culturally competent and sensitive to their needs.

REFERENCES

1. Wainright JL, Russell ST, Patterson CJ. Psychosocial adjustment, school outcomes, and romantic relationships of adolescents with same-sex parents. *Child Dev* 2004 Nov–Dec;75(6):1886–98.
2. James-Abra S, Tarasoff LA, Marvel S, Green D, Epstein R, Anderson S, Steele LS, Ross LE. Trans people's experiences with assisted reproduction services: A qualitative study. *Hum Reprod* 2015;30:1365–74.
3. Flores A. Examining variation in surveying attitudes on same-sex marriage: A meta-analysis. *Public Opin Q* 2015;2:580–93.
4. Gates GJ, Brown TNT. *Marriage and Same-Sex Couples after Obergefell*. The Williams Institute, UCLA School of Law 2015.
5. Gates GJ. Marriage and family: LGBT individuals and same-sex couples. *Future Child* 2015;2:67–87.
6. Gates GJ. *Demographics of Married and Unmarried Same-Sex Couples: Analysis of the 2013 American Community Survey*. The Williams Institute, UCLA School of Law, 2014.
7. The Ethics Committee of the American Society for Reproductive Medicine. Access to fertility treatment by gays, lesbians, and unmarried persons: A committee opinion. *Fertil Steril* 2013 Dec;100(6):1524–7.
8. The Ethics Committee of the American Society for Reproductive Medicine. Access to fertility services by transgender persons: An ethics committee opinion. *Fertil Steril* 2015 Nov;104(5):1111–5.
9. Committee on Health Care for Underserved Women. Committee Opinion No. 525: Health care for lesbians and bisexual women. *Obstet Gynecol* 2012 May;119(5):1077–80.
10. Food and Drug Administration. Eligibility determination for donors of human cells, tissues and cellular and tissue-based products, final rule. *Fed Regist* 2004;69(101):29785–834.
11. Chen M, Wei S, Hu J, Quan S. Can comprehensive chromosomal screening technology improve IVF/ICSI outcomes? A meta-analysis. *PLoS ONE* 2015;10(10):e0140779. doi: 10.3071/journal.pone.0140779.
12. The Practice Committees of the American Society for Reproductive Medicine and the Society for Assisted Reproductive Technology. Mature oocyte cryopreservation: A guideline. *Fertil Steril* 2013;99:37–43.

11

Evaluation and Management of Male Infertility

Stephen Lazarou

Introduction

Approximately 15% of couples are unable to conceive after 1 year of unprotected intercourse. A male factor is responsible in about 20% of infertile couples and contributory in another 30%–40% [1]. Male infertility is generally determined by the finding of an abnormal semen analysis, although other factors may play a role in the setting of a normal semen analysis.

Male infertility can be attributed to a variety of conditions. Some of these conditions are potentially reversible, such as obstruction of the vas deferens and hormonal imbalances. Other conditions are not reversible, such as bilateral testicular atrophy secondary to a viral infection.

Treatment of various conditions may improve male infertility and allow for conception through intercourse. Even men who have absent sperm on their semen analyses (azoospermia) may have sperm production by their testicles. Detection of conditions for which there are no treatments spares couples the distress of attempting therapies that are not effective. Identifying certain genetic causes of male infertility allows couples to be informed about the potential to transmit genetic conditions that may affect the health of offspring. Therefore, a comprehensive evaluation of the male partner allows the couple to better understand the basis of their infertility and to obtain genetic counseling where necessary. Male infertility may be the presenting manifestation of an underlying life-threatening condition, such as testicular or pituitary tumors [2].

If corrective treatment is not available, assisted reproductive techniques (ARTs) such as testicular or epididymal sperm retrieval in combination with in vitro fertilization (IVF)/intracytoplasmic sperm injection (ICSI) may be utilized. Other options for couples include donor insemination or adoption.

When to Evaluate the Male

A couple attempting to conceive should have an evaluation for infertility if pregnancy does not occur within 1 year of regular unprotected intercourse. An evaluation should be done before 1 year if male infertility risk factors, such as a history of bilateral cryptorchidism (undescended testes) or chemotherapy, are known to be present. Other reasons may include female infertility risk factors, including advancing female age (over the age of 35) or a couple that questions the male partner's fertility potential. While a man may have a history of previous involvement in a pregnancy, this does not exclude the possibility of a newly acquired factor preventing normal fertility (secondary infertility). Men with secondary infertility should be evaluated in the same comprehensive way as men who have never initiated a pregnancy.

Evaluation of the Infertile Male

The evaluation of the infertile male should be performed by a urologist and include a complete reproductive and medical history, physical examination, and at least two semen analyses ideally separated by at least a week. The reproductive and medical history should include coital frequency and timing, duration of infertility and prior fertility, childhood illnesses and developmental history, medications, systemic medical illnesses (e.g., diabetes mellitus and upper respiratory diseases) and prior surgeries (e.g., hernia repair), sexual history including sexually transmitted infections, and exposure to toxins from heat, chemicals, and radiation, including smoking and family reproductive history, review of systems, and allergies.

Physical Examination

A general physical examination is an essential part of the evaluation. In addition to the general physical examination, particular attention is made to the genitalia including (1) examination of the penis including the location of the urethral meatus or presence of plaque/lesion; (2) palpation of the testes and measurement of their size; (3) presence and consistency of both the vasa and epididymides; (4) presence of a varicocele; (5) secondary sex characteristics including body habitus, hair distribution, and breast development; and (6) digital rectal exam.

Based on the results of the full evaluation, the urologist may recommend other procedures and tests to determine the cause of a patient's infertility. These tests may include additional semen analyses, hormone evaluation, post-ejaculatory urinalysis, ultrasonography, specialized tests of semen, and genetic screening.

Semen Analysis

A semen analysis is the principal laboratory evaluation of the infertile male and helps to define the severity of the male factor. An abstinence period of 2 to 3 days is necessary before semen can be collected by masturbation or by intercourse using special semen collection condoms that do not contain substances detrimental to sperm (i.e., lubricants/spermicide). The specimen may be collected at home or at the laboratory. The specimen should be kept at room temperature or, ideally, body temperature during transport and examined within 1 hour of collection.

The semen analysis provides information on semen volume as well as sperm concentration, motility, and morphology (Table 11.1). Values that fall outside these ranges indicate the need for consideration of additional clinical/laboratory evaluation of the patient. It is important to note that reference values for semen parameters are not the same as the minimum values needed for conception and that men with semen variables outside the reference ranges may be fertile. In a study comparing 765 infertile couples with 696 fertile couples (Table 11.2), the threshold values for sperm concentration, motility, and morphology were used to classify men as subfertile, of indeterminate fertility, or fertile. None of the

TABLE 11.1

Normal Reference Values for Semen Analysis

Ejaculatory volume	2.0–5.0 mL
pH	>7.2
Sperm concentration	>20 million/mL
Total sperm number	>40 million/ejaculate
% Motile	>50%
Forward progression	>2 (scale 0–4)
Normal morphology	>4% normal Strict Kruger morphology (WHO 2010)

TABLE 11.2

Fertile, Indeterminate, and Subfertile Ranges for Sperm Measurements and Corresponding Odds Ratios for Infertility

Variable	Semen Measurement		
	Concentration ($\times 10^6$/mL)	Motility (%)	Morphology (% normal)
Fertile range	>48.0	>63	>12
Indeterminate range	13.5–48.0	32–63	9–12
Univariate odds ratio for infertility (95% CI)	1.5 (1.2–1.8)	1.7 (1.5–2.2)	1.8 (1.4–2.4)
Subfertile range	<13.5	<32	<9
Univariate odds ratio for infertility (95% CI)	5.3 (3.3–8.3)	5.6 (3.5–8.3)	3.8 (3.0–5.0)

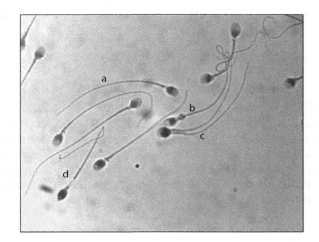

FIGURE 11.1 Examples of varied sperm morphology: (a) normal; (b) mid-piece defect; (c) tail defect; (d) tapered head.

measures, however, were entirely diagnostic of infertility. In fact, patients with values within the reference range may still be subfertile [3].

Absent sperm in the ejaculate, or azoospermia, is not diagnosed unless the specimen is centrifuged and the pellet is examined. The evaluation of sperm morphology (shape) has changed considerably over time. Sperm morphology assessment by strict (Kruger) criteria has been used to identify couples who have a poor chance of fertilization with standard IVF [4,5] or a better chance of fertilization with ICSI [6,7]. True reference ranges have not been established for semen parameters (Figure 11.1).

Endocrine Evaluation

Hormonal abnormalities of the hypothalamic–pituitary–testicular axis are well-known causes of male infertility. Endocrine laboratory work should be obtained if there is an abnormal semen analysis, impaired sexual function, or other clinical signs or symptoms suggestive of a specific endocrinopathy. The initial hormonal evaluation should consist of measurements of serum follicle-stimulating hormone (FSH), luteinizing hormone (LH), testosterone, and prolactin. The relationship of testosterone, LH, FSH, and prolactin helps identify various clinical conditions, such as primary steroidogenic/spermatogenic dysfunction or pituitary dysfunction. A normal serum FSH level does not guarantee the presence of intact spermatogenesis. However, an elevated FSH level even in the upper range of "normal" is indicative of an abnormality in spermatogenesis.

Post-Ejaculatory Urinalysis

Low-volume or absent ejaculate suggests retrograde ejaculation (semen going back into the bladder instead of out the urethra), lack of emission, ejaculatory duct obstruction, hypogonadism (low testosterone), or congenital bilateral absence of the vas deferens (CBAVD). Other explanations of low-volume ejaculate are incomplete collection and short periods (<2 days) of abstinence. Retrograde ejaculation can occur in men who have diabetes and those with testicular cancer who have undergone a lymph node dissection that can disrupt the sympathetic nerves. In order to diagnose possible retrograde ejaculation, a post-ejaculatory urinalysis (analysis of urine sample after ejaculation) should be performed for any man whose ejaculatory volume is low and who has not been diagnosed with hypogonadism or CBAVD.

The post-ejaculatory urinalysis is performed by centrifuging the specimen and microscopically inspecting the pellet. The presence of any sperm in a post-ejaculatory urinalysis of a patient with azoospermia is suggestive of retrograde ejaculation. Significant numbers of sperm must be found in the urine of patients with low ejaculate volume oligospermia in order to suggest the diagnosis of retrograde ejaculation.

Ultrasonography

Scrotal Ultrasonography

Most scrotal abnormalities are visible and palpable on physical examination. This includes varicoceles (dilated veins in the scrotum), spermatoceles (epididymal cysts), absence of the vas deferens, epididymal induration, and testicular masses. Scrotal ultrasonography may identify non-palpable varicoceles. Scrotal ultrasonography may be useful to clarify ambiguous findings on examination, such as may occur in patients with testes that are in the upper scrotum, small scrotal sacs, or other anatomy that makes physical examination difficult.

Transrectal Ultrasonography

The finding of dilated seminal vesicles, dilated ejaculatory ducts, and/or midline prostatic cystic structures on transrectal ultrasonography (TRUS) is suggestive of complete or partial ejaculatory duct obstruction [8]. Normal seminal vesicles are less than 2.0 cm in anteroposterior diameter [9]. Patients with complete ejaculatory duct obstruction produce low-volume, fructose-negative, acidic, azoospermic ejaculates and may have dilated seminal vesicles identified by ultrasound. Patients with CBAVD may also have these findings because they often have absent or atrophic seminal vesicles. Patients with partial ejaculatory duct obstruction often present with low-volume, diminished sperm concentration and/or poor motility. Cysts at the ejaculatory ducts may be identified by ultrasonography and are occasionally amenable to transurethral resection ("unroofing"), which may allow sperm to present in the ejaculate.

Specialized Clinical Tests on Semen and Sperm

In some cases, semen analyses fail to accurately predict a man's fertility. Specialized clinical tests should be reserved only for those cases in which identification of the cause of male infertility will direct treatment.

Strict Sperm Morphology

The clinical implications of poor morphology are controversial. Initial studies evaluating the utility of strict sperm morphology in predicting fertilization rates during IVF used a score of greater than 14% for normal. However, subsequent studies report fertilization rates being lowest for patients with morphology scores of less than 4%. Pregnancy rates have also been reported to be suboptimal with lower scores, but some recent studies have reported no relationship between morphology and IVF results [10,11]. The relationship between morphology scores and pregnancy rates with intrauterine insemination (IUI) and intercourse has been examined [12–16]. However, there is no consensus on the implications of poor morphology scores. Furthermore, the interpretation of sperm morphology varies from laboratory to laboratory. However, certain rare morphological abnormalities, such as sperm without acrosomes, are highly predictive of failure to fertilize eggs. Yet, in most cases, fertilization and pregnancy are possible even with very low morphology scores. Although most physicians utilize strict morphology in practice, most studies have not addressed the significance of isolated low morphology in patients with otherwise normal semen parameters.

DNA Integrity

DNA integrity testing refers to a variety of assays utilized to evaluate the degree of sperm DNA fragmentation. Assessment of sperm DNA integrity has been evaluated for correlation with the ability to conceive by intercourse, IUI, IVF, and IVF using ICSI. Studies demonstrate a statistically significant lower pregnancy rate in those patients with impaired sperm DNA integrity. Nonetheless, many couples with impaired sperm DNA integrity conceive by intercourse [16–18]. The tests are inadequate as screening tests for pregnancy by intercourse. One large study has suggested that abnormal DNA integrity in the sample used for IUI was predictive of pregnancy rates [19]. Most studies have examined the predictive value of sperm DNA integrity testing in routine IVF and IVF using ICSI. Meta-analysis of published studies has found a small, statistically significant predictive effect of DNA integrity results on pregnancy rates for IVF with or without ICSI [20,21]. Data suggest that DNA integrity testing may be of value in identifying those at risk for recurrent pregnancy loss [22]. The "TUNEL" assay is used to assess DNA fragmentation, and in a meta-analysis of miscarriage rates, the test had the highest associated risk ratio at nearly 4 compared with other tests [23]. However, at this time, there is insufficient evidence to warrant routine testing.

Reactive Oxygen Species

Elevated reactive oxygen species (ROS) have been implicated as a cause of male infertility. Both sperm and white blood cells in the semen can produce ROS. ROS may interfere with sperm function by peroxidation of sperm lipid membranes and creation of toxic fatty acid peroxides. Controversy exists regarding the best method of testing for ROS and whether therapies are effective at reducing seminal ROS and improving fecundity. Routine clinical testing and treatment of ROS are not indicated at this time.

Quantitation of Leukocytes in Semen

An elevated number of leukocytes (white blood cells) in the semen has been associated with decreased sperm function and motility. Under microscopy, both leukocytes and immature germ cells appear similar and are properly termed "round cells." The laboratory must make sure that the two types of cells are evaluated to differentiate between a possible infection and immature sperm. A variety of assays are available to differentiate leukocytes from immature germ cells [24]. Men with true pyospermia (greater than 1 million leukocytes per milliliter) should be evaluated for a genital tract infection or inflammation. A semen culture may also be of value to determine the presence of microorganisms.

Tests for Antisperm Antibodies

Pregnancy rates may be reduced by antisperm antibodies (ASA) in the semen [25]. Risk factors for ASA include ductal obstruction, prior genital infection, testicular trauma, and prior vasectomy and reversal. ASA testing may be considered when there is isolated poor motility with normal sperm concentration, sperm agglutination, or an abnormal postcoital test. Some physicians recommend ASA testing for couples with unexplained infertility. ASA testing is not needed if sperm are to be used for ICSI.

Sperm Viability Tests

Sperm viability can be assessed by mixing fresh semen with a dye such as eosin or trypan blue, or by the use of the hypoosmotic swelling (HOS) test. These assays determine whether nonmotile sperm are viable by identifying which sperm have intact cell membranes. Nonmotile but viable sperm, as determined by the HOS test, may be used successfully for ICSI. In the HOS test, sperm are placed into two different media (first in a solution called polyvinylpyrrolidone (PVP), and then to the actual HOS medium itself consisting of sperm wash media and water) and then are left to sit for 30 seconds. At this point, the sperm are observed for the presence of a curled or kinked tails, which indicate viability. The viable sperm can then be extracted and used for ICSI.

Tests of Sperm–Cervical Mucus Interaction

The postcoital test is the microscopic examination of the cervical mucus performed before expected ovulation and within hours after intercourse to identify the presence of motile sperm in the mucus. It is used to identify cervical factors that contribute to infertility. Examination may reveal gross evidence of cervical inflammation that can be treated. Although its value has been seriously questioned, some physicians still consider it as a useful diagnostic test because it may help identify an ineffective coital technique or a cervical issue [26].

Zona Free Hamster Oocyte Penetration Test

Removal of the zona pellucida from hamster oocytes allows human sperm to fuse with hamster ova. This test is often termed a sperm penetration assay (SPA). For penetration to occur, sperm must undergo a series of reactions to integrate into the egg (capacitation, acrosome reaction, fusion with the oolemma, and incorporation into the ooplasm). SPAs have been used clinically, and the value of the test results depends on the experience of the laboratory performing the test [27]. Although this test was used in the past, it is very rarely used presently.

Computer-Aided Sperm Analysis

Computer-aided sperm analysis (CASA) requires sophisticated instruments for quantitative assessment of sperm from a microscopic image or from videotape. CASA is used to measure sperm numbers, motility, and morphology. CASA is useful for assessing sperm motility and motion, such as velocity or speed and head movement, which are important factors in determining sperm fertility potential. While the use of CASA may provide better standardization of semen analyses, it can be cost prohibitive for many centers.

Genetic Screening

Genetic abnormalities may cause infertility by affecting sperm production and/or transport. The three most common genetic factors known to be related to male infertility are cystic fibrosis gene mutations associated with CBAVD, chromosomal abnormalities resulting in impaired testicular function, and Y-chromosome microdeletions (YCMDs) associated with impaired spermatogenesis. Azoospermia and severe oligospermia (sperm concentration <5 million/mL) are more often associated with genetic abnormalities. Men with non-obstructive azoospermia (NOA) and severe oligospermia should be informed that they might have chromosomal abnormalities or YCMD. Genetic counseling should be offered whenever a genetic abnormality is found.

Cystic Fibrosis Gene Mutations

The most common cause of CBAVD is a mutation of the cystic fibrosis transmembrane conductance regulator (CFTR) gene. Almost all males with clinical cystic fibrosis have CBAVD. Approximately 70% of men with CBAVD and no clinical evidence of cystic fibrosis have an identifiable abnormality of the CFTR gene [28,29]. Since normal vasa are palpable within the scrotum, the diagnosis of vasal absence (agenesis), either bilateral or unilateral, is established by physical examination. Imaging studies and surgery are not necessary to confirm the diagnosis but may be useful for diagnosing abnormalities associated with vasal agenesis. Most patients with vasal agenesis also have malformed or absent seminal vesicles. Since the majority of semen is derived from the seminal vesicles, almost all patients with CBAVD have low semen volume.

In the azoospermic patient who has unilateral vasal agenesis, radiologic imaging with TRUS may be useful to evaluate the ampullary portion of the contralateral vas deferens and the seminal vesicles, because unilateral vasal agenesis can be associated with contralateral segmental abnormality of the vas deferens or seminal vesicle, resulting in obstructive azoospermia [30].

It is recommended that both partners undergo genetic counseling and testing of the CFTR gene to rule out abnormalities. Failure to identify a CFTR abnormality in a man with CBAVD, however, does not absolutely rule out the presence of a mutation, since many are undetectable by routine testing methods. It is important to test the partner for CFTR gene abnormalities before performing a treatment that utilizes his sperm because of the risk that she may be a carrier.

Genetic testing of the patient with CBAVD is important because of future health effects of CFTR mutations as well as counseling siblings about their risk of being carriers of CFTR mutations [31,32]. There is a strong association between unilateral vasal agenesis and kidney abnormalities owing to their common embryological origin. Interestingly, the association of renal anomalies and CBAVD is much weaker, with a prevalence of only 11%. However, for those patients who have CBAVD and CFTR mutations, the prevalence of renal anomalies is extremely rare [33]. Therefore, imaging of the kidneys with either ultrasound or CT scan is more likely to detect abnormalities in men with unilateral vasal agenesis or men with CBAVD who do not have mutations in CFTR.

Karyotype

A karyotype analyzes all chromosomes for the gain or loss of entire chromosomes as well as structural defects, including chromosome rearrangements (translocations), duplications, deletions, and inversions. Chromosomal abnormalities account for approximately 6% of all male infertility and the prevalence increases with poorer semen parameters (i.e., severe oligospermia and nonobstructive azoospermia). Paternal transmission of chromosome defects can result in pregnancy loss, birth defects, male infertility, and other syndromes. Karyotypes should be ordered in men with severe oligospermia (sperm concentrations less than 5 million/mL) and azoospermia.

Y-Chromosome Microdeletions

Approximately 13% of men with nonobstructive azoospermia or severe oligospermia have an underlying YCMD (deletion in the Y chromosome) [34]. YCMDs responsible for infertility (azoospermic factor/

AZF regions a, b, or c) are detected using sequence tagged sites (STS) and polymerase chain reaction (PCR) analysis. Successful testicular sperm extraction has not been reported in infertile men with either an AZFa or AZFb deletion, but the total number of reports is limited. In contrast, up to 80% of men with AZFc deletions have sperm that can be retrieved for ICSI. The couple must be counseled on the transmission of the gene to all male offspring [35–37].

Treatments for Male Infertility

There are several causes of infertility for which there is no treatment. For instance, there are no current treatments to stimulate sperm production when the seminiferous tubules have been severely damaged; examples include Klinefelter syndrome and YCMD.

In contrast, some azoospermic conditions, such as in those with obstruction, may have sperm that can be extracted from the seminiferous tubules of the testes. If mature sperm are obtained, they can be cryo-preserved or used immediately to fertilize oocytes through IVF. Even in cases with primary testicular failure, such as Klinefelter syndrome, sperm retrieval techniques can be employed along with ICSI [38]. There are important genetic ramifications for these procedures [39].

Specific endocrine treatment is available for men whose infertility results from hypogonadotropic hypogonadism, that is, from a pituitary/hypothalamic abnormality in which the pituitary gland does not properly release gonadotropic hormones that stimulate the testes. If hypogonadotropic hypogonadism results from hyperprolactinemia (elevated prolactin levels), the hypogonadism can often be corrected and fertility can be restored by lowering the serum prolactin concentration. If the hyperprolactinemia results from a medication, that medication should be discontinued. If the hyperprolactinemia results from a pituitary tumor identified by magnetic resonance imaging, the adenoma can be treated with a dopamine agonist, such as cabergoline or bromocriptine. Resumption of normal spermatogenesis usually does not occur for at least 3 to 6 months.

In some patients who have a large pituitary tumor (macroadenoma), the hypogonadotropic hypogonadism appears to be the result of permanent damage to the gonadotroph cells by the mass effect of the adenoma. Lowering the serum prolactin concentration and reducing the tumor in this setting may not be sufficient to increase the testosterone concentration and sperm count. Thus, if the serum testosterone concentration does not increase to normal within 6 months of the serum prolactin being reduced to normal, gonadotropin treatment may be considered.

Removal of Gonadotoxic Agents

A wide range of chemical substances can affect sperm quality or quantity, including medications. The medications listed below are not exhaustive, but are commonly associated with male infertility and should be avoided:

- Anabolic steroids
- Anti-androgens (e.g., nilutamide, bicalutamide, flutamide)
- Antihypertensives (e.g., spironolactone)
- Allopurinol
- Chemotherapeutic agents (e.g., cyclophosphamide)
- Colchicine
- Cyclosporine
- Dilantin
- Antibiotics (e.g., gentamycin, nitrofurantoin, erythromycin, tetracycline)
- Opiates
- Anti-psychotics

Radiation

Testes directly exposed to ionizing radiation suffer germ cell loss and Leydig cell dysfunction. The chances of having future offspring are lessened by radiation doses to the testes of 7.5 Gy and above. Injury to the testis may occur even if not directly irradiated.

Treatment with Human Chorionic Gonadotropin and Human Menopausal Gonadotropin

Men who have hypogonadotropic hypogonadism owing to hypothalamic disease can be treated with gonadotropin-releasing hormone (GnRH). Treatment is initiated with human chorionic gonadotropin (hCG), 1500 to 2000 IU three times per week subcutaneously or intramuscularly for at least 6 months. hCG has the biologic activity of LH. The hCG dose is adjusted upward according to symptoms of hypogonadism, serum testosterone concentrations, and semen parameters. Some patients with acquired hypogonadotropic states can be stimulated with hCG alone to produce sufficient sperm. If after 6 months the patient remains azoospermic or severely oligospermic, then human menopausal gonadotropin or recombinant FSH may be added.

Pulsatile GnRH Treatment

Pulsatile subcutaneous or intravenous treatment with GnRH has also been successfully used to treat gonadotropin-deficient patients [39]. GnRH has to be delivered in pulses using a portable pump with an attached catheter and needle for many months or years; most patients find it inconvenient to use GnRH therapy for so long.

Treatment of Genital Infections

Infertile men rarely present with symptoms or signs of acute genital infections or prostatitis, but they are sometimes diagnosed as having infections of the urogenital tract by the presence of increased leukocytes in the semen. Unfortunately, specific organisms are rarely identified. It is unclear if the leukospermia plays a pathogenic role in the infertility. The presence of leukocytes may decrease sperm functional capacity by the release of ROS. Semen cultures should be obtained when there are more than 1 million leukocytes in the semen; however, the yield is usually poor and nondiagnostic [40].

Despite the absence of symptoms, patients who have leukospermia even if the culture is negative are treated with at least a 10-day course of antibiotics such as doxycycline or a quinolone. A second course of therapy is usually given if leukocytes persist in the semen after antibiotics. However, poor results make it difficult to demonstrate a cause-and-effect relationship between genital infections and male infertility. Exceptions are patients with a past history of gonorrhea, tuberculosis, and other specific sexually transmitted diseases, which lead to genital tract obstruction at the epididymis or vas deferens [41].

Treatment of Anti-Sperm Antibodies

The presence of sperm antibodies can be detected on the sperm surface or in the seminal fluid by the immunobead test or mixed antiglobulin reaction. Glucocorticoids have been used in such patients. Continuous or intermittent high doses of prednisone for up to 6 months have been shown in placebo-controlled trials to improve pregnancy significantly [42]. However, there are adverse effects of high-dose corticosteroid therapy including aseptic necrosis of the femoral head. As a result, most couples attempt an ART, such as ICSI.

Retrograde Ejaculation

Retrograde ejaculation (sperm backing up into the bladder) occurs in neurological conditions such as urogenital tract surgery, sympathetic denervation, and diabetes. IUI can be performed using semen collected after alkalinization of the urine and extensive washing of the sperm. The washed sperm can also be used for IVF or ICSI procedures. Concurrent use of alpha agonists, such as pseudoephedrine (Sudafed) beginning 1 week before producing a sample, may be helpful in closing the bladder neck and, more occasionally, converting retrograde ejaculation to antegrade ejaculation.

Varicocele

Varicoceles are dilated veins of the scrotum that are commonly associated with diminished semen parameters. They are thought to have deleterious effects by increasing the temperature of the scrotum and potentially creating back pressure and toxins [43,44]. Although the presence of varicoceles can be associated with normal semen parameters and normal fertility, many men with varicoceles have abnormal semen parameters including low sperm concentration and motility and abnormal morphology. In a World Health Organization (WHO) study of more than 9000 men who were partners in an infertile couple, a varicocele was much more common in men with abnormal semen (25.4% vs. 11.7% with normal semen) [45]. When patients are carefully screened, and the goals as well as the time frame to achieve pregnancy are clearly determined, varicocele repair may significantly improve semen parameters and thereby improve the success of conceiving naturally or with assisted reproduction.

Atrophic testes, elevated serum FSH levels, and severe oligospermia or azoospermia indicate severe damage and are associated with a diminished likelihood of fertility after varicocele repair. A subinguinal approach has been shown to be effective treatment with low chance of adverse events. In some centers, laparoscopic varicocelectomy or vascular catheter embolization of spermatic veins is utilized [46]. An alternative to varicocele ligation or embolization is an ART. Subfertile men with varicoceles should be offered repair with the understanding that it may take anywhere from 3 to 12 months before there may be an improvement in semen parameters. Furthermore, couples may still require IUI or IVF in the future, depending on a variety of cofactors.

Obstructive Azoospermia

Obstructive azoospermia is determined by finding testes of normal size, normal serum FSH concentration, and absent sperm in the ejaculate. Both surgery and assisted reproduction techniques may be beneficial in such patients. As an example, obstruction of the epididymis or ejaculatory duct can be treated surgically. Azoospermia owing to obstruction in the epididymis can be treated by surgical end-to-end anastomosis of the epididymal duct to the vas deferens. These procedures may lead to the presence of ejaculated sperm, but the results are variable and depend on the site of connection (reanastomosis), the skill of the surgeon, and the duration of obstruction. Patients should have the opportunity for sperm extraction and cryopreservation at the time of the reversal in the event they wish to proceed immediately with assisted reproduction, or in the event of reversal failure and obstruction.

The results are best when obstructive azoospermia is attributed to a vasectomy [47]. The appearance of sperm after a vasectomy reversal can be over 85% resulting in pregnancy in over 50% of males and their partners. The success rate depends in part on the duration between vasectomy and the reversal procedure (Table 11.3). In general, the more time that has elapsed after a vasectomy, the poorer the pregnancy rates with reversal [48].

Ejaculatory duct obstruction presents with decreased semen volume and azoospermia or severe oligo/asthenospermia. TRUS demonstrates dilated seminal vesicles, and aspiration of the seminal vesicles shows spermatozoa, suggesting obstruction. This condition may be treated by transurethral resection

TABLE 11.3

Patency and Pregnancy Rates for Vasectomy Reversals as a Function of Time

Time Since Vasectomy	Patency Rate (Sperm Returning to the Semen)	Pregnancy Rate
<3 years	97%	76%
3–8 years	88%	53%
9–14 years	79%	44%
>15 years	71%	30%

(opening via the urethra) of the ejaculatory ducts with resulting improved semen quality and pregnancy in the partner [49,50].

ARTs can be combined to use sperm from men who have obstructive azoospermia to fertilize ova of their partners and achieve pregnancy. Sperm obtained by microsurgical aspiration from the epididymis (MESA) or from the testes by biopsy or fine needle aspiration can be used with eggs aspirated from the female partner for IVF or ICSI [51]. The fertilization rate of microsurgical sperm aspiration along with ICSI, despite epididymal or testicular sperm of low quality, is approximately 50%, and the pregnancy rate is about 40% per cycle and 20% per microsurgical aspiration [52].

For obstruction attributed to other epididymal lesions, or absent vas deferens, the results of surgical anastomosis are not as effective as those with aspiration and ICSI. Given the continuous improvements in sperm retrieval and ICSI techniques, surgical reversal versus ART must be discussed before an informed decision can be made [53].

Testicular Microdissection

New surgical techniques have been introduced to extract sperm from patients with NOA. A technique called microdissection of the testis to extract sperm (microTESE) from the seminiferous tubules has been successful in obtaining sperm in more than 50% of patients with nonobstructive azoospermia, including patients with Klinefelter syndrome [54–56]. Despite the chromosomal imbalance, the chance of transmission to an offspring is low.

Empirical Therapy

Many treatments have been used empirically for male infertility, including clomiphene citrate and other hormones as well as vitamins [57]. However, when placebo-controlled prospective clinical trials have been performed with adequate numbers of subjects in randomized placebo-controlled trials, none of these methods (including clomiphene citrate and human recombinant FSH) has been proven effective in oligospermia or azoospermia of unknown etiology. Some data suggest that aromatase inhibitors (e.g., anastrozole) may improve sperm concentrations in men with severe oligospermia or azoospermia before sperm retrieval for ICSI [58].

Another recommendation often made to infertile men is to wear boxer undershorts instead of jockey style and not to take hot showers or baths. The rationale is that increased scrotal temperature may impair sperm production. However, a 12-month study of men who wore tight athletic supporters found a slight increase in scrotal temperature but no change in semen quality. The wearing of ordinary brief underwear had no effect on scrotal temperature compared to boxer-style underwear [59]. Similarly, no change in semen parameters were found in men taking frequent saunas or hot baths.

Assisted Reproductive Techniques

ARTs are commonly used for the treatment of the female partner of men with severe oligospermia and azoospermia. IUI consists of washing an ejaculated semen specimen to remove prostaglandins, concentrating the sperm in a small volume of culture media, and injecting the sperm suspension directly into the upper uterine cavity using a small catheter through the cervix. The insemination is timed to take place just before ovulation. In couples with mild male infertility, IUI improves pregnancy rates when compared to intracervical insemination or timed natural cycles. However, in cases of moderate to severe oligospermia, IUI treatments are rarely successful [60].

IVF with ICSI

ICSI has revolutionized treatment and improved the prognosis for infertile men with severe oligospermia, asthenospermia (low sperm motility), teratospermia (a higher rate of abnormal sperm morphology), and even azoospermia. This technique involves the direct injection of a single sperm into the cytoplasm of a human oocyte, usually obtained from follicles produced under controlled ovarian hyperstimulation. This technique has also been successful in some men with Klinefelter syndrome where sperm are obtained from testicular biopsies [61,62]. The overall fertilization rate is approximately 60% and the clinical pregnancy rate per cycle is about 20% while the multiple pregnancy rate is about 29% to 38%. The ICSI results are not influenced by either the cause of the azoospermia or the origin of the spermatozoa.

When there are no sperm in the ejaculate but there are sperm-producing cells (Sertoli cells) in the testes, ICSI can be performed with sperm isolated from testicular extraction [63,64]. Success is dependent on retrieving adequate numbers of sperm. Successful pregnancy can occur using injection of fresh or cryopreserved (frozen) sperm, but not with spermatocytes (immature sperm). Extracted testicular sperm may fertilize oocytes even in azoospermic men with maturation arrest, defective spermatogenesis, Klinefelter syndrome, and long-standing azoospermia after chemotherapy [65–69].

The ability of sperm from men with severe sperm abnormality and genetic disorders to fertilize human oocytes raises the issue of chromosomal abnormalities and congenital malformations in pregnancies from ICSI.

Artificial Insemination with Donor Semen

The alternative to ART for many couples is artificial insemination with donor sperm. This method has a very high success rate in otherwise normal females with close to 50% pregnancy rate within six cycles of insemination.

Conclusion

It is important to realize that infertility is often secondary to a male factor. In the past, men with infertility had relatively few options for treatment. In this era, however, it is often possible to determine the etiology of male subfertility and provide treatment options that offer help to many couples. Men with abnormal semen parameters or other known infertility risks factors should have a urological evaluation.

REFERENCES

1. Thonneau P, Marchand S, Tallec A et al. Incidence and main causes of infertility in a resident population (1,850,000) of three French regions (1988–1989). *Hum Reprod* 1991;6:811–6.
2. Honig SC, Lipshultz LI, Jarow J. Significant medical pathology uncovered by a comprehensive male infertility evaluation. *Fertil Steril* 1994;62:1028–34.
3. Guzick DS, Overstreet JW, Factor-Litvak P et al. Sperm morphology, motility, and concentration in fertile and infertile men. *N Engl J Med* 2001;345:1388–93.
4. Kruger TF, Acosta AA, Simmons KF et al. Predictive value of abnormal sperm morphology in in vitro fertilization. *Fertil Steril* 1988;49:112–7.

5. Menkveld R, Stander FS, Kotze TJ et al. The evaluation of morphological characteristics of human spermatozoa according to stricter criteria. *Hum Reprod* 1990;5:586–92.
6. WHO laboratory manual for the examination of human semen and sperm—Cervical mucus interaction; Cambridge University Press, 2010.
7. Pisarska MD, Casson PR, Cisneros PL et al. Fertilization after standard in vitro fertilization versus intracytoplasmic sperm injection in subfertile males using sibling oocytes. *Fertil Steril* 1999;71:627–32.
8. Carter SS, Shinohara K, Lipshultz LI. Transrectal ultrasonography in disorders of the seminal vesicles and ejaculatory ducts. *Urol Clin North Am* 1989;6:773–90.
9. Jarow JP. Transrectal ultrasonography of infertile men. *Fertil Steril* 1993;60:1035–9.
10. Coetzee K, Kruge TF, Lombard CJ. Predictive value of normal sperm morphology: A structured literature review. *Hum Reprod Update* 1998;4:73–82.
11. Keegan BR, Barton S, Sanchez X et al. Isolated teratozoospermia does not affect in vitro fertilization outcome and is not an indication for intracytoplasmic sperm injection. *Fertil Steril* 2007;88:1583–8.
12. Van Waart J, Kruger TF, Lombard CJ et al. Predictive value of normal sperm morphology in intrauterine insemination (IUI): A structured literature review. *Hum Reprod Update* 2001;7:495–500.
13. Spiessens C, Vanderschueren D, Meuleman C et al. Isolated teratozoospermia and intrauterine insemination. *Fertil Steril* 2003;80:1185–9.
14. Shibahara H, Obara H, Ayustawati et al. Prediction of pregnancy by intrauterine insemination using CASA estimates and strict criteria in patients with male factor infertility. *Int J Androl* 2004;27:63–8.
15. Gunalp S, Onculoglu C, Gurgan T et al. A study of semen parameters with emphasis on sperm morphology in a fertile population: An attempt to develop clinical thresholds. *Hum Reprod* 2001;16:110–4.
16. Evenson DP, Jost LK, Marshall D et al. Utility of the sperm chromatin structure assay as a diagnostic and prognostic tool in the human fertility clinic. *Hum Reprod* 1999;14:1039–49.
17. Spano M, Bonde JP, Hjollund HI et al. Sperm chromatin damage impairs human fertility. The Danish First Pregnancy Planner Study Team. *Fertil Steril* 2000;73:43–50.
18. Evenson DP, Wixon R. Data analysis of two in vivo fertility studies using Sperm Chromatin Structure Assay-derived DNA fragmentation index vs. pregnancy outcome. *Fertil Steril* 2008;90:1229–31.
19. Bungum M, Humaidan P, Axmon A et al. Sperm DNA integrity assessment in prediction of assisted reproduction technology outcome. *Hum Reprod* 2007;22:174–9.
20. Collins JA, Barnhart KT, Schlegel PN. Do sperm DNA integrity tests predict pregnancy with in vitro fertilization? *Fertil Steril* 2008;89:823–31.
21. Zini A, Sigman M. Are tests of sperm DNA damage clinically useful? Pros and cons. *J Androl* 2009;30:219–29.
22. Zini A, Boman JM, Belzile E et al. Sperm DNA damage is associated with an increased risk of pregnancy loss after IVF and ICSI: Systematic review and meta-analysis. *Hum Reprod* 2008;23:2663–8.
23. Sakkas D, Alvarez JG. Sperm DNA fragmentation: Mechanisms of origin, impact on reproductive outcome, and analysis. *Fertil Steril* 2010 Mar 1;93(4):1027–36.
24. Wolff H, Anderson DJ. Immunohistologic characterization and quantitation of leukocyte subpopulations in human semen. *Fertil Steril* 1988;49:497–504.
25. Ayvaliotis B, Bronson R, Rosenfeld D et al. Conception rates in couples where autoimmunity to sperm is detected. *Fertil Steril* 1985;43:739–42.
26. Oei SG, Helmerhorst FM, Bloemenkamp KM et al. Effectiveness of the postcoital test: Randomised controlled trial. *BMJ* 1998;317:502–5.
27. Liu de Y, Liu ML, Garrett C et al. Comparison of the frequency of defective sperm–zona pellucida (ZP) binding and the ZP-induced acrosome reaction between subfertile men with normal and abnormal semen. *Hum Reprod* 2007;22:1878–84.
28. Anguiano A, Oates RD, Amos JA et al. Congenital bilateral absence of the vas deferens. A primarily genital form of cystic fibrosis. *JAMA* 1992;267:1794–7.
29. Chillon M, Casals T, Mercier B et al. Mutations in the cystic fibrosis gene in patients with congenital absence of the vas deferens. *New Engl J Med* 1995;332:1475–80.
30. Hall S, Oates RD. Unilateral absence of the scrotal vas deferens associated with contralateral mesonephric duct anomalies resulting in infertility: Laboratory, physical and radiographic findings, and therapeutic alternatives. *J Urol* 1993;150:1161–4.
31. Castellani C, Bonizzato A, Pradal U et al. Evidence of mild respiratory disease in men with congenital absence of the vas deferens. *Respir Med* 1999;93:869–75.

32. Gilljam M, Moltyaner Y, Downey GP et al. Airway inflammation and infection in congenital absence of the vas deferens. *Am J Respir Crit Care Med* 2004;169:174–9.

33. Schlegel PN, Shin D, Goldstein M. Urogenital anomalies in men with congenital absence of the vas deferens. *J Urol* 1996;155:1644–8.

34. Reijo R, Alagappan RK, Patrizio P et al. Severe oligozoospermia resulting from deletions of azoospermia factor gene on Y chromosome. *Lancet* 1996;347:1290–3.

35. Silber SJ, Repping S. Transmission of male infertility to future generations: Lessons from the Y chromosome. *Hum Reprod Update* 2002;8:217–29.

36. Foresta C, Moro E, Ferlin A. Y chromosome microdeletions and alterations of spermatogenesis. *Endocr Rev* 2001;22:226–39.

37. Schiff JD, Palermo GD, Veeck LL et al. Success of testicular sperm extraction and intracytoplasmic sperm injection in men with Klinefelter syndrome. *J Clin Endocrinol Metab* 2005;90:6263–7.

38. Lanfranco F, Kamischke A, Zitzmann M, Nieschlag E. Klinefelter's syndrome. *Lancet* 2004;364:273–83.

39. Crowley WF Jr, Filicori M, Spratt DI, Santoro NF. The physiology of gonadotropin-releasing hormone (GnRH) secretion in men and women. *Recent Prog Horm Res* 1985;41:473–531.

40. Hua VN, Schaeffer AJ. Acute and chronic prostatitis. *Med Clin North Am* 2004;88:483–94.

41. Bar-Chama N, Goluboff E, Fisch H. Infection and pyospermia in male infertility. Is it really a problem? *Urol Clin North Am* 1994;21:469–75.

42. Hendry WF, Hughes L, Scammell G et al. Comparison of prednisolone and placebo in subfertile men with antibodies to spermatozoa. *Lancet* 1990;335:85–8.

43. The influence of varicocele on parameters of fertility in a large group of men presenting to infertility clinics. World Health Organization. *Fertil Steril* 1992;57:1289–93.

44. Saypol DC, Howards SS, Turner TT, Miller ED Jr. Influence of surgically induced varicocele on testicular blood flow, temperature, and histology in adult rats and dogs. *J Clin Invest* 1981;68:39–45.

45. Mieusset R, Bujan L, Mondinat C et al. Association of scrotal hyperthermia with impaired spermatogenesis in infertile men. *Fertil Steril* 1987;48:1006–1011.

46. White RI. Radiologic management of varicoceles using embolotherapy. In: Whitehead ED, Nagler HM (eds.). *Management of Impotence and Infertility*. Philadelphia: JB Lippincott, 1994, p. 228.

47. Southwick GJ, Temple-Smith PD. Epididymal microsurgery: Current techniques and new horizons. *Microsurgery* 1988;9:266–77.

48. Belker AM, Thomas AJ Jr, Fuchs EF et al. Results of 1,469 microsurgical vasectomy reversals by the Vasovasostomy Study Group. *J Urol* 1991;145:505–11.

49. Meacham RB, Hellerstein DK, Lipshultz LI. Evaluation and treatment of ejaculatory duct obstruction in the infertile male. *Fertil Steril* 1993;59:393–7.

50. Jarow, JP. Transrectal ultrasonography in the diagnosis and management of ejaculatory duct obstruction. *J Androl* 1996;17:467–72.

51. Silber SJ, Ord T, Balmaceda J et al. Congenital absence of the vas deferens. The fertilizing capacity of human epididymal sperm. *N Engl J Med* 1990;323:1788–92.

52. Silber SJ, Devroey P, Tournaye H, Van Steirteghem AC. Fertilizing capacity of epididymal and testicular sperm using intracytoplasmic sperm injection (ICSI). *Reprod Fertil Dev* 1995;7:281–92.

53. Robb P, Sandlow JI. Cost-effectiveness of vasectomy reversal. *Urol Clin North Am* 2009;36:391–6.

54. Donoso P, Tournaye H, Devroey P. Which is the best sperm retrieval technique for non-obstructive azoospermia? A systematic review. *Hum Reprod Update* 2007;13:539–49.

55. Ramasamy R, Ricci JA, Palermo GD et al. Successful fertility treatment for Klinefelter's syndrome. *J Urol* 2009;182:1108–13.

56. Schlegel PN. Nonobstructive azoospermia: A revolutionary surgical approach and results. *Semin Reprod Med* 2009;27:165–70.

57. Schill WB. Survey of medical therapy in andrology. *Int J Androl* 1995;18 Suppl 2:56–62.

58. Kim HH, Schlegel PN. Endocrine manipulation in male infertility. *Urol Clin North Am* 2008;35:303–18.

59. Munkelwitz R, Gilbert BR. Are boxer shorts really better? A critical analysis of the role of underwear type in male subfertility. *J Urol* 1998;160:1329–33.

60. Van Voorhis BJ, Barnett M, Sparks AE, Syrop CH, Rosenthal G, Dawson J. Effect of the total motile sperm count on the efficacy and cost-effectiveness of intrauterine insemination and in vitro fertilization. *Fertil Steril* 2001 Apr;75(4):661–8.

61. Palermo GD, Schlegel PN, Sills ES et al. Births after intracytoplasmic injection of sperm obtained by testicular extraction from men with nonmosaic Klinefelter's syndrome. *N Engl J Med* 1998;338:588–90.

62. Reubinoff BE, Abeliovich D, Werner M et al. A birth in non-mosaic Klinefelter's syndrome after testicular fine needle aspiration, intracytoplasmic sperm injection and preimplantation genetic diagnosis. *Hum Reprod* 1998;13:1887–92.

63. Tournaye H, Camus M, Goossens A et al. Recent concepts in the management of infertility because of non-obstructive azoospermia. *Hum Reprod* 1995;10 Suppl 1:115–9.

64. Schlegel PN, Palermo GD, Goldstein M et al. Testicular sperm extraction with intracytoplasmic sperm injection for nonobstructive azoospermia. *Urology* 1997;49:435–40.

65. Silber SJ, van Steirteghem A, Nagy Z et al. Normal pregnancies resulting from testicular sperm extraction and intracytoplasmic sperm injection for azoospermia due to maturation arrest. *Fertil Steril* 1996;66:110–7.

66. Chen SU, Ho HN, Chen HF et al. Fertilization and embryo cleavage after intracytoplasmic spermatid injection in an obstructive azoospermic patient with defective spermiogenesis. *Fertil Steril* 1996;66:157–60.

67. Mulhall JP, Reijo R, Alagappan R et al. Azoospermic men with deletion of the DAZ gene cluster are capable of completing spermatogenesis: Fertilization, normal embryonic development and pregnancy occur when retrieved testicular spermatozoa are used for intracytoplasmic sperm injection. *Hum Reprod* 1997;12:503–8.

68. Tournaye H, Staessen C, Liebaers I et al. Testicular sperm recovery in nine 47,XXY Klinefelter patients. *Hum Reprod* 1996;11:1644–9.

69. Chan PT, Palermo GD, Veeck LL et al. Testicular sperm extraction combined with intracytoplasmic sperm injection in the treatment of men with persistent azoospermia postchemotherapy. *Cancer* 2001;92:1632–7.

12

Preimplantation Genetic Testing

Kim L. Thornton

Preimplantation genetic testing (PGT) includes preimplantation genetic screening (PGS) and preimplantation genetic diagnosis (PGD), which are techniques that provide testing of the embryos before their transfer into the uterus. PGS identifies those embryos with numerical chromosomal aberrations whereas PGD is a directed molecular diagnostic test for a particular gene of interest. In couples using PGT, accurate and reliable determination of single gene defects, chromosome structure, and chromosome number is used to guide embryo selection before transfer. For many, this is a far more desirable option than awaiting fetal diagnosis in the first or second trimester of pregnancy via chorionic villus sampling (CVS) or amniocentesis. While continuing to rapidly expand, PGS is being offered to many couples undergoing in vitro fertilization (IVF) but may be especially helpful for those who have had repeated IVF failure (RIF) or recurrent pregnancy loss (RPL), or for women of advanced maternal age.

Techniques

Embryo Biopsy

The technique of obtaining cellular material for genetic analysis has evolved such that a trophecto-derm (TE) biopsy taken from a blastocyst has been validated as the most appropriate technique to ensure that there is no negative impact on embryo viability or reproductive potential and that there is adequate cellular material to analyze to ensure that the results mirror the actual genetic composition of the embryo with the highest accuracy. Other methods of obtaining cellular material from the embryo include blastomere biopsy of day 3 cleavage stage embryos at the 6–10 cell stage. Polar body biopsy of the oocyte before the completion of fertilization is another technique that has been employed in the past.

TE Biopsy

TE biopsy at the blastocyst stage is performed on day 5 or 6 of development when the embryo is composed of 200–300 cells. The zona is typically penetrated, mechanically generating a fenestration through which 5–10 herniated TE cells are removed (Figure 12.1). The advantage of TE biopsy in contrast to removing a single cell from a day 3 embryo is that more DNA is available for analysis, which results in a more accurate and reliable genetic assessment. The more robust analysis has demonstrated that TE mosaicism is seen in only 3%–5% of blastocysts; thus, TE is more accurate in obtaining a true representation of the majority of cells that exist within a given embryo. Another advantage is that TE biopsy allows for only the most developmentally competent embryos to be tested and thus proves to be a more cost-effective approach as compared to biopsy of cleavage stage embryos. TE biopsy has been shown not to impact blastocyst reproductive potential as compared to blastomere biopsy, in which a 39% reduction in implantation rate has been reported. Blastocysts that undergo TE biopsy are then cryopreserved pending the genetic analysis and then transferred in a subsequent cycle.

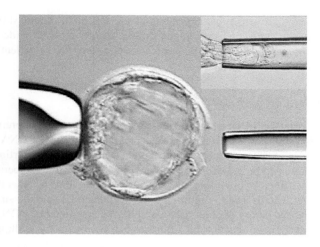

FIGURE 12.1 Performance of a trophectoderm biopsy. A pipette on the left holds the blastocyst in place. An opening has been created in the zona pellucida with a laser. A smaller pipette is used to take a biopsy of 8–10 cells, which is then submitted for testing.

Blastomere Biopsy

Blastomere biopsy of cleavage stage embryos is a much less commonly employed method to obtain genetic material for PGT because embryo viability has been shown to be compromised in embryos biopsied at the cellular stage. Blastomere biopsy is performed on day 3 of embryo development at the 6–10 cell stage when embryonic cells are totipotent and have not begun the process of compaction. One or two blastomeres, if less than 25% of total embryo cellular material, can be removed from the embryo. High error rates, noninformative biopsies, and embryo damage from biopsy highlight the importance of an experienced embryologist to produce reliable results. Removed blastomeres are subsequently analyzed for gene mutations or chromosomal abnormalities while the biopsied embryos continue to be observed in the laboratory. Once PGT results are available, normal embryos that have become blastocysts are selected for transfer on day 5. Not all blastomeres of a single embryo share identical chromosomal constitution, and this variance, termed mosaicism, poses an unavoidable limitation of blastomere analysis. Studies that have analyzed blastomeres from embryos at the cleavage stage with follow-up blastomere analysis at the blastocyst stage have confirmed that mosaicism may be present in upward of 50% of embryos and may contribute to an error rate of 5%. Laboratory expertise in embryo biopsy may also vary and no diagnosis results may occur in up to 10% of cells biopsied. These factors are a major limitation of blastomere biopsy.

Polar Body Biopsy

Polar body biopsy involves the removal of one or both of the polar bodies that are generated and extruded during the oocyte divisions that complete meiosis at ovulation and fertilization. Polar bodies may be safely removed after mechanical or chemical penetration of the zona pellucida surrounding the oocyte without disrupting the oocyte or embryo. Analysis of oocyte polar bodies strictly involves maternally derived genetic material, and therefore, paternally derived genetic or chromosomal abnormalities are not evaluated. In cases of maternally transmitted genetic disease or aneuploidy related to oocyte age, polar body PGD is 95%–98% accurate.

Genetic Analysis

Embryonic cellular material obtained via biopsy can be analyzed for specific gene sequences to diagnose single gene defects or for chromosomal enumeration to screen for aneuploidy or chromosomal structural abnormalities. For aneuploidy screening, the technology has evolved for all platforms to provide whole chromosome aneuploidy screening; depending on the specific technology, they can also identify large segmental deletions or duplications and mitochondrial copy number. Providers should have a clear understanding of the limitations of the particular technology to optimize patient's expectation of the potential clinical outcome.

Polymerase Chain Reaction

The polymerase chain reaction (PCR) technique provides the ability to screen preimplantation embryos for single gene defects with known mutation sequences. After extraction of DNA from biopsied cells, oligonucleotide primers specific for the gene region of interest are used as the starting point for DNA replication by a temperature-specific polymerase. Through repeated specific temperature cycles, selected gene regions are amplified, thereby providing sufficient DNA to determine whether the normal or mutated gene sequence is present. Challenges to optimizing this technique include the small initial amount of DNA available from embryo biopsy and the risk of amplifying contaminating DNA. Nested PCR technique or simultaneous PCR amplification of different gene fragments by multiplex PCR or qPCR is routinely used to enhance the reliability in this setting, allowing comparisons across the genome. Whole genome amplification by PCR can also be employed for analysis by comparative genomic hybridization (CGH) or single nucleotide polymorphism (SNP) microarrays but can be especially sensitive to the same challenges of small starting genetic material and risk of contamination. In some cases, Y chromosome amplification may not have as high fidelity as with other chromosomes and more stringent PCR conditions are necessary for accurate results. Allele dropout and partial amplification can lead to misdiagnosis and are major limitations of any PCR-based molecular technique.

Array Comparative Genomic Hybridization

Array comparative genomic hybridization (aCGH) is a technique that allows simultaneous and complete enumeration of chromosomes from a single biopsied cell without cellular fixation. With aCGH, labeled DNA from both test and normal DNA samples are hybridized to a DNA microarray that includes approximately 4000 markers spaced throughout the entire genome. aCGH does not directly visualize chromosomes but determines the relative copy number of chromosome between the test DNA and a control normal DNA after concurrent PCR amplification (Figure 12.2). The technique is capable of screening biopsied cells for chromosome copy number (aneuploidy) and unbalanced chromosome translocations. aCGH can also be used for diagnosis of some translocations, inversions, and other chromosome abnormalities where there is a gain or loss of chromatin. Depending on the size of probes used (bacterial artificial chromosome or oligonucleotide), some clinically important microdeletion or microduplication disorders may also be detected. It will not differentiate balanced translocations unless there are subtle differences in DNA copy numbers that occasionally occur in these and other chromosomal structural rearrangements such as inversions. aCGH will also not differentiate whole genome ploidy states such as polyploidy (e.g., 69,XX) or monoploidy (23,X) as there is equal representation of all chromosomes. It is also unable to detect uniparental disomy. This technique has limited ability to identify mosaicisms only if the platform has been previously validated against a mosaic cell sample. aCGH platforms are able to amplify DNA and complete the analysis in 12–15 hours, thus lending itself to fresh or frozen transfers.

SNP Microarray

SNPs are highly conserved variations at a single site in the DNA that exist in a frequency greater than 1% within a population. There are more than 40 million SNPs in the human genome that have been validated, making it a highly sensitive and specific genotyping marker for diagnosis. The microarray consists of a chip containing nucleotide acid sequences complementary to each SNP region of interest (density coverage may range from 600,000 to 2 million SNPs depending on the chip). The sample DNA obtained from PGD is amplified and hybridized to the chip. The hybridization signal detected can simultaneously provide information on DNA copy number important for aneuploidy screening and detection of clinically significant microdeletion and microduplications as well as determine parental origin,

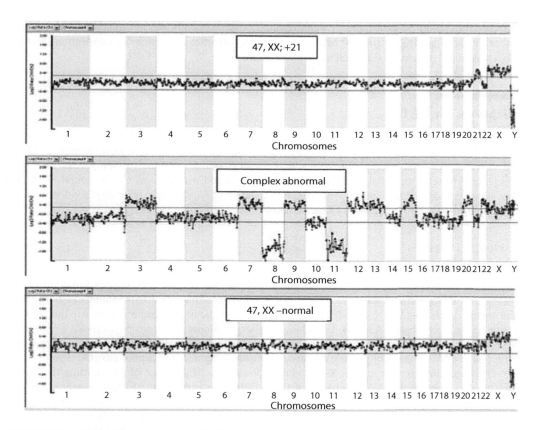

FIGURE 12.2 CGH results performed on biopsies taken from a day 3 embryo. (Courtesy of Dr. Mark Hughes, Genesis Genetics, Detroit, Michigan.)

presence of uniparental disomy, and loss of heterozygosity. It is a powerful molecular tool but with some limitations, specifically the inability to identify balanced translocations, whole genome polyploidy, and the fact that there may be many de novo structural chromosomal abnormalities that are below the resolution of the SNP array. Important to note again is that sensitivity of the assay, especially to detect low-level mosaicism, is variable, with the most experienced laboratories reporting a threshold detection of 10% mosaicism. SNP arrays take 30–40 hours to complete the analysis, thus lending itself only to frozen embryo transfers.

Next-Generation Sequencing

Next-generation sequencing (NGS) is a technology that uses optimized, high-throughput DNA amplification to sequence DNA. The process involves fragmenting DNA into millions of small fragments that are then fused with an adaptor and a barcode to create a DNA library. The library is then loaded into a flow cell where the fragments bind to a surface of complementary surface-bound oligonucleotides and then amplified to create distinct clonal clusters. High-throughput, paired-end reversible terminator-based sequencing of the fragments detects single bases as they are incorporated into the DNA template strands, reducing sequencing errors. Paired-end sequencing produces twice the number of reads that occur and the paired sequences are aligned as read pairs, further reducing the likelihood of errors in sequencing. The amplified fragments are aligned to a reference genome to detect differences between the fragment and the reference. The attachment of the barcode allows for multiple libraries to be run simultaneously and then sorted before final analysis. Advances in NGS have reduced time for library preparation and time for sequencing. The ability to multiplex allows for scalable instrumentation depending on the anticipated utilization. NGS will detect whole chromosome aneuploidy, mosaicism, triploidy, large deletions, or duplications greater than 50 Mb, some clinically significant deletions or duplications 800 b to 1 Mb, uniparental disomy, and mitochondrial copy number.

Indications for PGD

As the technology for PGD advances, the indications for genetic evaluation of embryos before transfer are expanding. At present, PGD is routinely used for couples affected by or carrying alleles for known sex-linked diseases or autosomal single gene defects. PGS is also commonly employed for patients at increased risk of chromosomal aneuploidy owing to advanced ovarian age, chromosomal rearrangements, repeated implantation failure with IVF, RPL, and severe male factor infertility. Evidence to support the routine use of PGS for many of these indications is still controversial.

Sex-Linked Diseases

Since the original reports of successful PGD pregnancies in 1990, the technology has been widely used to screen embryos at risk for sex-linked disorders. For patients with or carrying sex-linked disorders, knowledge of the specific genetic mutation is not required as carrier or disease status can be deduced based on sex determination. X-linked recessive disorders are the most common of the sex-linked disorders and include hemophilia A and B, Duchenne and Becker's muscular dystrophy, adrenal leukodystrophy, X-linked ichthyosis, and Lesch–Nyhan syndrome among others. Fathers affected by a sex-linked disorder have a 50% chance of passing on carrier status to daughters but cannot pass the disorder on to male offspring. Mothers carrying an X-linked disorder have a 50% chance of transmitting the disease state to male offspring and a 50% chance of transmitting the carrier state to female offspring. With the exception of Fragile X syndrome, which occurs 1 in 3600 males and 1 in 4000 to 6000 females, X-linked dominant disorders are less common. Here, affected mothers have a 50% chance of passing the disease onto their offspring, whereas affected fathers can only pass the disease state to female offspring. Inheritance counseling in FMR1-related disorders such as Fragile X syndrome is particularly unique because less than 1% of cases are attributed to deletions, missense mutations, or RNA splicing defects and follow the X-linked dominant inheritance patterns. The rest of Fragile X syndrome cases are attributed to full expansions (greater than 200) of CGG trinucleotide repeats inherited from a parent with the premutation (55 to 200 repeats). Expansion only occurs through inheritance of the affected maternal allele, i.e., all mothers of affected individuals are premutation carriers. These women are at risk of having a child with the full mutation but they are also at increased risk of developing premature ovarian failure and fragile X-associated tremor/ataxia syndrome. Male premutation carriers can only transmit the premutation to their offspring, but all children will be carriers.

There are even fewer Y-linked disorders, but they are especially significant in reproduction because they often involve male infertility. Preimplantation genetic diagnosis offers an option for these couples carrying sex chromosome–linked conditions to determine the embryo sex and transfer sex-selected embryos to avoid disease or carrier status in their children. Sex determination of biopsied embryos can be performed with PCR, aCGH, or NGS with excellent accuracy estimated at approximately 99%.

Single Gene Defects

With the completion of the Human Genome Project, the sequence information for single gene disorders has rapidly expanded, allowing the application of PGD to detect disease or carrier status in embryos. Autosomal recessive disorders are more common and many have been successfully screened by PGD including cystic fibrosis, Tay–Sachs disease, sickle cell anemia, β thalassemia, spinal muscular atrophy, and familial dysautonomia. Autosomal dominant disorders for which PGD has been applied include Huntington's disease, neurofibromatosis, retinitis pigmentosa, Marfan's syndrome, and familial adenomatous polyposis coli. Among the challenges of preimplantation diagnosis of monogenic diseases is the ability to screen for the various mutations leading to disease. For example, cystic fibrosis can be caused by more than 1000 known mutations in the cystic fibrosis transmembrane conductance regulator (CFTR) gene, of which 25 are routinely tested. With known sequence and mutation data, fluorescent and multiplex PCR can provide accurate diagnostic screening of biopsied embryo cells with an error rate of less than 5% (Table 12.1). Despite the applicability of PGD for single gene defects, it is still the standard of care to test parents for carrier status using conventional techniques and testing for that specific mutation in the offspring.

Aneuploidy

Even in the best prognosis patients, pregnancy success per cycle of IVF is, at best, 40%–50% and the chance of miscarriage is 15%–20%. The overwhelming majority of failed implantations and pregnancy loss is attributed to chromosomal nondisjunction resulting in nonviable aneuploid embryos. In part, because human oocytes are arrested in meiosis for the duration of a woman's life until the time of conception, it is believed that the chromosomal spindle apparatus and the chiasmata adhering paired chromosomes are particularly vulnerable to damage accumulating with age. Oocyte aneuploidy is therefore perhaps the greatest limitation of human reproduction and at present there are no potential methods to prevent or reverse this phenomenon. Unfortunately, the current grading of embryos by morphological analysis does not correlate with chromosomal status, and neither this, nor any other noninvasive method, can accurately predict euploid or aneuploid status in early embryos. PGS for chromosomal enumeration using currently accepted technologies is therefore a valuable technology to select chromosomally normal embryos before transfer.

While polar body biopsy evaluates only the maternal chromosomal contribution to the embryo, it is estimated that 90% of aneuploidy in embryos is maternal in origin and therefore polar body analysis can be used as a reliable approach. However, PGS of TE biopsies is favored by most fertility centers as both the paternal and maternal contribution is assessed. The current common indications for PGS include advanced maternal age, RIF, and RPL; however, a consensus regarding the attributable benefit of this screening in each of these conditions has not yet been established. Historically, large randomized controlled trials aimed at determining whether PGS by fluorescent in situ hybridization (FISH) could improve live birth rates have overall shown increased pregnancy rates but no change in live birth rates. Because of this, the European Society of Human Reproduction and Embryology (ESHRE) had established guidelines for the responsible use of PGS: (1) PGS may have more potential benefit for those of advanced maternal age greater than 37 years old, (2) PGS should only be performed if there are at least six embryos of normal morphology, (3) only highly experienced embryologists should perform the biopsies, and (4) limitations of FISH and availability of 24 chromosome screening made CGH or SNP microarrays the more desirable molecular approach. The Practice Committee of the American Society for Reproductive Medicine (ASRM) concluded after extensive review of the available literature in 2008 that there was insufficient evidence to advocate PGS by conventional FISH technology to improve live birth rates in women of advanced maternal age. Recently, there have been several randomized trials where 24 chromosomes screening after TE biopsy and fresh or frozen embryo transfer was compared to traditional IVF. Results demonstrate a significantly higher implantation rate with fresh and frozen embryo transfer as compared to assessment by morphology alone. Pregnancy rates and delivery rates were also improved compared to morphologic assessment alone. These studies were performed in good prognosis patients and may not be generalizable to all patients. However, the data regarding aneuploidy screening is promising when considering the goal to transition to elective single embryo transfer in clinical practice.

Advanced Maternal Age

As aneuploidy increases with maternal age, aneuploidy screening by PGS is an option for women of advanced reproductive age, generally considered to be 35 years and older. The original retrospective studies examining the effect of PGS on aneuploidy screening demonstrated a significant increase in

TABLE 12.1

Most Common Genetic Disorders Evaluated by PGD

Achondroplasia (FGFR3)

Adrenoleukodystrophy (ABCD1)

Agammaglobulinemia-Bruton (TyrsKnse)

Alpha thalassemia (HBA1)

Alpha-antitrypsin (AAT)

Alport syndrome (COL4A5)

Alzheimer's disease (very early onset-PSEN1)

Beta thalassemia (HBB)

Bloom syndrome (Blm)

Canavan disease (ASPA)

Charcot–Marie–Tooth neuropathy—2E

Charcot–Marie–Tooth neuropathy—1B

Choroideremia (CHM)

Chronic granulomatous disease (CYBB)

Citrullinemia (ASS)

Cleidocranial dysplasia (RUNX2)

Congenital adrenal hyperplasia (CYP31A2)

Congenital erythropoietic porphyria (UROS)

Crigler–Najjar syndrome (UGT1A1)

Cystic fibrosis (CFTR)

Darier disease (ATP2A2)

Diamond–Blackfan anemia (DBA-RSP19)

Diamond–Blackfan anemia (DBA2)

Duchenne muscular dystrophy (DMD)

Dystrophia myotonica (DMPK)

Emery–Dreifuss muscular dystrophy (EDMD1,2,4)

Epidermolytic hyperkeratosis (KRT10) factor

13 Deficiency (F13A1)

Familial adenomatous polyposis (APC)

Familial dysautonomia (IKBKAP)

Fanconi anemia A (FANCA)

Fanconi anemia C (FANCC)

Fanconi anemia F (FANCF)

Fanconia anemia G (FANCG)

Fragile X syndrome (FMR1)

Friedreich ataxia I (FRDA)

Gaucher disease (GBA)

Glutaric acidemia type 1 (GCDH)

Hemophilia A (F8)

Hemophilia B (F9)

HLA DR beta1 class II MHC (HLA DRB1*)

HLA-A class I MHC (HGNC HLA-A)

Hunter syndrome (IDS)

Huntington's disease (HD)

Hurler syndrome (MPSI-IDUA)

Hyper IgM (CD40-ligand; TNFSF5)

Hypophosphatasia (ALPL)

Incontinentia pigmenti (KBKG-NEMO)

Kennedy's disease (AR)

(Continued)

TABLE 12.1 (CONTINUED)

Most Common Genetic Disorders Evaluated by PGD

Krabbe disease (GALC)

Lesch–Nyhan syndrome (HPRT1)

Leukemia, acute lymphocytic (for HLA)

Leukemia, acute myelogenous (for HLA)

Leukemia, chronic myelogenous (for HLA)

Leukocyte adhesion deficiency (ITGB2)

Li–Fraumeni syndrome (TP53)

Lymphoproliferative disorder (X-linked)

Marfan syndrome (FBN1)

Menkes disease (ATP7A)

Metachromatic leukodystrophy (ARSA)

Mucolipidosis 2 (I-Cell)

Neurofibromatosis (NF1 and NF2)

Niemann–Pick disease type C (NPC1)

Ornithine transcarbamylase deficiency (OTC)

Osteogenesis imperfecta (COL1A1)

Pachyonychia congenita (KRT16 and KRT6A)

Periventricular heterotopia (PH)

Polycystic kidney disease, autosomal recessive (AR-PKD1)

Retinoblastoma 1 (RB1)

Rhesus blood group D (RHD)

Rhizomelic chondrodysplasia punctata (RCDP1)

Sacral agenesis (HLXB9)

Sanfilippo A disease (MPSIIIA)

SCID-X1 (severe combined immunodeficiency disease) (IL2RG)

Sexing for X-linked disease (AMELX/Y; ZFX/Y)

Shwachman–Diamond syndrome (SBDS)

Sickle cell anemia (HBB)

Smith–Lemli–Opitz syndrome (SLOS)

Spinal muscular atrophy (SMN1)

Spinocerebellar ataxia 3 (SCA3)

Spinocerebellar ataxia 2 (SCA2)

Tay–Sachs disease (HEXA)

Treacher Collins syndrome (TOCF1)

Tuberous sclerosis 1 (TSC1)

Wiskott–Aldrich syndrome (WAS)

implantation rate and decreased miscarriage rate. Randomized controlled and multicenter trials in the United States have been criticized by their insufficient power and confounding variables such as the type of biopsy technique, number of blastomeres removed, day of transfer, and low overall implantation rates. The largest and most strictly designed study examining the impact of PGS aneuploidy screening is a randomized controlled trial based in Belgium that failed to demonstrate a statistically significant difference in implantation, ongoing pregnancies, or pregnancy losses in 148 PGS subjects and 141 control subjects undergoing blastocyst transfer without PGS. Significantly fewer embryos were transferred in the PGS group and, though not statistically significant, the twin gestation rate was lower in the PGS group. In a recent retrospective review of TE biopsies, aneuploidy risk was evident with increasing female age. Another recent retrospective study comparing implantation rates in embryos screened for ploidy using TE biopsy versus unscreened embryos demonstrated that frozen euploid embryo transfer implantation rates were significantly greater than implantation rates of unscreened fresh or frozen embryo transfers. Increased implantation rates with enhanced embryo screening with

PGS in women with advanced maternal age encourages elective single embryo transfer, reducing the risk for multiple gestation. However, decreased number of available embryos in women of advanced age may limit the available of embryos to screen. While further data examining the clinical impact of PGS aneuploidy screening in this population is forthcoming, couples may find the added assurance of embryo chromosomal status invaluable for decisions regarding selection of embryos for transfer and cryopreservation.

Recurrent Pregnancy Loss

For couples with two or more previous spontaneous abortions, screening for aneuploidy, together with chromosomal translocations, may provide valuable information, enhance pregnancy success, and decrease pregnancy loss. On the basis of PGS studies in patients with a prior history of an aneuploidy loss, the risk of subsequent aneuploidy is increased, particularly in women aged greater than 35 years. For those women with RPL without aneuploidy, the data are less clear. Recent study indicates that in patients with idiopathic RPL, preimplantation genetic screening may decrease miscarriage rates, suggesting that aneuploidy may in fact be the most common cause of RPL in these patients. In women with recurrent loss and advanced maternal age greater than 40 years, the potential benefits are also variable owing to the decreased yield of embryos developing beyond day 3 and the known extremely high rate of aneuploidy in surviving embryos.

Repeated IVF Failure

Similar to RPL, it is presumed that a significant contributing etiology to failed IVF in poor prognosis patients is chromosomal aberrations. Some studies using CGH suggest that patients with RIF have more complex abnormalities. It has been difficult to compare studies because of the wide variation in definition and molecular technique used for screening. Mean aneuploidy rates may be as high as 70% in embryos of these couples. Randomized controlled trials of PGS in the setting of RIF only employed 7- to 9-probe FISH, and there was no significant difference between PGS and control groups in implantation or clinical pregnancy rates. Patients should be counseled on the inconclusive benefit of PGS in RIF if PGS is offered as a treatment option.

Chromosomal Translocations

PGS is also beneficial in couples where a parental chromosomal translocation is discovered during the evaluation for RPL or infertility. Patients who are carriers of balanced translocations or inversions are predisposed to having a higher proportion of chromosomally abnormal gametes. PGS may benefit in cases of specific types of rearrangements, for example, if the involved chromosomes are of greatly disparate sizes. Paracentric inversions only yield 50% viable gametes, but these are balanced, whereas pericentric inversions produce 100% viable gametes with 50% of them unbalanced. In this situation, PGS for pericentric inversion carriers may decrease miscarriage rates from aneuploidy and delivery of a child with an unbalanced karyotype. Reciprocal translocations result in one-third gametes with normal complement. The risk of unbalanced offspring in Robertsonian translocations (those involving acrocentric chromosomes) depends on the sex of the carrier parent and the chromosomes involved. Though data are not extensive, one report of nearly 500 patients undergoing PGS for parental Robertsonian and reciprocal translocations shows that the loss rate was significantly reduced to 2% with an overall probability of pregnancy of 20%–36%. PGS platforms to evaluate patients with translocations are limited by the resolution of the platform to detect small segmental imbalances. Thus, each couple must be evaluated to determine if the platform can detect all of the specific abnormalities that can be derived from any rearrangement before testing. PGS testing has been demonstrated in multiple trials to improve implantation rates and live birth rates and decrease miscarriage rates. In addition to diagnosing translocations, the ability of current platforms to assess aneuploidy unrelated to a translocation offers the added advantage of further improving the clinical outcomes in these patients. Genetic counseling is crucial before proceeding with PGD or PGS to determine the true risk in all these clinical scenarios.

Controversial Topics

Several important concerns have arisen from PGD/PGS technology. Ethical debates have been especially fierce in cases when PGD is used to select human leukocyte antigen (HLA)–compatible embryos to help treat a sibling affected by a disease amenable to cure with transplantation. Some patients struggle with decisions to donate unaffected non–HLA-matched embryos to other couples or for research or whether to discard them. Since the beginning of PGD, there have been precedent cases questioning if "designer" babies can morally be used for treatment of their older siblings and if parents can have sound conscience by not attempting every option available especially in situations when fatality would otherwise be inevitable.

Unique situations involving nondisclosure of parental genotype may occur if a parent at risk of an adult-onset disorder desires unaffected offspring without knowing his or her carrier status. While this is relatively infrequent, it has clear implications on expenses and risks involved in undergoing potentially unnecessary procedures in one or more IVF cycles for the emotional or mental benefit to the patient who does not desire to know his or her genotype.

Treatment for young cancer patients has improved dramatically. Patients with adult-onset cancers such as Li–Fraumeni syndrome, Von Hippel–Lindau syndrome, and BRCA-related breast cancers can look forward to longer survival. Longer survival and improved quality of life for these patients translate into realistic expectations to become parents. Although the American College of Medical Genetics and Genomics has clear guidelines on when persons at risk of developing one of these disorders should be tested, PGD to screen for carrier embryos is very controversial because transmission penetrance of most of these disorders is often less than 100%. Although it is not known which carrier embryo will ultimately develop the disease later in life, it is more acceptable for some parents to select against these embryos as their disease status may bias their decisions.

Finally, there were some early concerns regarding increased risk of congenital anomalies in embryos subjected to PGD techniques. Current data from the ESHRE PGD Consortium and more than 1000 cases in a large PGD program in Chicago do not suggest increased rates of congenital anomalies overall or in any one organ system. These groups continue to collect data on live born infants resulting from PGD so that individual groups can be more closely examined such as patients with or without infertility history, embryos that required ICSI, those embryos undergoing cryopreservation, and patients with prior poor IVF outcomes.

Future PGD Indications

Recent data from PGD performed in healthy and young egg donors indicate that the ratio of aneuploid to normal embryos is high, approximating more than 30%. These data have led some clinicians to consider whether couples using oocyte donation may benefit from PGD analysis. As more outcomes data become available, it is possible that PGD may be more widely applied to assess chromosomal status in donor cycles and perhaps all cycles in the future.

Selection and Counseling of Patients Who May Benefit from PGD/PGS

Clinicians can best identify those patients who are likely to benefit from PGD/PGS by obtaining a thorough genetic and obstetric history. Patients who may have or carry single gene defects may have a history of genetic disease in family members or a family history of unexplained pregnancy losses or neonatal deaths. A couple's family history may also reveal specific ethnicities that are associated with increased rates of genetic disease such as the association between sickle cell anemia and African American heritage or the association between cystic fibrosis and Northern European or Ashkenazi Jewish heritage. Couples with RPL or recurrent implantation failure are at increased risk of carrying a chromosomal translocation and would benefit from PGS. Women with poor pregnancy or IVF outcomes or those of advanced maternal age are more likely to produce aneuploid embryos and therefore should also be offered PGS.

It is our policy that all couples undergoing PGD/PGS meet with a genetic counselor so that they have a complete understanding of the genetic disorder of concern, as well as the limitations of PGD/PGS. When counseling couples, it is also important that they be made aware of alternative options including donor gametes. For those couples at risk of chromosomal or genetic abnormalities that do not undergo PGD/PGS and do become pregnant, noninvasive prenatal screening can be performed at 9–11 weeks and prenatal diagnosis can be performed later in pregnancy by CVS at 12–14 weeks or amniocentesis at 16–20 weeks. Those couples who desire preimplantation testing should also be made aware of the inherent limitations of the testing owing to a baseline error rate depending on the molecular technique used, the contribution of embryonic mosaicism, and the possibility of a reduced overall embryo yield per cycle. In addition, the ASRM guidelines for proper counseling of patients who choose preimplantation genetic testing include discussion of risks associated with IVF and embryo biopsy, genetic counseling regarding inheritance and expected outcomes based on diagnosis desired (single testing or tiered diagnosis with HLA testing, single gene detection, or sex selection), alternatives to preimplantation testing such as CVS, amniocentesis, options of donor gamete, and disposition of undesired embryos (affected and unaffected). Further, if pregnancy is achieved after PGD/PGS, we strongly recommend a CVS or amniocentesis to confirm the diagnosis.

Conclusions

In summary, PGD and PGS are a rapidly expanding technological advance that may greatly benefit couples at risk for transmitting genetic or chromosomal abnormalities to their offspring. As more published data become available, it is likely that the use of PGD and PGS will become more widespread and may prove to be beneficial to more if not all couples using assisted reproductive technologies.

RECOMMENDED READING

American Society for Reproductive Medicine. Preimplantation genetic testing: A practice committee opinion. *Fertil Steril* 2008;90:S136–43.

Baart EB, Martini E, van den Berg I, Macklon NS, Galjaard RJ, Fauser BC, Van Opstal D. Preimplantation genetic diagnosis reveals a high incidence of aneuploidy and mosaicism in embryos from young women undergoing IVF. *Human Reprod* 2006;21:223–33.

Braude P, Pickering S, Flinter F, Ogilivie CM. Preimplantation genetic diagnosis. *Nature Rev* 2002;3:941–53.

Brezina PR, Anchan R, Kearns WG. Preimplantation genetic testing for aneuploidy: What technology should you use and what are the differences. *J Assist Repro Genet* 2016;33:823–32.

Carp HA, Dirnfeld M, Dor J, Grudzinksas JG. ART in recurrent miscarriage: Preimplantation genetic diagnosis/screening or surrogacy? *Human Reprod* 2004;19:1502–5.

Dahdouh E, Balayla J, Audibert F. Technical update; preimplantation genetic diagnosis and screening. *J Obstet Gynaecol Can* 2015;37(5):451–63.

Demko ZP, Simon AL, McCoy RC, Petrov DA, Rabinowitz M. Effects of maternal age on euploidy rates in a large cohort of embryos analyzed with 24-chromosome single-nucleotide polymorphism-based preimplantation genetic screening. *Fertil Steril* 2016 May;105(5):1307–13.

Geraedts J, Sermon K. Preimplantation genetic screening 2.0: The theory. *Mol Hum Reprod* 2016;22(8):539–44.

Kuliev A, Verlinsky Y. Place of preimplantation diagnosis in genetic practice. *Am J Med Genet* 2005;134A:105–10.

Lee HL, McCulloh DH, Hodes-Wertz B, Adler A, McCaffrey C, Grifo JA. In vitro fertilization with preimplantation genetic screening improves implantation and live birth in women age 40 through 43. *J Assist Reprod Genet* 2015 Mar;32(3):435–44.

Morin SJ, Eccles J, Iturriaga A, Zimmerman RS. Translocations, inversions and other chromosome rearrangements. *Fertil Steril* 2017;107(1):19–26.

Munne S, Chen S, Fischer J, Colls P, Zheng X, Stevens J, Escudero T, Oter M, Schoolcraft B, Simpson JL, Cohen J. Preimplantation genetic diagnosis reduces pregnancy loss in women aged 35 years and older with a history of recurrent miscarriage. *Fertil Steril* 2005;84:331–5.

Murugappan G, Shahine LK, Perfetto CO, Hickok LR, Lathi RB. Intent to treat analysis of in vitro fertilization and preimplantation genetic screening versus expectant management in patients with recurrent pregnancy loss. *Hum Reprod* 2016 Aug;31(8):1668–74.

Northrop LE, Treff NR, Levy B, Scott RT Jr. SNP microarray-based 24 chromosome aneuploidy screening demonstrates that cleavage-stage FISH poorly predicts aneuploidy in embryos that develop to morphologically normal blastocysts. *Mol Hum Reprod* 2010;16:590–600.

Sermon K, Van Steirteghem A, Liebaers I. Preimplantation genetic diagnosis. *Lancet* 2004;363:1633–41.

Simpson JL. Preimplantation genetic diagnosis at 20 years. *Prenat Diagn* 2010;30:682–95.

Staessen C, Platteau P, Van Assche E, Michels A, Tournay H, Camus M, Devroey P, Liebars I, Van Steriteghem A. Comparison of blastocyst transfer with or without preimplantation genetic diagnosis for aneuploidy screening in couples with advanced maternal age: A prospective randomized controlled trial. *Hum Reprod* 2004;19:2849–58.

Ubaldi FM, Capalbo A, Colamaria S, Ferrero S, Maggiulli R, Vajta G, Sapienza F, Cimadomo D, Giuliani M, Gravotta E, Vaiarelli A, Rienzi L. Reduction of multiple pregnancies in the advanced maternal age population after implementation of an elective single embryo transfer policy coupled with enhanced embryo selection: Pre- and post-intervention study. *Hum Reprod* 2015 Sep;30(9):2097–106.

13

Endometriosis and Infertility

Daniel Griffin

Endometriosis is defined as the presence of endometrial glands and stroma outside of the uterine cavity. One of the challenges practitioners face is how best to treat patients with endometriosis who have difficulties conceiving a pregnancy. Endometriosis is prevalent in women who have infertility. It has been reported that 25% to 50% of women with infertility have endometriosis [1,2]. There are several mechanisms that have been proposed to cause infertility in women who have endometriosis. One clear mechanism is the presence of adhesive disease and distortion of the normal tubo-ovarian relationship. Adhesions from endometriosis affect the ability of the tube to pick up the oocyte properly [3]. Endometriosis alters the peritoneal environment and creates an inflammatory state within the peritoneal cavity, which may impact sperm transport, fertilization, fallopian tube, and embryo function. Several inflammatory cytokines have been shown to be increased in patients with endometriosis including interleukin-6 and tumor necrosis factor-α [4]. Alterations in humoral immunity including an increase in IgA and IgG antibodies as well as increased lymphocytes have been reported in the endometrium of women with endometriosis. This may contribute to decreased endometrial receptivity and impaired implantation [5]. Endometriosis has been associated with ovulatory dysfunction including luteal phase defects [2]. Endometriosis may also be associated with poor oocyte or embryo quality [6]. Because of the varying stages of endometriosis and the multiple mechanisms in which it may lead to subfertility, there are different treatment options that are used to achieve a pregnancy.

Diagnosis

A patient history and physical examination can be useful in determining the probability of finding endometriosis. Common symptoms of endometriosis include dysmenorrhea, dyspareunia, pelvic pain, and infertility. Bowel or bladder complaints may also point to involvement of endometriosis in those areas [7]. There may be physical signs of endometriosis including an adnexal mass or tenderness to palpation, uterosacral nodularity, or a fixed uterus on examination [8]. An ultrasound examination may also be useful in evaluating the ovaries for endometriomas [9]. The only way to definitively diagnose a patient with endometriosis is with a surgical procedure called a laparoscopy. A pathologic diagnosis by biopsy is recommended at the time of surgery should a diagnosis not be attained with visualization of endometriotic implants [2]. The correlation between visualizing endometriosis and pathologic diagnosis is good [10]. If a diagnosis is in doubt, then a biopsy should be performed. Pathologic criteria to make the diagnosis of endometriosis include the presence of endometrial glands and stroma along with hemosiderin-laden macrophages [10].

The decision to proceed with surgical evaluation should be undertaken based on a patient's symptoms or diagnostic findings rather than strictly for infertility. Many patients with infertility will have endometriosis at the time of laparoscopy; however, the clinical significance of these findings in relation to the patient's subfertility is debatable. Treating a patient's other symptoms (dysmenorrhea and dyspareunia) are better indications to proceed with surgery than infertility itself [11]. The American Society for Reproductive Medicine developed a staging system for endometriosis. The staging is based on the type of endometriotic implants, their size, location, and adhesive disease [12]. The stage of endometriosis begins with stage I (minimal), stage II (mild), stage III (moderate), up to stage IV (severe) disease. While staging of endometriosis is important for surgical evaluation and research purposes, there is no good correlation between the stage of disease with chances of pregnancy (spontaneous or with assisted reproductive treatment).

Surgical Management

There is a significant although minimal increase in live birth in patients with stage I/II disease who are treated surgically. A prospective randomized trial was performed in women with stage I/II endometriosis in which, during laparoscopy, one group was treated with ablation/excision and one group was not treated. The results demonstrated a significant increase in the ongoing pregnancy rate with treatment (29%) compared to the untreated group (17%) [13]. However another prospective trial published by an Italian group failed to reproduce these findings and did not show a change in pregnancy rates in treated (20%) versus untreated women (22%) with stage I/II disease [14]. A meta-analysis that combined the results from the two trials demonstrated an odds ratio of 1.64 (95% CI, 1.05 to 2.57) with ongoing pregnancy in favor of treatment [15]. On the basis of this meta-analysis, the number of patients with endometriosis needed to treat with laparoscopy to achieve one live birth would be 12 [2]. If 50% of women with infertility have stage I/II endometriosis, then approximately 25 laparoscopies would need to be done in order to achieve one additional live birth. The benefits of performing a laparoscopy on patients with infertility without other symptoms affecting their quality of life appear to be minimal.

There are no randomized trials evaluating surgical treatment and effects on natural fecundity rates in patients with stage III/IV endometriosis. A prospective cohort study evaluating laparoscopic surgical treatment of endometriosis showed a pregnancy rate of 67.2% in patients with stage III disease and 68.6% in patients with stage IV disease [16]. Another large prospective cohort study showed a pregnancy rate of 46% with stage III and 44% with stage IV endometriosis within 3 years of laparoscopic surgical management [17]. These results may be difficult to extrapolate to other populations because of the expertise of the surgical groups in these studies. Surgery in moderate to severe endometriosis may be helpful, especially in patients who do not want to pursue assisted reproductive treatment.

After surgical management of endometriosis, medical suppressive treatment should not be used in order to enhance fertility [2,9]. These medical options include leuprolide acetate, oral contraceptive pills, depot medroxyprogesterone acetate, and others. Treating patients with medical agents only delays attempts at conception and has not been shown to improve the fecundity rates in clinical studies. In fact, it may be detrimental to achieving a pregnancy especially in women of advanced maternal age or with a diminished ovarian reserve [2].

Ovulation Induction/Intrauterine Insemination

In general, patients with minimal/mild endometriosis should be treated in a similar way to those with unexplained infertility. The combination of ovulation induction with intrauterine insemination (IUI) treatment is the best initial treatment. The usual starting medication is clomiphene citrate (CC) in combination with an IUI. The use of CC and IUI treatment was evaluated in a crossover randomized controlled trial in patients with endometriosis and unexplained infertility. The pregnancy rate was 9.5% per cycle in the IUI group compared to 3.3% per cycle in the timed intercourse group [18]. Another study evaluated couples with infertility including endometriosis and the fecundity rate per cycle with CC and IUI [19]. This study evaluated a total of 3381 CC–IUI cycles with a cumulative clinical pregnancy rate of 9.2%. In the first cycle, the clinical pregnancy rate was 10.4%, and after four total cycles, the pregnancy rate dropped to 2.2% or less in subsequent cycles ($p = 0.001$) [19]. This study suggests that after four failed cycles of CC with IUI, pregnancies are unlikely to occur and other options should be considered.

If a pregnancy has not occurred after three to four treatment cycles, then moving forward with gonadotropin treatment with IUI may be appropriate. In those patients who have not had a prior laparoscopy and are having symptoms suggestive of endometriosis, they can be offered a diagnostic laparoscopy after treatment failure. Gonadotropin with IUI treatment has been evaluated in patients with infertility including stage I/II endometriosis [20]. This study evaluated a total of 932 couples in four different treatment arms. The groups consisted of group 1, intracervical insemination; group 2, IUI; group 3, gonadotropin superovulation with intracervical insemination; and group 4, gonadotropin superovulation with IUI. Each group was treated with up to four treatment cycles to achieve a pregnancy. The cumulative pregnancy rates per couple were 10% for group 1, 18% for group 2, 19% for group 3, and 33% for group 4. The pregnancy rate of group 4 was significantly higher compared to every other group ($p < 0.001$) [20]. The risk of multiples with gonadotropin superovulation was >20% in this study, with seven sets of high-order multiples [20].

A recent randomized trial compared CC, letrozole, and gonadotropins with IUI treatment in patients with unexplained infertility [21]. The study evaluated a total of 900 couples with infertility. The groups were treated up to four cycles. The live birth rates were 32.2% after gonadotropin treatment, 23.3% after CC treatment, and 18.7% after letrozole treatment. The live birth rate was significantly higher in the gonadotropin compared to the clomiphene ($p = 0.02$) and the letrozole ($p < 0.001$) group. The difference in live birth rates between CC and letrozole was not statistically significant [21]. The risk of multiples was significantly higher in the gonadotropin (32%) than in the CC (5.7%) or letrozole (14.3%) group ($p = 0.001$). There was no significant difference in the risk of multiples between letrozole and CC. Letrozole may be a better choice in patients who have had intolerable side effects with CC or in patients who have had a thin endometrial lining with CC. Treatment with letrozole may be used up to three to four treatment cycles before moving onto other options.

A randomized clinical trial compared time to pregnancy and health care costs in unexplained fertility patients with an accelerated treatment strategy of three clomiphene/IUI cycles followed by in vitro fertilization (IVF) versus a stepwise treatment of three clomiphene/IUI cycles, three gonadotropin/IUI cycles, and then IVF [22]. The time to pregnancy was significantly shorter in the accelerated arm (8 months) compared to the conventional arm (11 months) ($p = 0.045$). Health care costs were also lower in the accelerated arm group compared to the conventional arm ($2624 savings in charges per couple).

After a patient has failed three to four CC or letrozole with IUI treatment cycles, it may be appropriate to move onto IVF treatment. If the patient is >35 years old, has a diminished ovarian reserve, has a male factor, has a tubal factor present, or has stage III/IV endometriosis, it may be appropriate to move onto IVF rather than using superovulation with gonadotropins. IVF provides a superior pregnancy rate as well as a lower risk of multiples, especially high-order multiples, compared to gonadotropin and IUI treatment. If there are financial or other ethical/religious reasons that would prevent a patient to not proceed with IVF, then gonadotropins with IUI or surgery may be a better choice.

In Vitro Fertilization

The presence of endometriosis having an adverse effect on IVF success remains a controversial topic. An analysis from the SART database showed no difference in the live birth rates between endometriosis and other infertility diagnoses [23]. Another meta-analysis using the SART database reviewed women with endometriosis and another concomitant infertility diagnosis versus women with unexplained or tubal infertility and IVF success rates [24]. In this meta-analysis, women with endometriosis had a higher live birth rate compared to other diagnoses (RR, 1.13; $p = 0.0001$). Women who have endometriosis plus another infertility diagnosis had a lower live birth rate compared to other diagnoses (RR, 0.84; $p = 0.0001$). Women with endometriosis appeared to have a lower oocyte yield and lower implantation rates compared to other diagnoses [24]. The addition of endometriosis with another infertility diagnosis (diminished ovarian reserve, male factor, or tubal factor) appeared to have a negative impact on IVF success rather than endometriosis itself.

Ovarian stimulation protocols in patients with endometriosis have been evaluated in several studies. A prospective trial compared patients with stage I or stage II endometriosis undergoing IVF with gonadotropin-releasing hormone (GnRH) agonist versus antagonist protocols [25]. There were no significant differences in implantation rate or clinical pregnancy rate between GnRH agonist versus antagonist [25]. Another prospective trial evaluated women with endometriosis who underwent a 3-month course of a GnRH agonist before IVF stimulation [26]. All of the patients in this study had endometriosis and a normal ovarian reserve and did not have an endometrioma present. One group had 3 months of GnRH agonist ($n = 25$) before undergoing IVF, and the control group went directly into an IVF cycle ($n = 26$). The group treated with a GnRH agonist for 3 months before IVF had a significantly higher ongoing pregnancy rate compared to the control group (80% vs. 53.85%, $p < 0.05$). Because of the high ongoing pregnancy rate in this study, it may be difficult to extrapolate the findings to the general endometriosis population. Treating patients with a diminished ovarian reserve or over the age of 35 years with 3 months of a GnRH agonist before stimulation may have an adverse effect on pregnancy rates because of the delay in treatment. Overall, there does not appear to be a superior IVF stimulation protocol in women with endometriosis.

Endometriomas

Ovarian endometriomas are a benign cyst of endometriosis that can be diagnosed by pelvic ultrasound. They are complex in appearance and classically have a "ground glass" appearance on ultrasound. They can vary widely in size. Endometriomas may pose a treatment dilemma for the clinician. Different surgical approaches have been used for endometriomas. A meta-analysis comparing drainage and ablation of the endometrioma versus cystectomy was performed. In this meta-analysis, there was a significant reduction in recurrence of dysmenorrhea, dyspareunia, and pelvic pain in the cystectomy group [27]. Also, there was a reduction in recurrence of the endometrioma and risk of reoperation [27]. Patients who have a cystectomy had a higher chance of natural conception versus drainage and ablation (OR, 5.21; 95% CI, 2.04 to 13.29) [27]. If a patient is symptomatic, then removal of an endometrioma is indicated. Other benefits of removal of an endometrioma include reducing potential endometrioma rupture as well as spillage during an oocyte retrieval, reducing possible contamination of endometrioma contents in follicular fluid, and confirming a definitive pathologic diagnosis [2]. A pooled analysis of case–control studies showed an increased odds ratio of ovarian cancer in women with endometriosis, specifically clear cell, endometrioid, and serous histologic types [28]. The disadvantages to treating an endometrioma are surgical risk including adhesion formation, surgical cost, and the removal or destruction of normal ovarian tissue leading to a diminished ovarian reserve. A case–control study comparing women with diminished ovarian reserve after removal of an endometrioma compared to women with idiopathic diminished ovarian reserve showed a significantly lower implantation rate (7.2% vs. 13.5%, $p = 0.03$) and lower pregnancy rate in women who had an endometrioma removed (11.6% vs. 20.6%, $p = 0.02$) [29]. These findings are in agreement with the meta-analysis described earlier [24] that the combination of endometriosis with another infertility factor (diminished ovarian reserve) leads to poorer IVF outcomes. A systematic review evaluated the effects of cystectomy for treatment of endometriomas on anti-Müllerian hormone (AMH) before and after surgery showing a significant decline in AMH levels postoperatively [30]. Another systematic review showed a postoperative change in AMH levels of -1.13 ng/mL (95% CI, -0.37 to -1.88) after ovarian cystectomy for an endometrioma [31]. A meta-analysis also showed no difference in live birth rate in patients with and without endometriomas who were undergoing IVF treatment [32]. The analysis also showed no difference in IVF outcomes in endometriomas that had been treated before compared to no treatment [32].

A combined technique has also been described for treating endometriomas with a partial cystectomy, but the cyst wall near the ovarian hilum was ablated [33]. The combined technique may have an advantage over cystectomy by causing less damage to normal ovarian tissue; however, this requires further study. Overall, the treatment of endometriomas should be individualized based on the clinical situation. If a patient has symptoms or the diagnosis is in doubt, then removal is indicated. Otherwise, removal of endometrioma is not necessary to proceed forward with fertility treatment and may be detrimental to a patient's ovarian reserve and subsequent treatment success.

Summary

A diagnostic algorithm is outlined in Figure 13.1. Patients who have symptoms that may be attributed to endometriosis and that may be affecting their quality of life should be offered diagnostic laparoscopy. In patients that have stage I or stage II endometriosis, surgical treatment with ablation or excision of lesions can improve the chances of natural conception. In patients with endometriosis (stage I or stage II) or unexplained infertility, treatment with CC and IUI up to four cycles should be offered initially. If CC and IUI treatment fails, then patients should be offered gonadotropin stimulation and IUI treatment or IVF treatment. Patients who have not had surgical evaluation after treatment failure should be offered a diagnostic laparoscopic evaluation. If a patient has stage III or stage IV endometriosis with a disrupted tubo-ovarian relationship, he or she may benefit from IVF treatment. Patients with endometriomas should have removal if they are symptomatic or the diagnosis is uncertain; otherwise, removal of an endometrioma may be detrimental and may lead to diminished ovarian reserve. A diminished ovarian reserve can subsequently lead to less of an ovarian response to gonadotropin stimulation and decrease the overall success of treatment. Endometriosis is a common cause of infertility and there are many treatment options that can be successful in helping patients achieve a pregnancy. In women who are >35 years old, have advanced stage endometriosis, or have a diminished ovarian reserve, aggressive fertility treatment such as IVF should not be delayed.

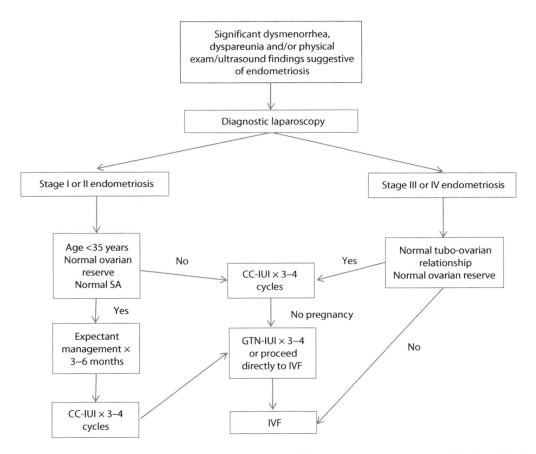

FIGURE 13.1   Treatment algorithm for endometriosis. CC, clomiphene citrate; GTN, gonadotropin injections; IUI, intra-uterine insemination; IVF, in vitro fertilization; SA, semen analysis.

REFERENCES

1. Verkauf BS. Incidence, symptoms, and signs of endometriosis in fertile and infertile women. *J Fla Med Assoc* 1987;74(9):671–5.
2. Practice Committee of the American Society for Reproductive M. Endometriosis and infertility: A committee opinion. *Fertil Steril* 2012;98(3):591–8.
3. Schenken RS, Asch RH, Williams RF, Hodgen GD. Etiology of infertility in monkeys with endometriosis: Luteinized unruptured follicles, luteal phase defects, pelvic adhesions, and spontaneous abortions. *Fertil Steril* 1984;41(1):122–30.
4. Bedaiwy MA, Falcone T, Sharma RK, Goldberg JM, Attaran M, Nelson DR et al. Prediction of endometriosis with serum and peritoneal fluid markers: A prospective controlled trial. *Hum Reprod* 2002;17(2):426–31.
5. Lebovic DI, Mueller MD, Taylor RN. Immunobiology of endometriosis. *Fertil Steril* 2001;75(1):1–10.
6. Garrido N, Navarro J, Garcia-Velasco J, Remoh J, Pellice A, Simon C. The endometrium versus embryonic quality in endometriosis-related infertility. *Hum Reprod Update* 2002;8(1):95–103.
7. Ballard KD, Seaman HE, de Vries CS, Wright JT. Can symptomatology help in the diagnosis of endometriosis? Findings from a national case-control study—Part 1. *BJOG* 2008;115(11):1382–91.
8. Hickey M, Ballard K, Farquhar C. Endometriosis. *BMJ* 2014;348:g1752.
9. Dunselman GA, Vermeulen N, Becker C, Calhaz-Jorge C, D'Hooghe T, De Bie B et al. ESHRE guideline: Management of women with endometriosis. *Hum Reprod* 2014;29(3):400–12.
10. Nisolle M, Paindaveine B, Bourdon A, Berliere M, Casanas-Roux F, Donnez J. Histologic study of peritoneal endometriosis in infertile women. *Fertil Steril* 1990;53(6):984–8.
11. Smith S, Pfeifer SM, Collins JA. Diagnosis and management of female infertility. *JAMA* 2003;290(13):1767–70.
12. Revised American Society for Reproductive Medicine classification of endometriosis: 1996. *Fertil Steril* 1997;67(5):817–21.
13. Marcoux S, Maheux R, Berube S. Laparoscopic surgery in infertile women with minimal or mild endometriosis. Canadian Collaborative Group on Endometriosis. *N Engl J Med* 1997;337(4):217–22.
14. Parazzini F. Ablation of lesions or no treatment in minimal-mild endometriosis in infertile women: A randomized trial. Gruppo Italiano per lo Studio dell'Endometriosi. *Hum Reprod* 1999;14(5):1332–4.
15. Jacobson TZ, Duffy JM, Barlow D, Farquhar C, Koninckx PR, Olive D. Laparoscopic surgery for subfertility associated with endometriosis. *Cochrane Database Syst Rev* 2010;(1):CD001398.
16. Nezhat C, Crowgey S, Nezhat F. Videolaseroscopy for the treatment of endometriosis associated with infertility. *Fertil Steril* 1989;51(2):237–40.
17. Vercellini P, Fedele L, Aimi G, De Giorgi O, Consonni D, Crosignani PG. Reproductive performance, pain recurrence and disease relapse after conservative surgical treatment for endometriosis: The predictive value of the current classification system. *Hum Reprod* 2006;21(10):2679–85.
18. Deaton JL, Gibson M, Blackmer KM, Nakajima ST, Badger GJ, Brumsted JR. A randomized, controlled trial of clomiphene citrate and intrauterine insemination in couples with unexplained infertility or surgically corrected endometriosis. *Fertil Steril* 1990;54(6):1083–8.
19. Dickey RP, Taylor SN, Lu PY, Sartor BM, Rye PH, Pyrzak R. Effect of diagnosis, age, sperm quality, and number of preovulatory follicles on the outcome of multiple cycles of clomiphene citrate-intrauterine insemination. *Fertil Steril* 2002;78(5):1088–95.
20. Guzick DS, Carson SA, Coutifaris C, Overstreet JW, Factor-Litvak P, Steinkampf MP et al. Efficacy of superovulation and intrauterine insemination in the treatment of infertility. National Cooperative Reproductive Medicine Network. *N Engl J Med* 1999;340(3):177–83.
21. Diamond MP, Legro RS, Coutifaris C, Alvero R, Robinson RD, Casson P et al. Letrozole, gonadotropin, or clomiphene for unexplained infertility. *N Engl J Med* 2015;373(13):1230–40.
22. Reindollar RH, Regan MM, Neumann PJ, Levine BS, Thornton KL, Alper MM et al. A randomized clinical trial to evaluate optimal treatment for unexplained infertility: The fast track and standard treatment (FASTT) trial. *Fertil Steril* 2010;94(3):888–99.
23. Stern JE, Brown MB, Wantman E, Kalra SK, Luke B. Live birth rates and birth outcomes by diagnosis using linked cycles from the SART CORS database. *J Assist Reprod Genet* 2013;30(11):1445–50.

24. Senapati S, Sammel MD, Morse C, Barnhart KT. Impact of endometriosis on in vitro fertilization outcomes: An evaluation of the Society for Assisted Reproductive Technologies Database. *Fertil Steril* 2016;106(1):164–71 e1.

25. Pabuccu R, Onalan G, Kaya C. GnRH agonist and antagonist protocols for stage I–II endometriosis and endometrioma in in vitro fertilization/intracytoplasmic sperm injection cycles. *Fertil Steril* 2007;88(4):832–9.

26. Surrey ES, Silverberg KM, Surrey MW, Schoolcraft WB. Effect of prolonged gonadotropin-releasing hormone agonist therapy on the outcome of in vitro fertilization-embryo transfer in patients with endometriosis. *Fertil Steril* 2002;78(4):699–704.

27. Hart RJ, Hickey M, Maouris P, Buckett W. Excisional surgery versus ablative surgery for ovarian endometriomata. *Cochrane Database Syst Rev* 2008(2):CD004992.

28. Pearce CL, Templeman C, Rossing MA, Lee A, Near AM, Webb PM et al. Association between endometriosis and risk of histological subtypes of ovarian cancer: A pooled analysis of case-control studies. *Lancet Oncol* 2012;13(4):385–94.

29. Roustan A, Perrin J, Debals-Gonthier M, Paulmyer-Lacroix O, Agostini A, Courbiere B. Surgical diminished ovarian reserve after endometrioma cystectomy versus idiopathic DOR: Comparison of in vitro fertilization outcome. *Hum Reprod* 2015;30(4):840–7.

30. Somigliana E, Berlanda N, Benaglia L, Vigano P, Vercellini P, Fedele L. Surgical excision of endometriomas and ovarian reserve: A systematic review on serum antimullerian hormone level modifications. *Fertil Steril* 2012;98(6):1531–8.

31. Raffi F, Metwally M, Amer S. The impact of excision of ovarian endometrioma on ovarian reserve: A systematic review and meta-analysis. *J Clin Endocrinol Metab* 2012;97(9):3146–54.

32. Hamdan M, Dunselman G, Li TC, Cheong Y. The impact of endometrioma on IVF/ICSI outcomes: A systematic review and meta-analysis. *Hum Reprod Update* 2015;21(6):809–25.

33. Donnez J, Lousse JC, Jadoul P, Donnez O, Squifflet J. Laparoscopic management of endometriomas using a combined technique of excisional (cystectomy) and ablative surgery. *Fertil Steril* 2010;94(1):28–32.

14

Polycystic Ovary Syndrome

Rita M. Sneeringer and Kristen Page Wright

Introduction

Polycystic ovary syndrome (PCOS) is the most common endocrinopathy of reproductive-age women and the most frequent cause of anovulatory infertility. As a syndrome, it is a collection of specific signs and symptoms rather than a well-defined disorder. As such, it can include variable clinical presentations. Depending on the criteria used for diagnosis, the prevalence ranges from 9% to 18% [1]. The etiology remains largely unknown. PCOS is associated with long-term health complications, including diabetes, obesity, heart disease, and endometrial hyperplasia or cancer. Accurate diagnosis allows for directed treatment and prevention of comorbidities. Diagnostic criteria, clinical presentation, potential pathophysiology, and evidence-based treatments are summarized here.

Diagnosis

Stein and Leventhal first described the syndrome of PCOS in 1935 as the combination of polycystic ovaries and amenorrhea. Since then, the definition and, hence, diagnosis of PCOS have evolved. Much controversy exists because of the varied presentation. In the past decades, several different diagnostic criteria have been developed for the classification of PCOS (Table 14.1). The initial diagnostic criteria were developed during a consensus meeting at the National Institutes of Health (NIH) in 1990. The NIH criteria required both chronic anovulation and clinical or biochemical signs of hyperandrogenism [2]. Notably, polycystic ovaries were not required for the diagnosis of PCOS. In 2003, a consensus workshop held jointly by the European Society of Human Reproduction and Embryology (ESHRE) and the American Society for Reproductive Medicine (ASRM) in Rotterdam revised the diagnostic criteria. For the Rotterdam criteria, two out of the following three symptoms are required: oligo-ovulation and/or anovulation, clinical and/or biochemical signs of hyperandrogenism, and polycystic ovaries [3]. The Rotterdam criteria broadened the clinical spectrum of PCOS by including two additional groups of women who did not previously meet the NIH definition: women with only hirsutism and polycystic ovaries, but regular menstrual cycles; and women with oligomenorrhea and polycystic ovaries, but without hyperandrogenism. Finally, in 2006, the Androgen Excess Society (AES) Task Force developed consensus guidelines that placed a greater emphasis on the elevated androgens that characterize this syndrome. In the AES criteria, PCOS can be diagnosed after documented hyperandrogenism (hirsutism and/or hyperandrogenemia) and ovarian dysfunction (oligo-ovulation and/or anovulation and/or polycystic ovaries) [4]. Women with ultrasound appearance of polycystic ovaries and ovulatory dysfunction in the absence of hyperandrogenism would not meet the AES criteria for the diagnosis of PCOS. Further, the AES and NIH criteria are quite similar with some minor modifications to include women with hyperandrogenism and polycystic ovaries in the absence of menstrual irregularity.

Despite historical controversy, the current internationally accepted criteria for PCOS are the Rotterdam criteria. This definition has now been endorsed by the Australian Guideline Committee [5], the NIH

TABLE 14.1

Diagnostic Criteria for PCOS and Associated Variable Phenotypes

Criteria	Hyperandrogenism (Clinical or Biochemical)	Menstrual Irregularity/ Anovulation	Polycystic Appearing Ovaries on Ultrasound
NIH	✓	✓	
Rotterdam	✓	✓	
	✓		✓
		✓	✓
	✓	✓	✓
Androgen Excess Society	✓	✓	
	✓		✓
	✓	✓	✓

in the United States [6], the US Endocrine Society Practice Guideline [7], the European Society for Endocrinology position statement [8], and the World Health Organization [9].

Importantly, the Rotterdam criteria, in addition to the NIH and AES criteria, require the exclusion of other etiologies of menstrual irregularities and hyperandrogenism. Possible other diagnoses include adrenal or ovarian androgen-secreting neoplasm, hyperprolactinemia, syndromes of severe insulin resistance, thyroid dysfunction, congenital adrenal hyperplasia, Cushing's syndrome, and acromegaly. Typically, the measurement of thyroid-stimulating hormone, prolactin, glucose, insulin, and an androgen panel (DHEA-S, testosterone, and 17-OH progesterone) is sufficient to exclude other major causes if normal levels are noted. Specific testing for Cushing's syndrome and acromegaly is done if suspected based on history or phenotypic changes noted on physical exam (e.g., striae, round face, dorsal fat pad, central obesity, uncontrolled hypertension, increased glove or shoe size). For patients who have either severe or rapid onset of hyperandrogenic symptoms, an alternative diagnosis should be suspected as this is atypical for PCOS. Virilization (clitoromegaly, male-pattern frontal balding, or increased musculature) may also suggest tumor development. An androgen-secreting tumor would typically contribute to serum testosterone levels greater than 150–200 ng/dL or DHEA-S levels above 700 μg/dL in premenopausal women. Congenital adrenal hyperplasia is suspected if 17-OH progesterone level is elevated. Further assessment with an ACTH stimulation test should be performed when a morning 17-OH progesterone level performed in the follicular phase is >200 ng/dL.

Additional testing that is consistent with the diagnosis of PCOS but is not part of any criteria includes an elevated luteinizing hormone (LH)/follicle-stimulating hormone (FSH) ratio (>3:1) and hyperinsulinemia. These factors have been linked to PCOS, possibly secondary to underlying etiology (see below), but are not necessary for the diagnosis of PCOS. It is also important to emphasize that PCOS is a syndrome, a collection of features rather than a definitive disease that may actually represent multiple underlying disorders.

Clinical Presentation and Evaluation

Patients with PCOS usually present to care for three primary reasons: menstrual disturbances, hyperandrogenism, and infertility. Additional hallmarks of PCOS include obesity and metabolic disorders such as diabetes. There can also be a strong family history. A few distinct subgroups may present without the "typical phenotype" including women with lean PCOS and adolescents. The clinical characteristics of PCOS and suggested evaluation are described here (Table 14.2).

Menstrual disturbances are found in the majority of PCOS patients. The type of menstrual disorder can vary, but the underlying etiology is the same, anovulatory cycles. Most patients present with oligoovulation or anovulation leading to oligomenorrhea or amenorrhea. However, some women appear to have spontaneous menses with abnormal flow. This excessive bleeding could be the result of an absent

TABLE 14.2

Suggested Evaluation of PCOS/Chronic Anovulation

History and Physical
    Menstrual history, galactorrhea
    BMI, blood pressure, waist circumference, hirsuitism, acanthosis nigricans, thyroid
    Striae, round face, dorsal fat pad, hypertension, central obesity (Cushing's symptoms)
    Enlarged hands and feet, prominent facial features (acromegaly)
Confirm the Diagnosis of PCOS
    Ultrasound of the ovaries and endometrial stripe
    Androgens (mildly elevated) and sex hormone binding globulin
    Consider luteal progesterone
Exclude Other Endocrinopathies/Causes of Chronic Anovulation
    hCG (pregnancy)
    Total testosterone (ovarian/adrenal tumor)
    DHEA-S (adrenal tumor)
    Morning 17-OH progesterone (congenital adrenal hyperplasia)
    FSH/LH (ovarian failure)
    TSH (thyroid disorder)
    Prolactin (hyperprolactinemia)
    Dexamethasone suppression test (Cushing's syndrome, only if suspected)
    IGF-1 (acromegaly, only if suspected)
Evaluate for Comorbidities of PCOS
    HgbA1C (diabetes/glucose intolerance)
    Endometrial biopsy for prolonged anovulation (endometrial hyperplasia/cancer)
    Lipid profile (hyperlipidemia, metabolic syndrome)

luteal phase, causing heavy, prolonged bleeding owing to unopposed effects of estrogen. Thus, for women who have any irregularity of their menses (cycles <21 days or >35 days, highly variable cycle length, or abnormal flow), PCOS is a potential diagnosis. Additional testing, such as a luteal progesterone level, can help determine if cycles are anovulatory. A progesterone level of >3 ng/mL is confirmation of ovulation.

Ultrasound assessment may reveal polycystic ovaries that are associated with chronic anovulation and can be a sign of the ovarian dysfunction in PCOS. However, this finding is not specific and can be seen in patients with multiple etiologies for anovulation. Further, polycystic ovaries can be a normal isolated finding in approximately one-third of ovulating women without metabolic sequelae typical for PCOS [10]. Therefore, it is important to correlate the presence of polycystic ovaries with other clinical findings. The specific parameters for the diagnosis of PCO-appearing ovaries according to the Rotterdam criteria are as follows: ≥12 follicles in each ovary that measure 2–9 mm or ovarian volume ≥10 cc (Figure 14.1). Recent studies have suggested that higher-resolution ultrasound machines detect a great number of follicles and that a higher threshold of antral follicles should be considered to diagnose a polycystic ovary [11]. However, there is currently no consensus as to what that number should be. Ultrasound evaluation is not valid if a dominant follicle is present.

Anti-Müllerian hormone (AMH) level correlates with number of antral follicles and is frequently elevated in women with PCOS. While AMH can be considered a biochemical marker for polycystic ovaries, normative ranges for AMH have yet to be established, and there is significant overlap between ovulatory women and women with PCOS [9,11].

Hyperandrogenism is the other major component of PCOS. Hirsutism (excessive hair growth) is dependent [12,13]. The Ferriman–Gallwey score has been the gold standard in assessing the degree of hirsutism. A modified Ferriman–Gallwey scoring system has been recently proposed (Figure 14.2). This scale assesses the density and distribution of hair growth on multiple areas of the body. Generally, a summation score of greater than 3 is consistent with hirsutism. Acne, oily skin, and male-pattern alopecia are less specific features and should not be considered clinical evidence of hyperandrogenemia [14]. Biochemical markers of hyperandrogenism include elevated testosterone or DHEA-S levels.

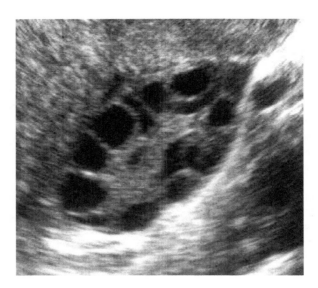

FIGURE 14.1   PCO morphology parameters: ≥12 follicles per ovary that measure 2–9 mm or ovarian volume ≥10 cc. The ultrasound evaluation is not valid if a dominant follicle is present. PCO morphology can be seen in only one ovary. PCO morphology alone is not sufficient for the diagnosis of PCOS and can be a normal finding of 20% of fertile women.

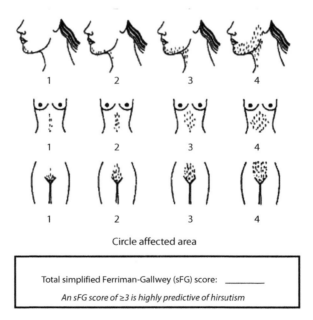

FIGURE 14.2   Modified Ferriman–Gallwey Score for the clinical assessment of hirsutism. A summation score of ≥3 is consistent with hirsutism. (Reprinted from Cook H, Brennan K, Azziz R. Reanalyzing the modified Ferriman–Gallwey score: is there a simpler method for assessing the extent of hirsutism? *Fertil Steril* 2011;96:1266–70, with permission from the American Society for Reproductive Medicine.)

In addition to the diagnostic symptoms, many patients with PCOS have metabolic abnormalities that should be recognized in order to mediate future health risks. Insulin resistance (and hence hyperinsulinemia) is an important finding in many PCOS patients and is suspected particularly among patients with acanthosis nigricans on physical exam. Acanthosis nigricans is a pigmented, velvety skin lesion that is noted most commonly on the back of the neck, axilla and groin. PCOS patients are at an increased risk for glucose intolerance or diabetes with up to 45% of patients affected [15] and approximately 16% of patients developing glucose intolerance annually [16]. Centripetal obesity is found in the majority of patients with PCOS and is considered part of the typical phenotype. It likely exacerbates risk of other comorbidities. The metabolic syndrome characterized by abdominal obesity, hypertension, high triglycerides, inflammatory factors, and increased thrombophilic factor is twice as likely to occur in patients with PCOS and is associated with an increased risk of cardiovascular disease [17]. Clearly, these associated metabolic conditions have significant long-term consequences and all patients with PCOS should be screened with regular assessment of glucose tolerance testing, blood pressure, waist/hip measurement, body mass index (BMI), and lipid panel (including triglycerides, total cholesterol, and HDL). HbA1C testing can be considered in lieu of glucose tolerance testing [9].

Reproductive potential is affected greatly by anovulation. Issues of subfertility and infertility are central to the presentation of PCOS patients, as are concerns about pregnancy outcomes and health risks to their offspring. The precise risks of infertility and spontaneous abortion rates are controversial, with varying degrees of risk reported in multiple studies. Some increased risk is likely, especially among obese patients, manifesting as increased time to conception, reduced efficacy of infertility treatments, and increased risk of miscarriage. In addition, obstetric risks, including pregnancy-induced hypertension, gestational diabetes, and preterm birth, are increased among patients with PCOS. These obstetric risks are also further exacerbated by obesity.

A higher incidence of endometrial abnormalities secondary to chronic anovulation is found in some patients with PCOS. Hyperplasia can occur and rarely endometrial cancer is encountered. Pathology evaluation of the endometrium is warranted in anovulatory patients regardless of age. However, an endometrium of <5 mm noted on vaginal ultrasound exam is rarely associated with endometrial hyperplasia and therefore an endometrial biopsy is not necessary in this circumstance.

PCOS can be associated with a significant psychological impact that is often overlooked. The feminine identity and body image are primarily affected, as patients suffer from obesity, acne, oily skin, and excess hair growth, not to mention infertility and several other health care issues. The data are limited but evidence exists that PCOS patients are more prone to also develop several psychiatric disorders, including major depression, anxiety, low self-esteem, negative body image, and psychosexual dysfunction [18,19]. As a result, patients whose lives and moods are significantly affected by the syndrome might also have a tougher time complying with lifestyle and treatment recommendations, all issues that need to be recognized and explored by clinicians.

Some patients do not fit the usual profile of PCOS. A special subset of patients are the lean PCOS patients. They represent between 10% and 50% of all PCOS patients [20] and present a challenging clinical conundrum. Despite having a normal BMI, these patients have greater insulin resistance compared to weight-matched controls [21]. They also manifest various metabolic abnormalities such as dyslipidemia [22], pro-thrombotic tendency, and increased pro-inflammatory markers. Unfortunately, their diagnosis is often delayed or missed altogether because they do not exhibit the typical obese PCOS phenotype.

Adolescents are a second atypical group and there is no overall consensus about how to diagnose PCOS in adolescence. A majority of young women have anovulatory menstrual cycles during the first 1–3 years after menarche and hirsuitism is less common in adolescence as this feature tends to develop over time. Biochemical markers of hyperandrogenemia and increased ovarian volume on ultrasound may therefore be more sensitive markers for the diagnosis of PCOS in adolescents [14]. Often, the diagnosis is delayed or oral contraceptives are initiated without a complete evaluation for PCOS. However, adolescents still have significant risks of metabolic comorbidities that could be mediated by early intervention and prevention strategies. This includes initiating weight management before severe obesity develops. Thus, it is important to complete a clinical assessment on adolescent patients who exhibit possible features of PCOS.

Pathophysiology/Etiology

The exact etiology of PCOS remains unclear. Several theories have been proposed, two of which have significant supporting research. These include theories of LH dysregulation and hyperinsulinemia. As

PCOS is a heterogeneous disorder with varied presentations, it is possible that both of these theories are correct but simply apply to different populations of patients. Alternatively, they could represent components of the same complex physiologic pathway. Specific research findings and potential explanations for the clinical presentation of PCOS for each theory are described.

The dysregulation of LH in PCOS patients has been reported in multiple studies and may account for many of the clinical symptoms of PCOS. Increased pulsatile GnRH secretion leads to increased LH pulse frequency. The primary cause of increased GnRH is unclear; it could be an intrinsic abnormality of the pulse generator or secondary to other factors such as chronically low levels of progesterone (from anovulation) or hyperinsulinemia [23–25]. Women with PCOS have reduced hypothalamic sensitivity to ovarian sex steroids [26] and enhanced pituitary sensitivity to GnRH, which likely contributes to the increased LH secretion and pulse amplitude. The increased LH secretion relative to FSH stimulates ovarian androgen (testosterone and androstenedione) production, leading to clinical hyperandrogenism. Anovulation results from insufficient selection of a dominant follicle in the setting of hyperthecosis.

Other research suggests hyperinsulinemia as the primary insult through direct and indirect effects [22]. Insulin augments LH stimulation of ovarian androgen production and inhibits hepatic sex hormone binding globulin (SHBG) production, which increases free androgen and estrogen levels. IGF-1 acts directly on the ovary to stimulate androgen production. Insulin at sufficiently high levels may cross-react with ovarian IGF receptors, enhance IGF action by up-regulating IGF receptors, and inhibit IGF-binding protein-1 production, leading to increased IGF-1 [24]. The end result of insulin action on the ovary is the preferential production of androgens with higher free levels owing to reduced SHBG. This explains how PCOS patients have hyperandrogenic symptoms despite normal androgen levels. The strong correlation of PCOS with hyperinsulinemia (see clinical presentation above) supports hyperinsulinemia as a possible central etiology.

Other physiologic effects are less well described, but may also play a role. For example, a reduction in ovarian aromatase activity has been proposed as a contributing factor to hyperandrogenism in PCOS, although this issue remains controversial [24].

Management

Several effective treatment strategies are available for patients with PCOS, including lifestyle modifications, medications, nonmedical treatments, and surgical intervention. Given the multifaceted approach to management, a multidisciplinary team is usually needed for best results. In addition, treatment should be tailored to a patient's specific needs, with attention to reproductive goals. Several treatments are contraindicated in patients who are pursuing fertility. The optimal management of PCOS incorporates healthy changes that can be maintained for a lifetime.

Lifestyle Interventions

Lifestyle changes should be the first-line approach for any PCOS patient, particularly those with obesity. Most importantly, lifestyle intervention should address weight loss or prevention of weight gain through dietary modifications and regular exercise. A body weight reduction of 5%–10% has been shown to exert a significant benefit on major psychological, reproductive (menstrual regulation, ovulation, fertility), and metabolic (hirsutism, insulin resistance, risk factors for diabetes, and cardiovascular disease) outcomes [27]. In addition, BMI is a clear prognostic factor for infertility treatments with reduced pregnancy rates among obese PCOS patients compared to normal weight PCOS patients. Consultation with a nutritionist who is familiar with the specific challenges of PCOS is recommended. In addition, regular exercise with a structured routine of at least 30 minutes a day can reduce cardiovascular risk associated with PCOS.

Bariatric surgery is sometimes considered in women with PCOS and obesity who are unsuccessful at weight loss after diet and exercise adjustments. Current guidelines state that bariatric surgery can be considered for women with BMI > 40 kg/m^2 or BMI > 35 kg/m^2 in the presence of obesity-related comorbidities such as type 2 diabetes. Bariatric surgery improves many features of PCOS including anovulation rate, hirsuitism, insulin resistance, and sexual libido. However, small for gestational age infants and preterm birth have emerged as complications associated with births after bariatric surgery owing to the resulting malabsorptive nutritional state of the mother. It is therefore unclear whether bariatric surgery improves overall maternal and fetal outcomes. Women with PCOS who become pregnant after bariatric surgery should be considered high risk and should be followed by a multidisciplinary health care team including a dietician [9]. Additionally, pregnancy should be avoided during periods of rapid weight loss and for at least 6–12 months after bariatric surgery.

Medical Therapies

Several medical therapies effectively treat the symptoms of PCOS (Table 14.3). The choice of medications depends on the specific symptoms and their severity. Medical therapies are often optimal when combined with lifestyle interventions or nonmedical therapies.

The symptoms of menstrual irregularity and hyperandrogenism can be improved through use of the oral contraceptive pill (OCP). The maximal benefit is achieved with combined estrogen-progestin pills, since these formulations take advantage of the first pass effect in the liver. As a result, levels of hepatic proteins, including SHBG, are significantly increased, thus reducing free circulating androgen concentrations. After initiation of OCP therapy, the regulation of the menstrual abnormality is usually immediate, but improvement in hyperandrogenic symptoms may not be appreciated for 4–6 months. Additionally, OCPs protect the endometrium from hyperplasia by providing progesterone exposure. For all patients who have prolonged anovulation, some form of progesterone exposure is needed. For most, OCPs offer the most convenient solution. For patients with contraindications to oral estrogen, progesterone administration alone for at least 10 days per month can be prescribed. Alternative routes of administration of progesterone such as the progestin-containing IUD, progesterone implant, and Depo-Provera injection will effectively protect the endometrium from hyperplasia but are less useful for improving symptoms of hyperandrogenism.

Several other medical treatments for hirsutism are also available for severe symptoms or symptoms not responsive to OCPs [28] (Table 14.3). As many of these medications work via an anti-androgen mechanism, which could be teratogenic, they are often combined with the use of OCPs. Hirsutism medical therapies include spironolactone, flutamide, finasteride, ketoconazole, and eflornithine. The choice of type of treatment must consider the side effect profile. Spironolactone (25–100 mg twice daily) acts as an androgen receptor blocker, preventing the action of androgens at the hair follicle. It is also a diuretic and should be avoided in patients with renal impairment owing to increased risk of hyperkalemia. Flutamide (125–250 mg/day) is a nonsteroidal anti-androgen, which is a teratogen and has been associated with hepatotoxicity rarely. Finasteride is a 5α-reductase inhibitor that prevents the formation of a potent androgen (DHT) that is the primary binding androgen at the hair follicle receptor. Finasteride is also a teratogen, but is associated with less renal or hepatic toxicity. Ketoconazole is an antifungal that inhibits steroid synthesis. Its use is limited by side effects of hypo-adrenalism and hepatotoxicity. Eflornithine is a topical treatment that is an irreversible inhibitor of ornithine decarboxylase, an enzyme that is important for the growth of hair. Optimal results are achieved when combined with mechanical removal of hair (see below). The above treatments for hirsutism offer moderate results over a long term of treatment. For most of the medications, response is often not noticeable until after months of treatment. Patients pursuing fertility are poor candidates for medical therapy given the potential for birth defect. They may choose alternative nonmedical therapies.

For patients with documented insulin resistance or glucose intolerance, insulin-sensitizing agents have been central to medical therapy. Metformin is a biguanide that acts by improving peripheral insulin sensitivity. It is currently approved by the Food and Drug Administration (FDA) for the treatment of type 2 diabetes mellitus (T2DM) but it has also been used extensively in the treatment of PCOS. Multiple studies have demonstrated an improvement in ovulation, menstrual cyclicity, and hirsutism with the initiation of metformin therapy [29]. In addition, metformin improves the cardiovascular and metabolic profiles of these

TABLE 14.3

Summary of Medical Treatments for PCOS

Medication and Dose	Mechanism	Indications	Contraindications and Side Effects
Oral contraceptives	Suppress ovulation and ovarian androgen production	Menstrual irregularity (prevention of endometrial disease); contraception; hirsuitism	Increased risk of thrombosis (low)
Spironolactone (50–100 mg twice daily)	Androgen receptor blocker and diuretic	Hirsuitism	Hepatic toxicity; renal dysfunction; potential teratogen; hyperkalemia (rare); hypotension; menstrual irregularity; polyuria
Finasteride (2.5–5.0 mg daily)	5α-Reductase inhibitor	Hirsuitism	Teratogen (can be absorbed through skin/do not handle); potential renal or hepatic toxicity (rare)
Flutamide (250–500 mg daily)	Anti-androgen	Hirsuitism	Hepatic toxicity (rare but could be severe); teratogen; yellow urine
Ketoconazole (400 mg daily)	Steroidogenesis inhibitor	Hirsuitism	Adrenal insufficiency; hepatotoxicity
Eflornithine (13.9% cream twice daily)	Ornithine decarboxylase inhibitor	Hirsuitism	Skin sensitivity
Clomiphene (50–150 mg × 5 days)	SERM/partial estrogen agonist at the pituitary	Ovulation induction	Multiple gestations (<10%); pituitary edema (rare) with visual changes; headache; hot flashes; mood lability
Letrozole (2.5–7.5 mg × 5 days)	Aromatase inhibitor	Ovulation induction	Contraindicated with hepatic disease; headaches, hot flashes
Metformin (500–2000 mg daily)	Biguanide; insulin-sensitizing agent	Ovulation induction (not first-line); diabetes prevention	Contraindicated with renal or hepatic disease; lactic acidosis (higher risk if renal disease); diarrhea

Note: Combined therapy with OCPs and anti-androgens is often utilized for higher efficacy with contraception for the teratogen risk.

patients, mainly reducing their risk of T2DM [30]. The recommended starting dose is 500 mg of the slow-release tablets once daily, followed by a gradual increase over weeks to months up to 2 g daily, if tolerated. Major side effects of metformin include gastrointestinal upset (diarrhea). Lactic acidosis is a significant but rare complication of metformin use and is almost exclusively encountered in patients with renal disease.

For infertility, ovulation induction with clomiphene citrate (CC) has been the traditional treatment for PCOS. CC is a nonsteroidal selective estrogen-receptor modulator (SERM) that acts on the pituitary to increase endogenous production of FSH. It was the first ovulation induction agent utilized in patients with oligomenorrhea and still remains the agent of choice for anovulatory infertility. The most recent joint ESHRE/ASRM recommendations suggest CC for up to six ovulatory cycles. When administered to anovulatory PCOS patients, it results in a 60%–80% ovulation rate and a 30%–40% pregnancy rate. The dose of CC is usually started at 50 mg for 5 days in the follicular phase and increased up to 150 mg as needed to achieve ovulation. The main side effects associated with CC include multiple gestation (5%–10%), hot flashes, and mood changes. Visual changes owing to pituitary edema are rarely encountered but warrant immediate discontinuation of the medication for symptom resolution.

Aromatase inhibitors (letrozole) may also be considered as treatment for ovulation induction [9]. Letrozole is also useful for patients who fail initial treatment with clomid either because of side effects, clomid resistance (no ovulation at highest dose), or unsuccessful cycles [31]. Aromatase inhibitors decrease serum estradiol concentrations, which decreases negative feedback to the pituitary, thereby increasing FSH. A recent multicenter randomized controlled trial conducted by the Reproductive Medicine Network compared CC to letrozole and demonstrated that letrozole resulted in higher ovulation rates and higher live birth rates than CC with no difference in pregnancy loss rate [32] (Figure 14.3). Importantly, the mean BMI in this study was 35 kg/m² and letrozole resulted in improved live birth rates

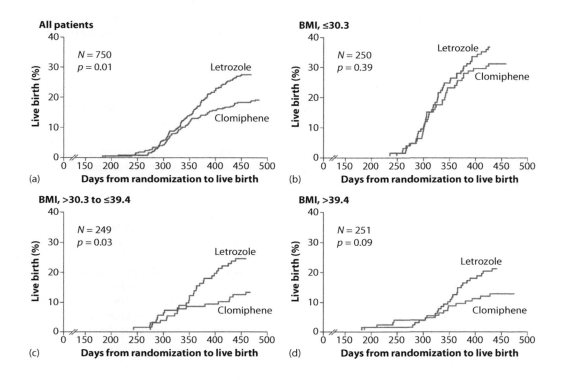

FIGURE 14.3 Kaplan–Meier curves for live birth. Live-birth rates are shown according to treatment group in panel (a) and according to treatment group and BMI, in thirds, in panels (b), (c), and (d). (Reprinted from Legro RS, Brzyski RG, Diamond MP et al. Letrozole versus clomiphene for infertility in the polycystic ovary syndrome. *N Engl J Med* 2007;356(6):119–129. Copyright 2014 Massachusetts Medical Society. All rights reserved.)

in all BMI quartiles, with a more pronounced effect in patients with BMI >30 kg/m². Treatment with letrozole is also associated with a reduction in multiple gestation risk because letrozole is associated with improved monofollicular ovulation compared to CC [33]. The dose of letrozole is usually started at 2.5 mg for 5 days in the follicular phase and increased up to 7.5 mg as needed to achieve ovulation. The most common side effects with letrozole are fatigue and headache. Letrozole is not currently FDA approved for ovulation induction. An analysis of the risk of birth defects in a large multicenter trial demonstrated no increased risk of birth defects in babies who were conceived via letrozole compared to CC [32].

Metformin has also been shown to increase ovulation in PCOS patients in several small observational studies. However, it does not appear to be as effective as clomiphene or letrozole for pregnancy and live birth. A randomized controlled trial by the Reproductive Medicine Network compared the efficacy of metformin and clomiphene [34]. Six hundred twenty-six PCOS patients were randomized to one of three treatment arms: clomiphene citrate (CC), metformin (M), or CC combined with M (CC/M). The cumulating pregnancy rates at the end of 6 months in the CC, M, and CC/M groups were 22.5%, 7.2%, and 26.8%, respectively. Although patients with metformin did ovulate, this did not translate to a comparable rate of live birth. Thus, metformin as a single agent for the treatment of infertility is not recommended. A subanalysis of this study confirmed the significant role of obesity in the prognosis of patients undergoing fertility treatments. For all groups, increased BMI was correlated with a reduced chance of a live birth [35]. There are conflicting reports as to whether metformin is useful as an adjuvant to CC in improving live birth rates but it may be useful in women with insulin resistance.

Gonadotropins or in vitro fertilization (IVF) offers good success rates, but can lead to an overresponse in PCOS patients, and therefore, close monitoring is essential. Patients most at risk are those with an elevated baseline AMH level or high antral follicle count [36]. Low-dose stimulation protocols are generally employed to mediate this risk. Advances in IVF protocols, including the use of leuprolide (Lupron) for ovulation trigger and embryo freeze-all cycles, have significantly reduced the risk of ovarian hyperstimulation syndrome in women with PCOS.

Nonmedical Therapies

Cosmetic procedures are frequently utilized for the treatment of hirsutism and are quite effective. These include bleaching, shaving, plucking, waxing, depilatory creams, electrolysis, light-assisted hair removal, and laser. Electrolysis and laser photothermolysis are among the most effective but also most expensive treatments. Laser therapy is most effective in patients with darker hair and lighter skin, where selective hair follicle damage is favored. These treatments can be used in combination with medical therapies.

Surgical Interventions

The surgical treatment for ovulation induction in patients with PCOS involves multiple ovarian punctures, i.e., "ovarian drilling." Before the advent of artificial reproductive technology, ovarian wedge resection was the only treatment that was offered to the PCOS patient, with ensuing postsurgery ovulation rates reported as high as 70%–80%. More recently, with laparoscopic advances, this procedure has progressed to laparoscopic ovarian diathermy (LOD) or laser. The main indication for surgical intervention is clomid or letrozole resistance in anovulatory PCOS patients. When compared with clomid–metformin combination treatment, LOD resulted in comparable ovulation and pregnancy rates [37]. A known complication of the procedure is adnexal adhesions. Long-term effects on ovarian function are unknown.

Summary

PCOS is a complex clinical syndrome that is characterized by hyperandrogenism and ovulatory dysfunction. For accurate diagnosis, other endocrinopathies must be excluded. Presentations can vary significantly, but often include comorbidities of obesity, glucose intolerance, and other metabolic derangements. Anovulatory infertility is another hallmark of this disorder. Management is directed toward specific symptoms experienced and includes lifetime monitoring for risk factors. A multidisciplinary approach with the inclusion of lifestyle modifications is the key to optimal health outcomes for PCOS patients.

REFERENCES

1. March WA, Moore VM, Willson KJ, Phillips DI, Normal RJ, Davies MJ. The prevalence of polycystic ovary syndrome in a community sample assessed under contrasting diagnostic criteria. *Hum Reprod* 2010;25(2):544–51.
2. Zawadski JK, Dunaif A. Diagnostic criteria for polycystic ovary syndrome; towards a rational approach. In: Dunaif A, Givens JR, Haseltine F (eds.) *Polycystic Ovary Syndrome*. Boston: Blackwell Scientific; 1992. pp. 377–84.
3. The Rotterdam ESHRE/ASRM-Sponsored PCOS Consensus Workshop Group. Revised 2003 consensus on diagnostic criteria and long-term health risks related to polycystic ovary syndrome (PCOS). *Fertil Steril* 2004;81(1):19–25.
4. Azziz R, Carmina E, Dewailly D, Diamanti-Kandarakis E, Escobar-Morreale HF, Futterweit W, Janssen OE, Legro RS, Norman RJ, Taylor AE, Witchel SF. Position statement: Criteria for defining polycystic ovary syndrome as a predominantly hyperandrogenic syndrome: An Androgen Excess Society guideline. *J Clin Endocrinol Metab* 2006;91(11):4237–45.
5. Teede HJ, Misso ML, Deeks AA, Moran LJ, Stuckey BG, Wong JL, Norman RJ, Costello MF. Assessment and management of polycystic ovary syndrome: Summary of an evidence-based guideline. *Med J Aust* 2011;195:S65–112.

6. Johnson T, Kaplan L, Ouyang P, Rizza R. National Institutes of Health. Evidence-based Methodology Workshop on Polycystic Ovary Syndrome. National Institutes of Health (NIH) Evidence-based Methodology Workshop 2012.

7. Legro RS, Arslanian SA, Ehrmann DA, Hoeger KM, Murad MH, Pasquali R, Welt CK, Endocrine S. Diagnosis and treatment of polycystic ovary syndrome: An Endocrine Society clinical practice guideline. *J Clin Endocrinol Metab* 2013;98:4565–92.

8. Conway G, Dewailly D, Diamanti-Kandarakis E, Escobar-Morreale HF, Franks S, Gambineri A, Kelestimur F, Macut D, Micic D, Pasquali R et al. Group EPSI. The polycystic ovary syndrome: A position statement from the European Society of Endocrinology. *Eur J Endocrinol* 2014;171:1–29.

9. Balen AH, Morley LC, Miso M, Franks S, Legro RS, Wijeyaratne CN, Stener-Victorin E, Fauser BCJM, Norman RJ, Teede H. The management of anovulatory infertility in women with polycystic ovary syndrome: Analysis of the evidence to support the development of global WHO guidance. *Hum Reprod Update* 2016:1–22.

10. Johnstone EB, Rosen MP, Neril R, Trevithick D, Sternfeld B, Murphy R, Addauan-Andersen C, McConnell D, Pera RR, Cedars MI. The polycystic ovary post-Rotterdam: A common, age-dependent finding in ovulatory women without metabolic significance. *J Clin Endocrinol Metab* 2010;95(11):4965–72.

11. Dewailly D, Lujan ME, Carmina E, Cedars MI, Laven J, Norman RJ, Escobar-Morreale HF. Definition and significance of polycystic ovarian morphology: A task force report from the Androgen Excess and Polycystic Ovary Syndrome Society. *Hum Reprod Update* 2014;20:334–352.

12. Yildiz BO, Bolour S, Woods K, Moore A, Azziz R. Visually scoring hirsutism. *Hum Reprod Update* 2010;16(1):51–64.

13. Ferriman D, Gallwey JD. Clinical assessment of body hair growth in women. *J Clin Endocrinol Metab* 1961;21:1440–47.

14. Fauser BC, Tarlatzis BC, Rebar RW, Legro RS, Balen AH, Lobo R, Carmina H, Chang RJ, Yildiz BO, Laven JS et al. Consensus on women's health aspects of polycystic ovary syndrome (PCOS). Amsterdam ESHRE/ASRM-Sponsored 3rd PCOS Consensus Workshop Group. *Hum Reprod* 2012 Jan;27(1):14–24.

15. Ehrmann DA, Barnes RB, Rosenfield RL, Cavaghan MK, Imperial J. Prevalence of impaired glucose tolerance and diabetes in women with polycystic ovary syndrome. *Diabetes Care* 1999 Jan;22(1):141–6.

16. Legro RS, Gnatuk CL, Kunselman AR, Dunaif A. Changes in glucose tolerance over time in women with polycystic ovary syndrome: A controlled study. *J Clin Endocrinol Metab* 2005 Jun;90(6):3236–42.

17. Apridonidze T, Essah PA, Iuorno MJ, Nestler JE. Prevalence and characteristics of the metabolic syndrome in women with polycystic ovary syndrome. *J Clin Endocrinol Metab* 2005 Apr;90(4):1929–35.

18. Rassi A, Veras AB, dos Reis M, Pastore DL, Bruno LM, Bruno RV, de Avila MA, Nardi AE. Prevalence of psychiatric disorders in patients with polycystic ovary syndrome. *Compr Psychiatry* 2010;51(6):599–602.

19. Deeks AA, Gibson-Helm ME, Teede HJ. Anxiety and depression in polycystic ovary syndrome: A comprehensive investigation. *Fertil Steril* 2010;93(7):2421–3.

20. Morales AJ, Laughlin GA, Bützow T, Maheshwari H, Baumann G, Yen SS. Insulin, somatotropic, and luteinizing hormone axes in lean and obese women with polycystic ovary syndrome: Common and distinct features. *J Clin Endocrinol Metab* 1996;81:2854–64.

21. Dunaif A, Segal KR, Futterweit W, Dobrjansky A. Profound peripheral insulin resistance, independent of obesity, in polycystic ovary syndrome. *Diabetes* 1989;38:1165–74.

22. Ehrmann, D.A. Medical progress: Polycystic ovary syndrome. *N Engl J Med* 2005;352:1223–36.

23. Eagleson CA et al. Polycystic ovarian syndrome: Evidence that flutamide restores sensitivity of the gonadotropin-releasing hormone pulse generator to inhibition by estradiol and progesterone. *J Clin Endocrinol Metab* 2000;85:4047–52.

24. Salehi M, Bravo-Vera R, Sheikh A, Gouller A, Poretsky L. Pathogenesis of polycystic ovary syndrome: What is the role of obesity? *Metab Clin Exp* 2004;53:358–76.

25. Daniels TL, Berga SL. Resistance of gonadotropin releasing hormone drive to sex steroid-induced suppression in hyperandrogenic anovulation. *J Clin Endocrinol Metab* 1997;82:4179–80.

26. Hall JE, Taylor AE, Hayes FJ, Crowley WF. Insights into hypothalamic–pituitary dysfunction in polycystic ovary syndrome. *J Endocrinol Invest* 1998;21:602–11.

27. Huber-Buchholz MM, Carey DG, Normal RJ. Restoration of reproductive potential by lifestyle modification in obese polycystic ovary syndrome: Role of insulin sensitivity and luteinizing hormone. *J Clin Endocrinol Metab* 1999;84:1470–4.

28. Moghetti P, Toscano V. Treatment of hirsutism and acne in hyperandrogenism. *Best Pract Res Clin Endocrinol Metab* 2006;20(2):221–34.
29. Tang T, Lord JM, Norman RJ, Yasmin E, Balen AH. Insulin-sensitising drugs for women with polycystic ovary syndrome, oligo amenorrhea and subfertility. *Cochrane Database Syst Rev* 2010;20(1).
30. Knowler WC, Barrett-Connor E, Fowler SE, Hamman RF, Lachin JM, Walker EA, Nathan DM. Diabetes Prevention Program Research Group. Reduction in the incidence of type 2 diabetes with lifestyle intervention or metformin. *N Engl J Med* 2002;346(6):393–403.
31. Palomba S, Falbo A, Zullo F. Management strategies for ovulation induction in women with polycystic ovary syndrome and known clomifene citrate resistance. *Curr Opin Obstet Gynecol* 2009;21:465–73.
32. Legro RS, Brzyski RG, Diamond MP, Coutifaris C, Schlaff WD, Casson P, Christman GM, Huang H, Yan Q, Alvero R et al. Network NRM Letrozole versus clomiphene for infertility in the polycystic ovary syndrome. *N Engl J Med* 2014;371:119–29.
33. Franik S, Kremer JA, Nelen WL, Farquhar C, Marjoribanks J. Aromatase inhibitors for subfertile women with polycystic ovary syndrome: Summary of a Cochrane Review. *Fertil Steril* 2015;103:353–5.
34. Legro RS, Barnhart HX, Schlaff WD, Carr BR, Diamond MP, Carson SA, Steinkampf MP, Coutifaris C, McGovern PG, Cataldo NA, Gosman GG, Nestler JE, Giucice LC, Leppert PC, Myers ER; Cooperative Multicenter Reproductive Medicine Network. Clomiphene, metformin, or both for infertility in the polycystic ovarian syndrome. *N Engl J Med* 2007;356(6):551–66.
35. Rausch ME, Legro RS, Barnhart HX, Schlaff WD, Carr BR, Diamond MP, Carson SA, Steinkampf MP, McGovern PG, Cataldo NA, Gosman GG, Nestler JE, Giudice LC, Leppert PC, Myers ER, Coutifaris C; Reproductive Medicine Network. Predictors of pregnancy in women with polycystic ovarian syndrome. *J Clin Endocrinol Metab* 2009;94(9):3183–4.
36. Nardo LG, Yates AP, Roberts SA, Pemberton P, Laing I. The relationships between AMH, androgens, insulin resistance and basal ovarian follicular status in non-obese subfertile women with and without polycystic ovary syndrome. *Hum Reprod* 2009;24:2917–23.
37. Abu Hashim H, El Lakany N, Sherief L. Combined metformin and clomiphene citrate versus laparoscopic ovarian diathermy for ovulation induction in clomiphene-resistant women with polycystic ovary syndrome: A randomized controlled trial. *J Obstet Gynaecol Res* 2011;37(3):169–77.

15

Recurrent Pregnancy Loss

Benjamin Lannon and Alison E. Zimon

The evaluation and management of couples with recurrent pregnancy loss (RPL) can often be challenging for both the clinician and the patient. For the patient, the devastation caused by a single pregnancy loss, let alone repeated losses, is emotionally straining and further burdensome because of uncertain causality and prognosis. The clinician is faced with addressing the psychosocial needs of the patient while embarking on a complex and sometimes ambiguous series of tests and treatment options that may not guarantee the desired outcome of a healthy live birth. Caring for the RPL patient requires responsiveness to the evolving diagnostic and treatment algorithms for RPL while focusing on the individual needs and therapy goals of the patient.

Defining Recurrent Pregnancy Loss

Traditionally, RPL has been defined by three or more losses. The Practice Committee of the American Society for Reproductive Medicine (ASRM) defines RPL as "... a disease distinct from infertility, defined by two or more failed pregnancies. When the cause is unknown, each pregnancy loss merits careful review to determine whether specific evaluation may be appropriate. After three or more losses, a thorough evaluation is warranted" [1]. The ASRM definition is restricted to clinically recognized pregnancy losses, with pregnancy confirmed by ultrasonography or histopathologic examination. In efforts to minimize the unnecessary hardship to patients who may suffer otherwise preventable pregnancy loss, most clinicians favor diagnosing RPL after two consecutive losses, despite recognition of the effort and cost associated with a full RPL diagnostic evaluation. It is important to note that many of the potential etiologies of RPL are not absolute, so the occurrence of interval live births does not preclude a diagnosis of RPL [2]. Certainly, each case of RPL should be considered individually and recommendations be based on the needs of the specific couple including their history of loss, prior live births, or other obstetric complications, rather than focus purely on the number of miscarriages [3].

Incidence

In young women, 15%–20% of clinically recognized pregnancies and upward of 50% of all pregnancies undergo spontaneous loss. These figures increase substantially with maternal age to as high as 40% and 85%, respectively, in women 40 years and older. The chance of having two consecutive losses is 5%, with 1% of couples experiencing three consecutive miscarriages [1].

Etiology

A number of etiologies have been proposed for RPL, and they may present alone or in combination. When counseling patients with RPL, it is helpful to present the potential etiologies in broad terms including

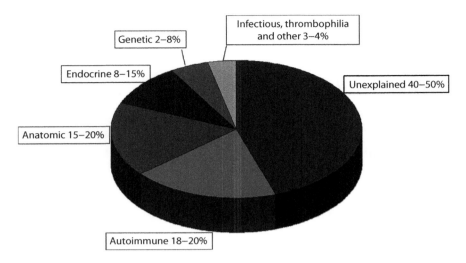

FIGURE 15.1   Causes of recurrent pregnancy loss.

anatomic factors, genetic variations, endocrinopathies, thrombophilias, autoimmune phenomena, and infectious etiologies. Despite these various potential causes, the majority of cases of RPL, around 50%, remain unexplained [4], a feature of this condition that is met with further frustration and helplessness for patients. In addition, because of the nonspecific nature of many of these etiologies, there is potential to attribute the cause of RPL to an incidental finding.

An important consideration in the evaluation of RPL is the age of the patient, as the rate of spontaneous miscarriage increases with maternal age. This is not included in the formal definition of RPL and other causes of RPL can occur at any age. However, the clinician must assess the role of declining oocyte quality and age-related spontaneous aneuploidy rates when beginning an assessment [2]. Another consideration is the timing of the miscarriage. If due to a specific etiology, RPL tends to occur at the same gestational age. Factors associated with embryonic loss, <10 weeks gestation, are different from those presenting with late RPL typically between 10 and 16 weeks gestation [5]. Likewise, there are obstetric factors, such as cervical insufficiency, that may contribute to late second trimester loss or extreme preterm delivery that are not included in this topic (Figure 15.1).

Anatomic Factors

Anatomic factors contributing to RPL are divided into congenital and acquired factors, and together account for 15%–25% of RPL. Congenital anomalies, including septate, bicornuate, unicornuate, and didelphic uteri, are found more commonly in women with RPL than the general population. Septate uterus is the most prevalent anomaly and also is the anomaly most tightly linked to reproductive failure, with an associated pregnancy loss rate as high as 79% [6]. An association between arcuate uterus and RPL is uncertain [7]. However, the specific contribution of these findings to RPL is difficult to quantify because of the varying diagnostic and management techniques reported in the literature. The pathophysiology is thought to be primarily a vascular phenomenon where there is reduced perfusion of the uterine septum and abnormal development of the overlying endometrium [5,8].

Acquired uterine factors such as fibroids, polyps, and Asherman's syndrome may also contribute to RPL. These factors may have some impact on embryonic implantation or uterine receptivity. The contribution of these pathologies to abnormal implantation, placentation, and pregnancy growth is speculative but is likely similarly related to aberrant vascularization and insufficient endometrial support of the pregnancy combined with alterations in the intrauterine immunological milieu favoring inflammation rather than growth [6].

Genetic Factors

In sporadic loss, chromosomal abnormalities account for at least 50% of clinically diagnosed spontaneous abortions and perhaps upward of 60%–75% of all pregnancy losses [9]. In RPL, 25%–51% of fetal losses are demonstrated to be aneuploid [3].

In sporadic pregnancy loss attributed to aneuploidy, age is certainly the major determining factor, with the chance of loss increasing directly with age from a 15%–20% prevalence in women less than 35 years of age to 40% in women over 40 years. This is attributable to the accumulated risk of acquired meiotic segregation errors, which lead to oocyte and embryonic aneuploidy. Interestingly, the correlation of age-related aneuploidy is similar in the sporadic and RPL populations, suggesting that some cases of RPL, particularly in women over the age of 35 years, are attributed to probability alone [9] or that additional factors, independent of age and aneuploidy, are also important in RPL [10].

Parental structural chromosome abnormalities are observed in 2.5%–8% of RPL [3,11,12]. Translocations account for the majority of these cases and include balanced reciprocal translocations, in which two different segments of parental autosomes are exchanged, and balanced Robertsonian translocations, in which the long arms of two acrocentric chromosomes (chromosomes 13, 14, 15, 21, and 22) join to form a single new chromosome. Chromosome inversions and other parental karyotypic abnormalities are seen as well. In some series, translocations are more commonly found in the female partner of a couple with RPL and are more likely to result in loss than male-derived translocations. Couples with a translocation may present with a history of prior live birth, RPL at an early age, or a family history of RPL [2]. Segregation genetics would suggest predictable rates of unbalanced, balanced, and normal chromosomes in conceptuses. Yet in reality, the distribution is skewed and a relatively lower rate of balanced and normal pregnancies is observed than would be expected, resulting in a higher embryo and pregnancy loss rate [9]. Nevertheless, both miscarriages and normal pregnancies are possible outcomes in cases of parental structural chromosomes, and a history of recurrent losses interspersed with normal full-term pregnancies should instigate parental chromosome testing.

Endocrinopathies

The primary endocrinopathies associated with RPL are thyroid dysfunction, hyperprolactinemia, diabetes mellitus, and the polycystic ovarian syndrome.

A euthyroid state is critical for optimal function in reproduction and pregnancy and poorly controlled thyroid disease has been associated with poor pregnancy outcome and RPL. The prevalence of abnormal thyroid function may be 3%–7% in the RPL population [3]. Further, even a subtle hypofunction of the thyroid, as in subclinical hypothyroidism, or euthyroidism in the presence of thyroid autoimmunity (the presence of thyroid peroxidase and thyroglobulin antibodies) may be associated with failed placentation and RPL [13]. While not confirmed, the etiology may relate to the increased demands of thyroid hormone in pregnancy, the resulting impact on placental growth, and a potentially detrimental effect of thyroid antibodies on the placenta [14]. A recent review of the literature elucidates the role of thyroid hormone and thyroid antibodies in gamete function, embryogenesis, embryo implantation, and placentation. Abnormal thyroid function may affect any of these key reproductive processes and ultimately lead to pregnancy complication or failure. However, the underlying pathobiology as well as specific treatment regimens remain unclear [15].

A connection between glycemic control and insulin resistance on maintaining an ongoing healthy pregnancy has been established. Well-controlled diabetes mellitus does not seem to increase the risk of pregnancy loss. However, poor control is associated with RPL, and this may be related to the impact of hyperglycemia toward worsening underlying vascular disease or the impact of insulin resistance on fibrinolysis during placentation [2]. The prevalence of previously undiagnosed frank diabetes is expected to be low (<1%) in the RPL population [3]. Higher rates of pregnancy loss in PCO lend further evidence that insulin resistance, alone or combined with hyperandrogenism, may have a negative impact on placental growth and maintenance of pregnancy, and among patients with RPL, the prevalence of PCO is as high as 36%–56% [7].

Abnormal prolactin levels can be associated with RPL potentially relating to an association with auto-immunity as in lupus or anti-phospholipid syndrome or alternatively as a marker of hypothalamic–pituitary dysfunction in the setting of neuroendocrine stress [7].

The impact of deficient production of progesterone in the luteal phase has been hypothesized as a cause of RPL, though substantial data to prove causality between progesterone deficiency or adequacy and pregnancy outcome have not been established [2,7,16].

Autoimmune Phenomena

The antiphospholipid antibodies are the most significant autoimmune phenomena associated with RPL occurring in between 18% and 20% of cases [3,10,17]. Antiphospholipid antibodies have been associated with both recurrent embryonic and fetal (>10 week) loss. In addition, they have been connected with other obstetric complications such as preeclampsia and growth restriction, as well as venous thrombo-embolism [18]. Specific diagnostic criteria for the antiphospholipid antibody syndrome are listed below as well as indications for testing. There is likely an overlap between patients with isolated positive anti-bodies and unrelated sporadic miscarriage, and therefore testing should be done with an appropriate history [19]. Likewise, given the potential for additional obstetric and maternal complications, treatment guidelines should be followed. The role of other antibody and rheumatologic testing such as phosphatidyl inositol, antinuclear antibody, and specific lymphocyte testing is uncertain.

Celiac disease is another autoimmune disorder that has been associated with several obstetric com-plications. A recent cohort study revealed a higher percentage of spontaneous abortions in women with celiac (50.6% vs. 40.6%), compared to controls. It is unclear if these results are mitigated by a gluten-free diet [20].

Immunomodulatory Factors

Immune modulation at the interface between the embryo and the maternal decidua is a critical factor in successful implantation and maintenance of pregnancy. Major shifts in the population of uterine natural killer (NK) cells are observed during the menstrual cycle with a preponderance of the CD56^{bright}CD16$^-$ NK cell subtype at the time of implantation, which is distinct from the NK cell profile of CD56^{dim}CD16$^+$ cells that predominate in peripheral blood, and it is believed that the uterine NK cells play an essential supportive role in implantation. Regulatory T cells (T_{reg}), macrophages, dendritic cells, and innate lym-phoid cells are also important in the uterine decidua and maintenance of pregnancy. Though widely hypothesized, it has not been clearly established whether abnormalities or modulation of uterine NK cells, T_{reg} cells, or other immune dysfunction are responsible for RPL [21,22].

Inherited Thrombophilias

Thrombophilia is defined by any disorder associated with an increased risk of thrombosis and venothrom-boembolism (VTE), and a number of inherited thrombophilias have been connected with RPL and other obstetric complications [19]. Specific inherited thrombophilias linked to adverse obstetric outcomes and pregnancy loss include Factor V Leiden mutation, prothrombin gene mutation, anti-thrombin III deficiency, protein C deficiency, and protein S deficiency. While early data suggested that methylene tetrahydrofolate reductase mutations and hyperhomocysteinemia caused VTE, more recent data have not validated this causality. Perhaps the most controversial of the etiologies, the association, causality, and treatment of inherited thrombophilias in patients with RPL is a source of debate in the field. Some studies demonstrate no increased prevalence of heritable thrombophilias in the RPL population [3]. The thrombosis of uteroplacental vessels underlies the theoretical pathobiology of these conditions and they are typically associated with late RPL, and the role of thrombophilias in early pregnancy and embryonic loss (<10 weeks) is unclear [23]. Likewise, the degree of risk for RPL and efficacy of treatment have been debated in the literature and in practice [24].

Infectious Etiologies

Based on associations with sporadic miscarriage, identification and treatment of certain microorganisms have been proposed in the evaluation of RPL. However, no studies have clearly identified infectious agents as a cause for RPL, and therefore, screening for *Chlamydia*, *Mycoplasma*, and *Ureaplasma* species is not recommended [2].

Lifestyle and Exposures

Lifestyle stress has been frequently implicated anecdotally and scientifically as an etiology for pregnancy loss and RPL. It is believed that stress-induced increased adrenocorticosteroids or stress-induced decreased immunity may negatively affect the ability to maintain a pregnancy. Dietary factors including high caffeine intake of the equivalent of over three cups of coffee a day or low antioxidant serum levels are associated with RPL [25]. Tobacco smoking and other toxic environmental exposures have also been associated with RPL. While the data are not conclusive, a possible link between these lifestyle factors cannot be completely excluded [26].

Insufficient levels of vitamin D may also be associated with RPL. This may be mediated by vitamin D's role in cellular immune function in which vitamin D inhibits the T cell activation of NK cells. In a retrospective study of women with RPL, almost half were found to have hypovitaminosis D. In addition, in vitro studies of these women revealed altered immune function with an increase in NK cell activity [27].

Sperm Factor

The sperm genome and sperm DNA integrity are known to be critical factors in embryo development and the maintenance of pregnancy, and high levels of sperm DNA fragmentation may be associated with poorer embryo quality and lower rates of conception and embryo survival. Increasing paternal age is associated with higher levels of DNA fragmentation and higher pregnancy loss rates. A recent meta-analysis of 16 cohort studies suggests that pregnancy loss may be increased twofold with increased sperm DNA fragmentation and that normal loss rates may be restored by applying methods to preselect normal sperm followed by intracytoplasmic sperm injection (ICSI) [28].

Other

Several additional rare or less well-defined conditions may be associated with spontaneous miscarriage and possibly RPL. These include obesity, diminished ovarian reserve, and teratospermia.

Evaluation and History

For patients and clinicians alike, the uncertainty of the etiology and the inability to predict recurrence of RPL create a strong incentive to identify a specific cause. While an extensive battery of testing could be performed, likely the best approach is to limit diagnostics to identify etiologies where causality and therapy options have been established by evidence-based research. The initial approach includes a thorough medical history and physical exam with attention to details of timing and outcomes of prior pregnancies and miscarriages, presence of uterine and pelvic factors, and evidence of associated medical conditions (Table 15.1).

Personal and Familial History

The personal history questionnaire should include symptoms and diagnoses related to endocrinopathies, autoimmune disorders, coagulopathies, obesity, infections, and lifestyle and environmental exposures.

TABLE 15.1

Diagnostic Testing for Recurrent Pregnancy Loss

Evaluation	Test
Uterine cavity defects and Mullerian anomalies	Hysterosalpingogram Saline-infused sonography 3D ultrasound or MRI Diagnostic hysteroscopy
Chromosomal abnormalities	Fetal tissue chromosome analysis by karyotype, FISH, or CGH Parental chromosome analysis by karyotype, FISH, or CGH
Endocrinopathies	TSH, FT4, anti-thyroid peroxidase antibodies, anti-thyroglobulin antibodies Fasting glucose, hemoglobin A1C% Prolactin Cycle day 3 FSH and estradiol
Antiphospholipid syndrome	Lupus anticoagulant, anticardiolipin IgG and IgM antibodies, anti-β2 glycoprotein-1 antibodies
Inherited thrombophilia	Factor V Leiden gene mutation, prothrombin G20210A gene mutation, protein C and protein S functional assay, anti-thrombin III levels
Infectious	Genital cultures (symptom-based)
Other	Screening for exposures, celiac disease, teratospermia, obesity

Note: CGH, comparative genomic hybridization; FISH, fluorescent in situ hybridization.

The reproductive history should include past uterine instrumentation, pelvic infection, total number of pregnancies, and outcomes. Pregnancy loss history should specify sequential or sporadic timing of pregnancy, the gestational age at diagnosis, whether fetal cardiac activity was documented, management, comorbidities, and fetal chromosome data if available. Familial history should include a thorough screening for RPL, stillbirth, or other fetal loss, as well as mental retardation, endocrinopathies, autoimmune disorders, coagulopathies, and obesity.

Physical Exam

Specific focus on the physical exam should be placed on identifying signs of thyroid disease, diabetes, lupus, rheumatoid arthritis, other autoimmune disorders, and pelvic anatomy.

Diagnostic Testing

It is recommended to initiate a diagnostic evaluation of RPL after two consecutive RPLs. This approach is favored over waiting for the classic definition of three consecutive losses in part to minimize further distress to a patient should a treatable etiology be identified. Further, the probability of identifying a pathoplysiological factor through testing is similar (40%) in patients with two and with three consecutive losses [3,19].

Uterine Examination

A hysterosalpingogram (HSG) is the preferred single uterine cavity study. This will allow accurate diagnosis of uterine anomalies and detection of intracavitary masses or lesions with a positive predictive value of upward of 85%. If HSG findings are not definitive, or if more specific testing is desired, a saline infused sonography (SIS) is recommended to detect intracavitary lesions with a positive predictive value of 95%. If definitive diagnosis is desired or intracavitary lesions are suspected based on prior radiological studies, hysteroscopy in the office or operative setting should be performed. If a congenital uterine anomaly is suspected based on HSG or SIS, a 3D ultrasound or pelvic magnetic resonance imaging can be performed.

Genetic Testing

A chromosomal analysis on both partners is recommended to assess for parental potential structural chromosomal abnormalities. In the patient with RPL, analysis of fetal chromosomes will prove extremely helpful, particularly as evidence of sporadic aneuploidy may be definitively diagnostic and obviate additional testing. The routine and traditional method of chromosome analysis is a metaphase spread karyotype on cultured parental blood lymphocytes or cultured chorionic villi cells. An additional option is employing newer comparative genomic hybridization (CGH) technologies, which, in the case of aneuploidy, identify the paternal or the maternal line as the source for the acquired or inherited defect (Figure 15.2).

Endocrine Testing

The panel of endocrine testing to screen for potential endocrinopathies associated with RPL includes tests to assess for underlying thyroid disease, hyperprolactinemia, diabetes, and diminished ovarian reserve.

Specifically, this serological testing panel includes thyroid-stimulating hormone (TSH), with or without free thyroxine (FT4), anti-thyroid peroxidase antibodies and anti-thyroglobulin antibodies, prolactin (PRL), fasting glucose or HgbA1C, and cycle day 3 follicle-stimulating hormone (FSH) and estradiol.

Diagnostic Testing for Antiphospholipid Syndrome

In order to fulfill the laboratory testing criteria for antiphospholipid syndrome (APS), it is required to demonstrate positive serum antiphosphopholipids at significant levels on two or more occasions and at least 12 weeks apart. Positive testing for antiphospholipid antibodies includes the detection of lupus anticoagulant, medium to high titers of anticardiolipin IgG or IgM antibodies, and titers of anti-B2 glycoprotein-1 antibodies upward of the 99th percentile [29]. Anti-phosphatidyl serine levels may also be

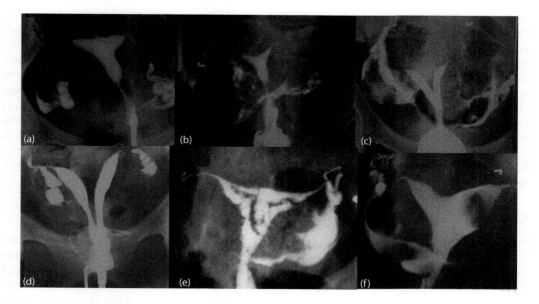

FIGURE 15.2 Hysterosalpingogram (HSG) images. The HSG is the preferred test to evaluate the uterine cavity in cases of RPL. The HSG images above are as follows: (a) normal uterine cavity; (b) arcuate cavity—note the slight depression impinging on the superior aspect of the cavity; this has no clinical significance; (c) uterine septum coming half way down the cavity; (d) a complete uterine septum; to differentiate a uterine septum versus bicornuate uterus, it is recommended to do a 3-D ultrasound or MRI; (e) Asherman's syndrome; and (f) intracavity uterine fibroid.

measured, but a correlation with RPL is less well established, and these antibodies are not included in the diagnostic criteria for APS.

Screening for Inherited Thrombophilia

The decision to include screening for inheritable thrombophilias in RPL is not straightforward. Causality between these conditions and adverse pregnancy outcomes early in gestation has not been established and the cost-effectiveness of ordering the thrombophilia testing panel in the RPL evaluation is questionable. Based on current opinions from ASRM and ACOG (American College of Obstetricians and Gynecologists), routine screening for inherited thrombophilias in women with RPL is not recommended. Nevertheless, one may consider inclusion of this laboratory screening in RPL, particularly when additional risk factors for coagulapathy are supported by the patients' personal or familial history or in patients with recurrent late fetal loss (>10 weeks) or with evidence of placental ischemia, infarction, or thrombosis. Testing should be limited to screening for abnormalities associated with thromboembolic events, and these include testing for Factor V Leiden gene mutation, prothrombin G20210A gene mutation, protein C and protein S deficiency via functional activity assays, and anti-thrombin III levels. Insufficient evidence exists to link hyperhomocysteinemia or methylene tetrahydrofolate reductase deficiency with RPL or VTE, and therefore testing for these is not currently recommended.

Management

Anatomic Factors

An improvement in obstetrical outcome after surgical correction of uterine anomalies has been best established in cases of uterine septi. Uterine septi are the most commonly diagnosed congenital uterine anomalies associated with early pregnancy loss and have been found to confer a risk of RPL of up to 79% [12]. Hysteroscopic metroplasty has been shown to decrease the chance of pregnancy loss to <15% and increase the chance of live birth from <20% to 35%–80% [6,11]. In cases of incidental diagnosis of uterine septi, it is not unreasonable to consider hysteroscopic myomectomy for prevention of pregnancy loss, though this approach is not universally advocated. Patients with Asherman's syndrome similarly benefit from surgical intervention via hysteroscopic adhesiolysis, which increases the chance for live birth and reduces rates of first- and second-trimester losses. The outcomes after hysteroscopic adhesiolysis are associated with severity of disease. The term pregnancy rate after surgical intervention may be upward of 81% and 66% for mild (American Fertility Society [AFS] Stage I) and moderate (AFS Stage II) disease, respectively. Given the partially irrecoverable losses to endometrial function in Asherman's syndrome, relatively high rates of pregnancy failure and relatively low chance for live birth (32% or less) are observed in patients with severe disease (AFS Stage III) after successful surgical resection [6]. In cases of polyps and fibroids, the link between etiology is less well established and decreased pregnancy loss rates have been demonstrated, but not consistently, in studies examining the impact of open myomectomy, hysteroscopic myomectomy, and hysteroscopic polypectomies on RPL (Table 15.2) [6].

Genetic Factors

Preimplantation genetic screening (PGS) is an option for couples with RPL as a result of aneuploidy, and recent major advances in embryo genetic screening platforms, trophoectoderm biopsy, and embryo vitrification have allowed marked increases in utilization and accuracy of this technology. The concept is to screen embryos at the blastocyst stage (embryo days 5–6) via biopsy to remove sample blastomeres and then test these cells for euploidy or aneuploidy by analyzing all 23 pairs of chromosomes via CGH, PCR, or next-generation sequencing (NGS) platform. Embryos are typically frozen and then euploid embryos are transferred in a subsequent endometrial preparation cycle. While complete outcomes data for newer PGS technologies suggest improved live birth rate, lower miscarriage rate, and shorter time to pregnancy in women over the age of 37 years, data for the RPL population are lacking. Of the limited

TABLE 15.2

Treatment Options for Recurrent Pregnancy Loss

Category	Diagnosis	Therapy
Uterine anomalies	Uterine septum	Hysteroscopic metroplasty
	Polyps	Polypectomy or myomectomy via laparoscopy
	Leiomyomas	or laparotomy
	Asherman's syndrome	Hysteroscopic adhesiolysis
Chromosomal abnormalities	Sporadic aneuploidy	Preimplantation genetic screening
	Parental chromosomal abnormality	
Endocrinopathies	Hypothyroidism	Levothyroxine
	Diabetes	Metformin, insulin, other
	Hyperprolactinemia	Bromocriptine or cabergoline
	Diminished ovarian reserve	Ovarian stimulation with FSH, IVF
Autoimmune	Antiphospholipid syndrome	Heparin (prophylactic dosing)
		Aspirin (low-dose)
Inherited thrombophilia	Factor V Leiden gene mutation	Anticoagulation in setting of VTE history
	Prothrombin G20210A gene mutation	
	Protein C deficiency	
	Protein S deficiency	
	Anti-thrombin III deficiency	
Infectious	Cervicitis	Antibiotics as appropriate
Other	Celiac disease	Treat underlying disorder
	Obesity	
	Teratospermia	

studies examining outcomes with PGS in RPL, most are retrospective, and limited prospective studies are available to date. PGS may in fact improve outcomes in RPL patients who successfully achieve a euploid embryo for transfer. However, when all cycle starts are considered, PGS may not improve the live birth rate per attempt given the high rate of PGS cancellation owing to insufficient embryo yield or blastulation, and in cases of low embryo yield, PGS may actually extend the time to pregnancy and live birth compared to those patients expectantly managed [30]. Biological and technical limitations of PGS include cellular mosaicism, the embryo's inherent ability to undergo some self-correction to demote aneuploid cells away from essential embryonic development pathways, and assay platform accuracy and precision. Nevertheless, the benefit of employing PGS in cases of RPL may include shortened time to pregnancy in patients with high oocyte and embryo yields, increased implantation rates, and decreased pregnancy loss rates. The psychological reassurance of transferring euploid rather than untested embryos is another benefit of PGS for RPL patients [31]. Cost-effectiveness studies have demonstrated a potential benefit of PGS when PGS is simply added to preexisting indications for IVF and when maternal age is 35 to 37 years or older, but PGS combined with IVF may prove to be cost-prohibitive for the patient or couple conceiving spontaneously without difficulty or in couples with advanced maternal age or those who have previously demonstrated high (>65%) embryonic aneuploidy [9]. Nevertheless, both RPL patients who chose PGS and those who opt for expectant management face a favorable prognostic outlook, with a 63%–71% chance of live birth without intervention. These data have been reproduced widely and support the benefits of natural selection as a viable option for RPL management [32].

In cases of increased male factor infertility, advanced paternal age, and increased sperm DNA fragmentation, the application of ICSI combined with various methods of preselection of normal sperm may improve embryo quality, increase the rates of ongoing pregnancy, and lower miscarriage [28].

Endocrinopathies

Though the extent to which endocrine dysfunction directly contributes to early pregnancy loss is not known, correction of underlying clinical or subclinical endocrinopathies is intuitive in the hope of not only minimizing the risk of early pregnancy loss but also optimizing general endocrine health as a woman embarks on a pregnancy. Hyperthyroid disease should be fully evaluated for underlying pathology including nodules, cancer, and Graves' disease and treated appropriately. In clinical hypothyroidism, levothyroxine treatment has been well established as a means to minimize adverse pregnancy outcomes of miscarriage and preterm birth. While not firmly established, levothyroxine treatment of autoimmune and subclinical hypothyroidism may also improve pregnancy outcomes and reduce pregnancy loss and RPL [13]. Levothyroxine dosing is based on weight and effect to achieve a TSH greater than 0.4 mIU/L and less than 2.5 mIU/L. Given the increased thyroid hormone demands of pregnancy, increasing the levothyroxine dose by 33% during early pregnancy is appropriate.

Dopamine agonists, bromocriptine, or cabergoline may be used to normalize elevated prolactin levels and discontinued once pregnancy occurs. Both medications appear to be non-teratogenic in pregnancy. As more pregnancy safety data are available, many providers favor bromocriptine use for treatment of hyperprolactinemia when pregnancy is anticipated.

Glucose intolerance and diabetes may be managed by diet and exercise and pharmacologically as needed to achieve normal fasting glucose levels and HbA1c levels before conception.

Thrombophilias

At this time, a connection between inherited thrombophilias and early pregnancy loss has not been firmly established, nor has a reduction in subsequent losses been demonstrated through anticoagulation. While still an area of debate, most guidelines, including ACOG's, dissuade from anticoagulation prophylaxis in cases of early RPL with underlying inheritable thrombophilia owing to the relative risk of treatment complication and the lack of proven benefit [18,33,34]. A recent systematic review of trials of low-molecular-weight heparin in women with placenta-mediated pregnancy complications failed to show a reduction of risk. The obstetric outcomes included preeclampsia, late pregnancy loss, placental abruption, and birth of a small-for-gestational-age neonate [35].

Autoimmune Phenomena

Substantial data have supported the benefits of anticoagulation in cases of antiphosphospholipid syndrome and prior adverse pregnancy outcomes including RPL. Based on randomized controlled trials and meta-analyses of available literature, the largest reduction in risk for RPL or other adverse pregnancy outcomes has been observed with a combination of heparin and aspirin. Therefore, at the present time, patients with APS should begin unfractionated or low-molecular-weight heparin at prophylactic dosing plus low-dose aspirin with the diagnosis of pregnancy [36–38]. The use of intravenous immunoglobulin or other immunomodulators for suspected autoimmune-mediated pregnancy loss is not recommended as a consistent benefit has not been demonstrated [39].

Immunotherapies

In attempts to foster implantation and to promote immunological tolerance of the embryo at the level of the maternal decidua, various immunotherapies, including intravenous immunoglobulin, granulocyte-macrophage colony stimulating factor, and intralipids (intravenous lipid emulsion), have been evaluated but none have consistently demonstrated increases in ongoing pregnancy or live birth. At the present time, immune-modulating therapies cannot be recommended for treatment of idiopathic RPL [40,41].

Counseling

RPL can be an emotionally and psychologically devastating condition for many patients. The uncertainty of etiology and potential for recurrence can be truly unsettling and may prevent individuals from attempting to conceive. It is equally likely for patients, in desperation, to adopt any number of superstitious behaviors or request unfounded testing or treatments. While many of these activities may provide some comfort, they also have potential for harm. It is essential to provide a careful explanation of what evidence exists for particular recommendations as well as to identify the patient's specific concerns and anxieties. It is also highly recommended that a mental health professional be available for additional counseling.

Prognosis

Fortunately, the majority of patients with RPL will achieve their goal of having a healthy child, with an overall chance of subsequent successful pregnancy of 65%. The challenge, no doubt, is helping patients through the difficult process of getting to that goal, while supporting those patients who must endure the potentially devastating impact of being in the 35% who are not successful.

REFERENCES

1. Practice Committee of American Society for Reproductive Medicine. Definitions of infertility and recurrent pregnancy loss. *Fertil Steril* 2008;90(5 Suppl):S60.
2. Rai R, Regan L. Recurrent miscarriage. *Lancet* 2006;368(9535):601–11.
3. Jaslow CR, Carney JL, Kutteh WH. Diagnostic factors identified in 1020 women with two versus three or more recurrent pregnancy losses. *Fertil Steril* 2010;93(4):1234–43.
4. Tang AW, Quenby S. Recent thoughts on management and prevention of recurrent early pregnancy loss. *Curr Opin Obstet Gynecol* 2010;22(6):446–51.
5. Branch DW, Gibson M, Silver RM. Clinical practice. Recurrent miscarriage. *N Engl J Med* 2010;363(18):1740–7.
6. Taylor E, Gomel V. The uterus and infertility. *Fertil Steril* 2008;89(1):1–16.
7. Porter TF, Scott JR. Evidence-based care of recurrent miscarriage. *Best Pract Res Clin Obstet Gynaecol* 2005;19(1):85–101.
8. Reichman DE, Laufer MR. Congenital uterine anomalies affecting reproduction. *Best Pract Res Clin Obstet Gynaecol* 2010;24:193–208.
9. Fritz MA, Speroff L. *Clinical Gynecologic Endocrinology and Infertility*, 8th ed. Philadelphia: Lippincott Williams & Wilkins; 2011. pp. 1191–1220.
10. Marquard K, Westphal LM, Milki AA, Lathi RB. Etiology of recurrent pregnancy loss in women over the age of 35 years. *Fertil Steril* 2010;94:1473–7.
11. Stephenson MD. Frequency of factors associated with habitual abortion in 197 couples. *Fertil Steril* 1996;66:24–9.
12. Ford HF, Schust DJ. Recurrent pregnancy loss: Etiology, diagnosis, and therapy. *Rev Obstet Gynecol* 2009;2(2):76–83.
13. Reid SM, Middleton P, Cossich MC, Crowther CA. Intervention for clinical and subclinical hypothyroidism in pregnancy. *Cochrane Database Syst Rev* 2010;7:CD007752.
14. Toulis KA, Goulis DG, Venetis CA et al. Risk of spontaneous miscarriage in euthyroid women with thyroid autoimmunity undergoing IVF: A meta-analysis. *Eur J Endocrinol* 2010;162(4);643–52.
15. Vissenberg R, Manders VD, Mastenbroek S, Fliers E, Afink GB, Ris-Stalpers C, Goddijn M, Bisschop PH. Pathophysiological aspects of thyroid hormone disorders/thyroid peroxidase autoantibodies and reproduction. *Hum Reprod Update* 2015 May–Jun;21(3):378–8.
16. Haas DM, Ramsey PS. Progesterone for preventing miscarriage. *Cochrane Database Syst Rev* 2008;16(2):CD003511.
17. Rey E, Kahn SR, David M, Shrier I. Thrombophilic disorders and fetal loss: A meta-analysis. *Lancet* 2003;361:901–8.
18. American College of Obstetricians and Gynecologists Committee on Practice Bulletins-Obstetrics. ACOG Practice Bulletin No. 118: Antiphospholipid syndrome. *Obstet Gynecol* 2011;117(1):192–9.
19. Said JM, Higgins JR, Moses EK et al. Inherited thrombophilia polymorphisms and pregnancy outcomes in nulliparous women. *Obstet Gynecol* 2010;115(1):5–13.
20. Moleski SM, Lindenmeyer CC, Veloski JJ et al. Increased rates of pregnancy complications in women with celiac disease. *Ann Gastroenterol* 2015;28(2):236–40.

21. Mori M, Bogdan A, Balassa T et al. The decidua—The maternal bed embracing the embryo—Maintains the pregnancy. *Semin Immunopathol* 2016;38(6):635–49.

22. Sharma S. Natural killer cells and regulatory T cells in early pregnancy loss. *Int J Dev Biol* 2014;58(0):219–29.

23. American College of Obstetricians and Gynecologists Committee on Practice Bulletins-Obstetrics. ACOG Practice Bulletin No. 138: Inherited thrombophilias in pregnancy. *Obstet Gynecol* 2013 Sep;122(3):706–17.

24. Branch DW. The truth about inherited thrombophilias and pregnancy. *Obstet Gynecol* 2010;115(1):2–4.

25. Ruder EH, Hartman TJ, Goldman MB. Impact on oxidative stress on female fertility. *Curr Opin Obstet Gynecol* 2009;21(3):219–22.

26. Parker VJ, Douglas AJ. Stress in early pregnancy: Maternal neuro-endocrine-immune response and effects. *J Reprod Immunol* 2010;85(1):86–92.

27. Ota K, Dambaeva S, Han AR, Beaman K, Gilman-Sachs A, Kwak-Kim J. Vitamin D deficiency may be a risk factor for recurrent pregnancy losses by increasing cellular immunity and autoimmunity. *Hum Reprod* 2014;29(2):208–9.

28. Robinson L, Gallos ID, Conner SJ, Rajkhowa M, Miller D, Lewis S, Kirkman-Brown J, Coomarasamy A. The effect of sperm DNA fragmentation on miscarriage rates: A systematic review and meta-analysis. *Hum Reprod* 2012 Oct;27(10):2908–17.

29. Lim W. Antiphospholipid antibody syndrome. *Hematology Am Soc Hematol Educ Program* 2009;233–39.

30. Murugappan G, Shahine LK, Perfetto CO, Hickok LR, Lathi RB. Intent to treat analysis of in vitro fertilization and preimplantation genetic screening versus expectant management in patients with recurrent pregnancy loss. *Hum Reprod* 2016 Aug;31(8):1668–74.

31. Fischer J, Colls P, Escudero T, Munne S. Preimplantation genetic diagnosis (PGS) improves pregnancy outcome for translocation carriers with a history of recurrent losses. *Fertil Steril* 2010;94(1):283–9.

32. Stephenson MD, Sierra S. Reproductive outcomes in recurrent pregnancy loss associated with a parental carrier of a structural chromosome rearrangement. *Hum Reprod* 2006;21(4):1076–82.

33. Benedetto C, Marozio L, Tavella AM et al. Coagulation disorders in pregnancy: Acquired and inherited thrombophilias. *Ann NY Acad Sci* 2010;1205:106–17.

34. Mantha S, Bauer KA, Zwicker JI. Low molecular weight heparin to achieve live birth following unexplained pregnancy loss: A systematic review. *J Thromb Haemost* 2010;8:263–8.

35. Rodger MA, Carrier M, Le Gal G et al. Low-molecular-weight heparin and recurrent placenta-mediated pregnancy complications: A meta-analysis of individual patient data from randomized controlled trials. *Lancet* 2016;388:2629–41.

36. Kaandorp SP, Goddijn M, van der Post JA et al. Aspirin plus heparin or aspirin alone in women with recurrent miscarriage. *N Engl J Med* 2010;362(17):1586–96.

37. Ziakas PD, Pavlou M, Voulgarelis M. Heparin treatment in antiphospholipid syndrome with recurrent pregnancy loss: A systematic review and meta-analysis. *Obstet Gynecol* 2010;115(6):1256–62.

38. Mak A, Cheung MW, Cheak AA, Ho RC. Combination of heparin and aspirin is superior to aspirin alone in enhancing live births in patients with recurrent pregnancy loss and positive anti-phospholipid antibodies: A meta-analysis of randomized controlled trials and meta-regression. *Rheumatology* 2010; 49:281–8.

39. Porter TF, LaCoursiere Y, Scott JR. Immunotherapy for recurrent miscarriage. *Cochrane Database Syst Rev* 2006;2:CD000112.

40. Wong LF, Porter TF, Scott JR. Immunotherapy for recurrent miscarriage. *Cochrane Database Syst Rev* 2014 Oct 21;(10):CD000112.

41. Christiansen OB, Larsen EC, Egerup P, Lunoee L, Egestad L, Nielsen HS. Intravenous immunoglobulin treatment for secondary recurrent miscarriage: A randomised, double-blind, placebo-controlled trial. *BJOG* 2015 Mar;122(4):500–8.

16

Fertility Preservation for Cancer Patients

David A. Ryley

In 2015, there were 810,170 new cases of cancer diagnosed in the United States among females, 29% of the total the result of breast cancer and, additionally, 60,290 new cases of breast carcinoma in situ. From 2009 to 2011, the probability of a cancer diagnosis among premenopausal women was 5.4% [1]. Improved cancer surveillance and treatment regimens have resulted in decreased mortality rates among this cohort, allowing these women to focus on survival and quality of life, including preservation of fertility. From 1975 to 2010, overall cancer 5-year survival rates among females increased by 19%, and breast cancer mortality among females has decreased by 35% in this period. Malignancies affecting younger women, such as breast cancer, cervical cancer, and lymphoma, have increased survival rates of greater than 70% as recorded from 2004 to 2010, significantly higher compared to the lower rates of 47%–75% recorded from 1975 to 1977, $p < 0.05$ [1].

In the United States, cancer is the second most common cause of death among children between the ages of 1 and 14 years, surpassed only by accidents [1]. In 2015, an estimated 10,380 children were diagnosed with cancer. The success of oncologic therapies is even more pronounced among cancers affecting these patients, including leukemia, cancers of the brain and nervous system, neuroblastomas, soft tissue sarcomas, renal tumors, and Hodgkin and non-Hodgkin lymphoma. The 5-year survival rate among children for all cancer sites combined improved from 58% for patients diagnosed in 1975–1977 to 83% in 2004–2010, $p < 0.05$ [1]. As of 2014, it was projected that 1 in 530 young adults (ages 20–39) were long-term survivors of a childhood malignancy [2].

Effects of Chemotherapy and Radiation on Fertility

Many treatments that have improved survival among both adults and children diagnosed with cancer are gonadotoxic, especially those that employ high doses of alkylating agents and radiation therapy directed near or toward the pelvis. The impact on the ovarian reserve is related to the accelerated depletion of the primordial germ cell pool resulting from these therapies.

Oogenesis is a process that begins in utero, approximately 3 weeks after conception, when the primordial germ cells derived from the endodermal yolk sac initiate their migration to the developing ovaries. These cells then undergo an inexorable differentiation to become primary oocytes, which, at the time of birth, are arrested in the prophase of the first meiotic division. At this time, there is no further differentiation of the germ cells, but a continuous apoptotic loss that depletes the supply from 1 to 2 million at birth to 300,000–500,000 at the time of puberty. Under the proper hormonal conditions, an ovum completes its first meiotic division in response to the maturation of the hypothalamic–pituitary–ovarian axis and the LH surge that causes the release of the oocyte on a monthly basis. Through ovulation and continued atresia of the nondominant follicles, the ovarian reserve is eventually depleted with an exponential loss of oocytes occurring at the age of 37 years up until the time of the menopause [3].

Alkylating agents (such as cyclophosphamide, ifosfamide, nitrosoureas, chlorambucil, melphalan, and busulfan), which are not cell cycle specific, confer their deleterious effect on the vast supply of primordial germ cells and carry the highest risk of ovarian failure. Anti-metabolites (such as methotrexate, bleomycin, 5-fluorouracil, actinomycin-D, mercaptopurine, and vincristine) affect the cells (granulosa and oocyte) of the metabolically active ovarian follicles and are considered to be low risk for gonadal dysfunction, while cisplatin appears to carry intermediate risk between the anti-metabolites and alkylating agents [4].

Women over the age of 40 years have a 90% chance of amenorrhea subsequent to multiagent chemotherapy, whereas the potential for premature ovarian failure in younger patients varies between 20% and 90% [5]. All patients exposed to chemotherapy will have a diminished ovarian reserve and, therefore, potential infertility with a significant predisposition for developing premature ovarian failure. Chemotherapy treatments may, in fact, be the leading cause of premature ovarian senescence, since 2% of the female population between the ages of 1 and 39 will be diagnosed with cancer, and half of these patients will require treatment with chemotherapy [1].

The tolerance of the ovary and uterus to radiation exposure is dependent on several factors including the age of the patient, the volume of irradiated tissue, the total dose of radiation, the risk of scatter, and the fractionation schedule. When applied conventionally, radiation doses of 24 Gy will result in ovarian failure. If the pelvis is included in the radiation field of an adult patient, the dose will typically exceed this level [6]. Doses of radiation between 14 and 30 Gy result in uterine dysfunction, increasing the risk of obstetric complications in future pregnancies [7].

The use of more precise radiation treatments has afforded oncologists the opportunity to decrease the exposure of the ovaries to the field of radiation. Three-dimensional computerized analysis of the dose of radiation received by the ovaries can allow more precise treatment and mitigate the gonadotoxic potential. For a given dose of radiotherapy at a known chronological age, oncologists can now predict the size of the surviving fraction of oocytes, and, therefore, the age at which ovarian failure can be expected for a patient [8]. These projections will serve the patient well as she and her physicians contemplate the timing and utility of fertility preservation strategies.

The greatest risk for developing premature ovarian failure occurs in the setting of the intensive multiagent chemotherapy and total body irradiation that is required for both adults and children who undergo bone marrow stem cell transplantation (BMSCT) for treatment of their malignancies. The doses required cause immediate ovarian failure in nearly all cases [5]. Chemotherapy treatments, most including cyclophosphamide, and BMSCT are also utilized in the treatment of benign and chronic diseases such as sickle-cell anemia, thalassemia, aplastic anemia, lupus, and autoimmune thrombocytopenia [9,10]. Additional benign indications for fertility preservation technologies include recurrent ovarian endometriosis, ovarian cysts, and the need for prophylactic oophorectomy in women affected by BRCA-1/2.

Fertility Preservation Guidelines

In March 2005, the Ethics Committee of the American Society for Reproductive Medicine (ASRM) published their guidelines for the preservation of fertility in cancer patients [11]. Faced with the prospect of gonadotoxic cancer therapies, individuals were counseled to consider the preservation of their fertility through the use of embryo cryopreservation from in vitro fertilization (IVF), and potentially with emerging techniques such as oocyte and ovarian tissue cryopreservation. At the time of their initial report in 2005, the Ethics Committee indicated that the only established methods of fertility preservation were sperm cryopreservation in males for use with intracytoplasmic sperm injection (ICSI) during IVF and embryo cryopreservation [11]. The guidelines were updated in November of 2013, reflecting the utility and increased efficiency of oocyte cryopreservation, a preferred option for fertility preservation for post-pubertal girls, single women, and those who have moral or ethical objections to embryo freezing [12]. The updated guidelines accounted for the designation by ASRM, announced in October 2012, that oocyte cryopreservation is no longer an experimental procedure, and, therefore, no longer requires the oversight of an Institutional Review Board (IRB) [13]. Their conclusions reviewed the data, including Level I evidence, that birth rates using frozen oocytes and ICSI are similar to fresh oocytes [14]. Additionally, an extensive review of the medical literature revealed that the birth outcomes of offspring derived from the thaw of previously cryopreserved oocytes were similar to fresh oocyte IVF and are not different from the general population [15]. It is important to note, however, that although oocyte cryopreservation for the purpose of fertility preservation is endorsed by ASRM for patients facing iatrogenic therapies that are gonadotoxic, it has not been supported for the sole purpose of circumventing childbearing ("social fertility preservation"). Their concerns are related to the lack of data reflecting the safety, efficacy, emotional burden, and cost-effectiveness of employing this technology for this group of women [13].

Ovarian tissue cryopreservation is deemed an experimental procedure and, as such, should only be offered with IRB oversight in a research setting. This experimental technology would theoretically be useful for women who are unable to delay cancer treatment, such as in the case of advanced stage blood-borne malignancies, to undergo controlled ovarian hyperstimulation (COH) for the purpose of oocyte or embryo cryopreservation.

The authors of the ASRM Ethics Committee Report express that concerns about the welfare of the potential offspring *should not* be cause for denying cancer patients assistance in reproducing. When raised in a loving and nurturing environment, children should be given the opportunity to thrive, despite the misfortune of an early death of one parent.

These recommendations parallel those initially published by the American Society of Clinical Oncology (ASCO) in 2006, which were updated in 2013 to reflect the advances and nonexperimental designation of oocyte cryopreservation [16,17]. The authors recommended that oncologists should consider the options for fertility preservation expediently, so as to facilitate discussions with reproductive specialists and advocacy groups that support these treatments. Established methods, in addition to embryo, oocyte, and sperm cryopreservation, include gonadal shielding and ovarian transposition in cases involving exposure of the pelvis to radiation therapies. Encouragingly, the ASCO guidelines confirm that there appears to be no increased risk of disease recurrence associated with use of the established treatments, even in tumors that might be hormonally sensitive, i.e., breast cancer. There is also no evidence of an increased risk of congenital abnormalities in the progeny of patients who have attempted to preserve their fertility, except in those cases that involve hereditary genetic syndromes [16,17].

Nonsurgical Fertility Preservation Techniques

Embryo Cryopreservation

Embryo cryopreservation, routinely performed in patients undergoing IVF, affords the patient an optimal chance to preserve her fertility, with excellent live birth rates resulting from the future thaw and transcervical uterine transfer of embryos/blastocysts, depending on the age of the patient at the time of her oocyte retrieval [18]. However, this approach requires a source of sperm, a problematic option for patients without a partner. Additionally, the treatment cannot be offered to prepubertal patients who have an undeveloped reproductive endocrine axis, or to adolescents who can neither provide consent nor use donor sperm. Concerns related to the oncogenic potential of supraphysiologic levels of gonadotropins and estradiol resulting from IVF on the course, prognosis, and treatment of estrogen-dependent neoplasms may decrease the utility of this treatment for certain patients [19]. Protocols for COH that include agents such as letrozole (aromatase inhibitor) and tamoxifen (selective estrogen receptor modulator) in conjunction with gonadotropins appear to yield high-quality embryos and counteract the potential impact of high estradiol levels [20]. When implemented in close collaboration with the patient's oncology team, these protocols can be completed for breast cancer patients during the 4- to 6-week interval that typically occurs between the patient's surgery and the initiation of chemotherapy.

Because of our enhanced understanding of the female hypothalamic–pituitary–gonadal axis, and the ability to use sophisticated COH treatment protocols, the timing and implementation of fertility preservation techniques can be done expediently. Traditional approaches required the initiation of fertility preservation treatment in the early follicular phase of the patient's menstrual cycle, adding time constraints that conferred unacceptable delays with respect to beginning chemotherapy or radiation treatments. The novel "cycle-independent" or "emergency" approach to COH for the purpose of oocyte retrieval and eventual embryo or oocyte cryopreservation can complete the process within 2–3 weeks of the patient's presentation to the reproductive endocrinologist [21]. Outcomes with regard to oocyte yields and fertilization rates, comparing the traditionally timed technique of COH versus the "cycle-independent" approach, show similar results. Encouragingly, a study of breast cancer patients in 2009, comparing the duration of time from a breast cancer diagnosis to the implementation of chemotherapy, revealed no significant difference between the patients undergoing COH for fertility preservation versus the group that was not utilizing this treatment [22]. These time frames allow the cancer patient and her oncology team the reassurance that unacceptable delays in cancer treatment have been avoided.

Oocyte Cryopreservation

Similar to embryo cryopreservation, oocyte cryopreservation results in elevated serum estradiol levels and requires a mature reproductive axis, the use of gonadotropins for COH, and delays in the timing of chemotherapy treatment. However, there is no need for a male partner or donor sperm, and issues related to the creation of surplus embryos are avoided. Oocyte freezing was heretofore considered an elusive and challenging technique owing to the unique properties of the human oocyte, particularly with its large water content and the fragility of the meiotic spindle [23,24]. Inefficiencies in the success of this technology were the result of increased ice crystal formation and hardening of the zona pellucida caused by the premature release of cortical granules, which, in turn, prevented the fertilization of the thawed oocyte [25]. More recently, with the use of cryoprotectants that limit osmolarity changes, rapid freezing techniques known as vitrification, and fertilization with ICSI, multiple clinics have reported increased success after the uterine transfer of embryos resulting from the fertilization of thawed oocytes [26,27]. At our center, a study from 2008 involved the cryopreservation of 140 metaphase II oocytes retrieved from eight anonymous donors. Of these, 118 (84.3%) survived the freeze–thaw process, and ICSI with partner sperm resulted in a fertilization rate of 79.7%. Ninety-two (97.9%) of the resulting embryos attained the cleavage stage, and 27 (43.5%) of the 62 biopsied embryos were determined to be euploid by preimplantation genetic analysis. The transfer of 12 of these blastocysts into 6 patients yielded a clinical pregnancy rate of 66.7% (4/6 patients) and 4 term deliveries (3 singletons and 1 set of twins) [26]. In a study of subjects undergoing the transfer of embryos derived from autologous and donor frozen/thawed oocytes, the pregnancy rates were similar to age-matched controls undergoing conventional IVF [21]. Finally, the randomized clinical trial from 2010, comparing the ongoing pregnancy rates between controls undergoing the transfer of embryos derived from fresh donor oocytes versus subjects receiving embryos derived from cryopreserved/thawed donor oocytes failed to show the superiority of the traditional fresh donor oocyte approach [14].

The aforementioned data, along with the publication of the reassuring birth outcomes of children derived from the fertilization of previously cryopreserved oocytes [15], have established this technology as a viable option for women seeking fertility preservation, similar to embryo cryopreservation.

In Vitro Maturation

As an alternative, in vitro maturation (IVM) of oocytes retrieved from unstimulated ovaries is an option for fertility preservation for young women that would not require the participation of a male partner or delays in cancer treatments. The IVM and freezing of these oocytes, similar to oocyte and ovarian tissue cryopreservation, are considered an experimental technique that has been typically used for the treatment of infertility in women with polycystic ovarian syndrome. This technology has been used in conjunction with ovarian tissue cryopreservation, allowing the aspiration of antral follicles before the cryobanking of ovarian tissue that has been surgically retrieved [28]. Live births have been reported from this procedure; its application is limited to specialized centers.

Ovarian Suppression with GnRH Analogs

The use of GnRH analog (GnRHa) therapy concomitant with chemotherapy/pelvic radiation has been purported to preserve ovarian function via down-regulation of the hypothalamic–pituitary–ovarian axis while the patient is undergoing gonadotoxic therapies [29]. The mechanism of this effect is unclear, and the data supporting its use are conflicting. Randomized controlled trials among cancer patients, including all cancer types as well as those confined to early stage breast cancer, have not consistently shown an advantage to the use of GnRHa during cancer treatments [30–33]. The present recommendations from ASCO regarding the utility of GnRHa treatments in conjunction with chemotherapy/radiation therapy instruct oncologists to inform patients that there is insufficient evidence regarding the effectiveness of GnRHa administration as a fertility preservation method [17]. The practical use of these medications can avert the development of menorrhagia during intensive chemotherapy, but side effects of their administration include the onset of vasomotor complaints as well as bone loss resulting from enhanced estrogen deprivation. Until the biologic plausibility of this treatment is established and well-designed studies show consistent results, both ASCO and the European Society for Medical Oncology suggest that GnRHa ovarian suppression for cancer patients be limited to treatments offered under the oversight of an IRB [17,34].

Surgical Fertility Preservation Techniques

Gynecologic Malignancies

Surgical techniques for the preservation of fertility among patients with early-stage cervical cancer allow preservation of the uterus and ovaries, and include *radical trachelectomy* with or without lymph node dissection [35]. Women diagnosed with microinvasive cervical cancer (stage 1A1) without lymphovascular space involvement are candidates for a cone biopsy [36]. Antepartum management for these women requires close observation for cervical incompetence and the potential need for prophylactic cerclage placement.

Oophoropexy and ovarian transposition, which limit gonadotoxicity induced by radiation exposure, are established surgical techniques offered to women who are undergoing radiation therapy for cancers involving the pelvis, such as cervical cancer, colon cancer, or metastatic Hodgkin lymphoma [37,38]. As mentioned above, uterine exposure to pelvic/abdominal radiation may require the use of gestational carriers in future pregnancies to eliminate the risk of obstetric complications related to these treatments.

Women with ovarian cancer, such as those with early-stage germ cell tumors, or select cases of Stage I epithelial ovarian cancers, are candidates for fertility preservation procedures that involve *unilateral salpingo-oophorectomy of the diseased ovary in conjunction with uterine preservation* [39].

Ovarian Tissue Cryopreservation

Ovarian tissue cryopreservation is an experimental option for women who, because of the need for immediate chemotherapy or radiation treatments, are not candidates for more established techniques such as oocyte cryopreservation or embryo cryopreservation from IVF. Typically, women diagnosed with blood-borne malignancies or those who face BMSCT for either primary or recurrent/metastatic disease (as well as certain benign conditions) would benefit from ovarian tissue cryopreservation. Prepubertal girls, who have yet to develop a mature hypothalamic–pituitary–ovarian axis, would also qualify for this novel procedure. As of 2013, 60 live births resulting from the reimplantation of previously cryopreserved ovarian tissue were reported in peer-reviewed journals and abstracts [40].

Concerns with the transplantation of cryopreserved–thawed ovarian tissue focus on the risk of disease recurrence emanating from the exposure of cancer survivors to diseased tissue that harbors malignant cells. Fortunately, the ovary is not considered to be a typical sanctuary for blood-borne malignancies [41,42]. In an Israeli study in 2008, 58 patients with hematologic malignancies, including non-Hodgkin lymphoma, acute leukemia, myelodysplastic syndrome, chronic myeloid leukemia (CML), and Hodgkin lymphoma, were evaluated for storage of ovarian tissue for fertility preservation. Two of the subjects were excluded from the study owing to preoperative imaging confirming the presence of macroscopic ovarian metastases. Of the remaining patients, post-thawing tissue analysis confirmed the presence of minimal residual disease in only one patient, retrieved from a patient with CML [43].

Conclusion

Cancer treatments, despite their gonadotoxicty, have allowed survivors to focus on an enhanced quality of life, including the ability to have a biologic child. Both established and experimental therapies can now be utilized to allow these women to overcome the infertility that may result from their chemotherapy and radiation therapies. Continued research into the surgical and nonsurgical approaches to fertility preservation is warranted.

REFERENCES

1. Siegel RL, Miller KD, Jemal A. Cancer statistics, 2015. *CA Cancer J Clin* 2015;65:5–29.
2. Ward E, DeSantis C, Robbins A, Kohler B, Jemal A. Childhood and adolescent cancer statistics, 2014. *CA Cancer J Clin* 2014;64:83–103.
3. Speroff L, Fritz M. *Clinical Gynecologic Endocrinology and Infertility.* 7th ed. Lippincott Williams and Wilkins; 2005.
4. Bokemeyer C, Schmoll HJ, van Rhee J, Kuczyk M, Schuppert F, Poliwoda H. Long-term gonadal toxicity after therapy for Hodgkin's and non-Hodgkin's lymphoma. *Ann Hematol* 1994;68(3):105–10.
5. Lobo RA. Potential options for preservation of fertility in women. *N Engl J Med* 2005;353(1):64–73.
6. Grigsby PW, Russell A, Bruner D et al. Late injury of cancer therapy on the female reproductive tract. *Int J Radiat Oncol Biol Phys* 1995;31(5):1281–99.
7. Crictchley H, Hamish B. Safety of pregnancy during and after cancer treatment. *J Nat Cancer Inst Monogr* 2005;34:64.
8. Wallace WH, Thomson AB, Saran F, Kelsey TW. Predicting age of ovarian failure after radiation to a field that includes the ovaries. *Int J Radiat Oncol Biol Phys* 2005;62(3):738–44.
9. Mattle V, Behringer K, Engert A, Wildt L. Female fertility after cytotoxic therapy—Protection of ovarian function during chemotherapy of malignant and non-malignant diseases. *Eur J Haematol Suppl* 2005;66(66):77–82.
10. Slavin S, Nagler A, Aker M, Shapira MY, Cividalli G, Or R. Non-myeloablative stem cell transplantation and donor lymphocyte infusion for the treatment of cancer and life-threatening non-malignant disorders. *Rev Clin Exp Hematol* 2001;5(2):135–46.
11. Ethics Committee of the American Society for Reproductive Medicine. Fertility preservation and reproduction in cancer patients. *Fertil Steril* 2005;83(6):1622–8.
12. Ethics Committee of the American Society for Reproductive Medicine. Fertility preservation and reproduction in patients facing gonadotoxic therapies: A committee opinion. *Fertil Steril* 2013;100:1224–31.
13. The Practice Committees of the American Society for Reproductive Medicine and the Society for Assisted Reproductive Technology. Mature oocyte cryopreservation: A guideline. *Fertil Steril* 2013;99:37–43.
14. Cobo A, Meseguer M, Remohi J, Pellicer A. Use of cryo-banked oocytes in an ovum donation programme: A prospective, randomized, controlled, clinical trial. *Hum Reprod* 2010;25:2239–46.
15. Noyes N, Porcu E, Borini A. Over 900 oocyte cryopreservation babies born with no apparent increase in congenital anomalies. *Reprod Biomed Online* 2009;18(6):769–76.
16. Lee SJ, Schover LR, Partridge AH et al. American Society of Clinical Oncology recommendations on fertility preservation in cancer patients. *J Clin Oncol* 2006;24(18):2917–31.
17. Loren AW, Mangu PB, Nohr Beck L, Brennan L, Magdalinski AJ, Partridge AH, Quinn G, Wallace WH, Otkay K. Fertility preservation for patients with cancer: American Society of Clinical Oncology clinical practice guideline update. *J Clin Oncol* 2013;31:2500–10.
18. Centers for Disease Control and Prevention. 2016 Assisted reproductive technology success rates: National summary and fertility clinic reports. http://www.sart.org.
19. Yue W, Santen RJ, Wang JP et al. Genotoxic metabolites of estradiol in breast: Potential mechanism of estradiol induced carcinogenesis. *J Steroid Biochem Mol Biol* 2003;86(3–5):477–86.
20. Oktay K, Hourvitz A, Sahin G et al. Letrozole reduces estrogen and gonadotropin exposure in women with breast cancer undergoing ovarian stimulation before chemotherapy. *J Clin Endocrinol Metab* 2006;91(10):3885–90.
21. Cakmak H, Katz A, Cedars MI, Rosen MP. Effective method for emergency fertility preservation: Random-start controlled ovarian stimulation. *Fertil Steril* 2013;100:1673–80.
22. Baynosa J, Westphal LM, Madrigrano A, Wapnir I. Timing of breast cancer treatments with oocyte retrieval and embryo cryopreservation. *J Am Coll Surg* 2009;209:603–7.
23. Porcu E, Venturoli S. Progress with oocyte cryopreservation. *Curr Opin Obstet Gynecol* 2006;18(3):273–9.
24. Chen SU, Lien YR, Chao KH, Ho HN, Yang YS, Lee TY. Effects of cryopreservation on meiotic spindles of oocytes and its dynamics after thawing: Clinical implications in oocyte freezing—A review article. *Mol Cell Endocrinol* 2003;202(1–2):101–7.
25. Vincent C, Pickering SJ, Johnson MH. The hardening effect of dimethylsulphoxide on the mouse zona pellucida requires the presence of an oocyte and is associated with a reduction in the number of cortical granules present. *J Reprod Fertil* 1990;89(1):253–9.

26. Kinzer D, Alper M, Barrett B. Abstract P-045. The American Society for Reproductive Medicine Annual Meeting. October 2008: San Francisco.

27. Grifo JA, Noyes N. Delivery rate using cryopreserved oocytes is comparable to conventional in vitro fertilization using fresh oocytes: Potential fertility preservation for female cancer patients. *Fertil Steril* 2010;93(2):391–6.

28. Huang JY, Tulandi T, Holzer H, Tan SL, Chian RC. Combining ovarian tissue cryobanking with retrieval of immature oocytes followed by in vitro maturation and vitrification: An additional strategy of fertility preservation. *Fertil Steril* 2008;89(3):567–72.

29. Blumenfeld Z, Avivi I, Eckman A, Epelbaum R, Rowe JM, Dann EJ. Gonadotropin-releasing hormone agonist decreases chemotherapy-induced gonadotoxicity and premature ovarian failure in young female patients with Hodgkin lymphoma. *Fertil Steril* 2008;89:166–73.

30. Badawy A, Elnashar A, El-Ashry M, Shahat M. Gonadotropin-releasing hormone agonists for prevention of chemotherapy-induced ovarian damage: Prospective randomized study. *Fertil Steril* 2009;91:694–7.

31. Elgindy EA, El-Haieg DO, Khorshid OM, Ismail EL, Abdelgawad M, Sallam HN, Abou-Setta AM. Gonadotropin suppression to prevent chemotherapy-induced ovarian damage: A randomized controlled trial. *Obstet Gynecol* 2013;121(1):78–86.

32. Lambertini M, Boni L, Michelotti A, Gamucci T, Scotto T, Gori S, Giordano M, Garrone O, Levaggi A, Poggio F, Girvadi S, Bighin C, Vecchio C, Sertoli MR, Pronzato P, DelMastro L, GIM Study Group. Ovarian suppression with Triptorelin during adjuvant breast cancer chemotherapy and long-term ovarian function, pregnancies, and disease-free survival: A randomized clinical trial. *JAMA* 2015;314(24):2632–40.

33. Moore HC, Unger JM, Phillips KA, Boyle F, Hitr E, Porter D, Francis PA, Goldstein LJ, Gomez HL, Vallejos CS, Partridge AH, Dakhil SR, Garcia AA, Gralow J, Lombard JM, Forbes JF, Martino S, Barlow WE, Fabian CJ, Minasian L, Meyskens FL, Gelber RD, Hortobagyi GN, Albain KS, POEMS/S0230 Investigators. Goserelin for ovarian protection during breast-cancer adjuvant chemotherapy. *NEJM* 2015;372(10):923–32.

34. Peccatori FA, Azim HA, Orecchia R, Hoekstra HJ, Pavlidis N, Kesic V, Pentheroudakis G, ESMO Guidelines Working Group. Cancer, pregnancy and fertility: ESMO clinical practice guidelines for diagnosis, treatment and follow-up. *Ann Oncol* 2013;24(suppl 6):vi160–70.

35. Plante M, Renaud MC, Francois H, Roy M. Vaginal radical trachelectomy: An oncologically safe fertility-preserving surgery. An updated series of 72 cases and review of the literature. *Gynecol Oncol* 2004; 94(3):614–23.

36. Bisseling KC, Bekkers RL, Rome RM, Quinn MA. Treatment of microinvasive adenocarcinoma of the uterine cervix: A retrospective study and review of the literature. *Gynecol Oncol* 2007;107(3):424–30.

37. Scott SM, Schlaff W. Laparoscopic medial oophoropexy prior to radiation therapy in an adolescent with Hodgkin's disease. *J Pediatr Adolesc Gynecol* 2005;18(5):355–7.

38. Morice P, Juncker L, Rey A, El-Hassan J, Haie-Meder C, Castaigne D. Ovarian transposition for patients with cervical carcinoma treated by radiosurgical combination. *Fertil Steril* 2000;74(4):743–8.

39. Schilder JM, Thompson AM, DePriest PD et al. Outcome of reproductive age women with stage IA or IC invasive epithelial ovarian cancer treated with fertility-sparing therapy. *Gynecol Oncol* 2002;87(1):1–7.

40. Donnez J, Dolmans MM, Pellicer A, Diaz-Garcia C, Sanchez Serrano M, Schmidt KT et al. Restoration of ovarian activity and pregnancy after transplantation of cryopreserved ovarian tissue: A review of 60 cases of reimplantation. *Fertil Steril* 2013;99:1503–13.

41. Khan MA, Dahill SW, Stewart KS. Primary Hodgkin's disease of the ovary. Case report. *Br J Obstet Gynaecol* 1986;93(12):1300–1.

42. Osborne BM, Robboy SJ. Lymphomas or leukemia presenting as ovarian tumors. An analysis of 42 cases. *Cancer* 1983;52(10):1933–43.

43. Meirow D, Hardan I, Dor J et al. Searching for evidence of disease and malignant cell contamination in ovarian tissue stored from hematologic cancer patients. *Hum Reprod* 2008;23(5):1007–13.

BIBLIOGRAPHY

Ethics Committee of the American Society for Reproductive Medicine. Fertility preservation and reproduction in patients facing gonadotoxic therapies: A committee opinion. *Fertil Steril* 2013;100:1224–31.

Loren AW, Mangu PB, Nohr Beck L, Brennan L, Magdalinski AJ, Partridge AH, Quinn G, Wallace WH, Otkay K. Fertility preservation for patients with cancer: American Society of Clinical Oncology clinical practice guideline update. *J Clin Oncol* 2013;31:2500–10.

17

Elective Egg Freezing

Samuel A. Pauli and Kerri L. Luzzo

Oocyte cryopreservation is one of the newest advancement in the field of in vitro fertilization (IVF). The laboratory technique to freeze oocytes has been perfected such that we have confidence that eggs that have been frozen have a high probability of surviving the thaw, can be fertilized, and result in a pregnancy. This chapter provides an overview of the application of this new technology.

Oocyte Cryopreservation Technology

Cryopreservation, a process in which tissues are cooled to subzero temperatures placing the cell in an arrested biologic state, allows women to freeze oocytes at a particular reproductive age to preserve for potential future use. This rapidly developing technology has progressed over the last couple of decades with improvements in cooling techniques and alterations in cryoprotectants. These changes led to the first human birth from cryopreserved oocytes in 1986 [1]. Challenges with initial methods of oocyte cryopreservation included cellular damage related to oocyte plasma membrane stability, osmotic damage, changes in salt concentrations, cellular ice formation, and meiotic spindle sensitivity to dehydration and rehydration. The two methods of cryopreservation, slow freezing and vitrification, use different concentrations of cryoprotectants and differing rates of cooling and warming. Vitrification, the most current method of cryopreservation, utilizes high concentrations of cryoprotectant and rapid cooling and warming, resulting in a solid glass-like cell that is free of ice crystals. Comparing vitrification and slow freeze success rates, data collected from 2009 to 2014 from the Italian National Assisted Reproductive Technology Register showed higher survival, implantation, and pregnancy rates with oocyte vitrification compared to cryopreservation via slow freezing [2]. A Cochrane review in 2014 suggested higher clinical pregnancy rates with oocyte vitrification versus slow freezing (RR, 3.86; 95% CI, 1.63–9.11; $p = 0.002$) [3]. A 2013 meta-analysis of 10 studies and 2265 oocyte cryopreservation cycles with slow freeze and vitrification revealed lower oocyte survival and fertilization rates as well as lower implantation and live birth rates with slow freezing [4].

Indications

Oocyte cryopreservation has various indications including preserving fertility in women facing gonadotoxic treatment with chemotherapy or radiation, minimizing the formation of excess embryos because of religious/legal concerns, or in the setting of IVF when sperm is unobtainable. As more women delay childbearing for social reasons, elective oocyte cryopreservation is increasing as a method to potentially preserve reproductive potential.

Oncology

In the United States, approximately 125,000 women under age 50 are diagnosed with cancer each year [5], and from 2002 to 2012, survival rates were 83% in women younger than 45 years [6]. The mainstay of cancer treatment is typically surgery, chemotherapy, or radiation. Over the last four decades, advancements in cancer therapies have led to dramatic improvements in survival. As survival rates increase in patients with cancer, subsequent quality of life, including potential adverse effects on reproduction, is an important part of overall counseling and care. For women undergoing gonadotoxic therapy, the potential negative outcomes include irregular menses, premature ovarian failure, or infertility. These potential outcomes are dependent on patient age, type of treatment (agent, dose, and duration), and primary diagnosis. The American Society of Clinical Oncology recommends that health care providers address fertility preservation before cancer treatment, to discuss the possibility of infertility and fertility preservation options or refer to reproductive specialists [7]. The psychological impact of cancer treatment and potential infertility should not be underestimated. Though many cancer survivors report wanting children in the future and report anxiety because of potential treatment-related infertility, only approximately 47%–60% are informed about fertility preservation options, despite counseling being associated with less regret and greater posttreatment quality of life [8–11].

Fertility preservation options for women include embryo cryopreservation, oocyte cryopreservation, and ovarian tissue cryopreservation. Treatments are individualized based on age, health and comorbidities, type of cancer/tumor and potential for ovarian metastases, type of planned treatment, time available, and partner status [12]. The natural ovarian aging process is an extremely important factor to consider when counseling patients on the potential effects of cancer treatment and chance of success with oocyte/embryo cryopreservation. The extent of radiotherapy damage to oocytes is based on the age of the patient, cumulative dose, concomitant use of chemotherapy, and site. Radiation is extremely toxic to the oocyte, causing a dose-related primordial ovarian follicle loss and cortical damage. A dose of 6 Gy can cause ovarian failure, a dose of 2–4 Gy can destroy 50% of the oocytes, and a dose of 16.5 Gy at age 20 years will lead to ovarian failure in 97.5% of women [13,14]. The extent of gonadotoxicity is variable, potentially causing delayed puberty, oligomenorrhea, amenorrhea, premature ovarian failure, or infertility. Chemotherapy agents, particularly alkylating agents, have the potential to invoke irreversible damage to both the steroid-producing granulosa and theca cells, along with the oocyte. Factors that contribute to toxicity include age, pretreatment fertility status and ovarian reserve, drug class, and cumulative dose. Similar to radiation therapy, chemotherapy-induced ovarian damage can lead to amenorrhea, premature ovarian failure, or infertility [14].

Oocyte Cryopreservation Outcomes

Regarding fertility preservation options, embryo cryopreservation is a well-established, reliable technology with a predictable likelihood of success based on patient age [15]. Since the first human births from a slow freeze embryo in 1984 and from vitrification in 1990, live birth rates have increased over the last decade [16]. However embryo cryopreservation requires a partner or donor sperm, is not suitable for adolescents with cancer, and has ethical, legal, and religious concerns in some countries. The advantages of oocyte cryopreservation include greater control over future gamete disposition and eliminating any ethical issues involved with the creation of excess embryos for storage and possible disposal. In 2012, the American Society for Reproductive Medicine (ASRM) removed the experimental label from oocyte cryopreservation and stated that "in the case of patients facing infertility due to chemotherapy or other gonadotoxic therapies, oocyte cryopreservation may be one of the few options available and therefore is recommended with appropriate counseling" [17].

Early experience with oocyte cryopreservation reported pregnancy rates between 8% and 33%. Outcomes from a 2006 meta-analysis comparing 26 slow freezing studies to IVF using fresh oocytes showed a live birth rate of 21.6% for frozen oocyte and 60.4% for fresh IVF cycles [18]. However, a subsequent study reported ongoing pregnancy/delivery rates of 57% of women using cryopreserved oocytes, similar to age-matched controls using fresh oocytes [19]. Studies examining outcomes from frozen donor oocyte cycles show that frozen oocytes have a similar potential to fresh oocytes. Survival rates range from 89% to 96.7%, fertilization rates range between 76% and 84.4%, no reported differences exist in blastocyst formation or embryo quality, pregnancy rates range from 55.6% to 65.2%, and live birth rates are approximately 47.2% [20–22]. A large randomized controlled trial comparing fresh and frozen vitrified oocytes in 600 patients revealed similar ongoing pregnancy rates between oocyte vitrification and fresh oocytes (43.7% vs. 41.7%, respectively; 95% CI, 0.667–1.274; $p = 0.744$), thus failing to confirm that fresh oocytes are superior to frozen ones [23].

A recent retrospective cohort examined oocyte vitrification outcomes for indications including elective fertility preservation, limiting excess embryo creation, or cases in which sperm sample was not obtainable on day of oocyte retrieval. Comparing fresh oocyte with vitrified oocytes, they found similar fertilization rates and higher implantation and pregnancy rates for vitrified versus fresh oocyte cycles, but no differences in live birth rates between fresh and frozen cycles. The overall per-oocyte live birth rate, or efficiency, which is important with regard to the number of oocytes to freeze and proper patient counseling, of 6.4% was dependent on maternal age [24]. A meta-analysis in 2013 reporting age-specific probability of live birth with oocyte cryopreservation showed that live birth declines with age regardless of slow freeze or vitrification technique [4]. Overall, the literature suggests that fresh and frozen oocytes are similar with respect to fertilization and pregnancy rates and, with appropriate counseling, should be considered in patients facing gonadotoxic treatments.

Oocyte Cryopreservation in Cancer Patients

Specific concerns regarding ovarian stimulation in patients with cancer include treatment delay, possible estrogen exposure stimulating tumor growth, possible increase in cancer recurrence rates, ovarian hyperstimulation, and pregnancy outcomes. While a typical IVF cycle can take 2–6 weeks depending on the menstrual cycle, using a random start (late follicular or luteal phase start protocol) can decrease the total time for IVF cycle without negatively affecting oocyte yield, maturity, or fertilization rates [25]. For patients with estrogen-sensitive breast tumors, aromatase inhibitors, which inhibit the rate-limiting step in the conversion of androgens to estrogens, are used in certain cases to avoid supraphysiologic rise in serum estradiol that is typically seen during an ovarian stimulation cycle. A review of the literature in 2012 indicated that using aromatase inhibitors in women with breast cancer is safe and effective in conjunction with gonadotropins and that the risk of breast cancer recurrence in the short term does not appear to increase [26]. Another approach to optimizing protocols in women with cancer is prevention of ovarian hyperstimulation syndrome, which can delay and complicate cancer treatment; this complication is minimized with an antagonist cycle with a Lupron trigger.

There has been concern that ovarian response in patients with cancer may be altered because of the type of malignancy and the systemic condition. One meta-analysis of seven retrospective case–control studies revealed that ovarian response, cycle cancelation, and fertilization rates were similar in patients with cancer compared to those without; however, patients with cancer had fewer number of oocytes retrieved (11.7 vs. 13.5, $p = 0.002$) [27]. However, many others have reported no differences in the amount of gonadotropins used [28–30], in number of oocytes obtained [28–30], fertilization rate [28,30], or number of embryos cryopreserved in patients with and without cancer undergoing IVF [30]. More recent studies suggest that the type of cancer may influence ovarian response [31,32]. Of note, the BRCA-1 mutation has been associated with risks of low ovarian response (33% vs. 3%, $p = 0.014$) and lower number of oocytes (7.4 vs. 12.4) compared to women with breast cancer without the mutation. This is possibly attributed to DNA repair deficiencies leading to DNA damage, clinically manifesting as diminished ovarian reserve and primary ovarian insufficiency [33]. These are important counseling points to consider when counseling oncology patients on oocyte cryopreservation.

Information regarding outcomes of oocyte vitrification in cancer patients is sparse owing to the fact that many patients have not come back to use their oocytes. One case report from 2011 describes a live birth after vitrification of seven oocytes for 9 years in a patient with chronic myeloid leukemia [34] and another study reported a live birth after slow freezing oocytes [35]. Other vitrification data for cancer patients include a case report of twins born after ovarian tissue cryopreservation, treatment with chemotherapy and radiation, followed by ovarian cortical transplantation and controlled ovarian hyperstimulation for oocyte vitrification [36]. Of the 102 oocyte vitrification cycles examined by Doyle and colleagues in 2015, two of the three cancer patients who returned had a live birth/ongoing pregnancy [24]. In a retrospective multicenter study in 2013 of both oncology and non-oncology patients (355 oocyte vitrification cycles for cancer), pregnancies were achieved in two of the four cancer patients who returned to use their oocytes [37]. Another study of pregnancy outcomes in women who underwent oocyte cryopreservation via vitrification before oncologic treatment revealed pregnancy in 7 of 11, and live birth in 4 of 7 of those who returned for treatment [38].

Neonatal Outcomes of Oocyte Cryopreservation

Though few patients with cancer have returned to use frozen oocytes, the data thus far suggest that oocyte cryopreservation does not increase perinatal/neonatal risk. A 2013 observational study and comparative analysis of obstetric and neonatal outcomes from pregnancies achieved with fresh or cryopreserved oocytes showed no differences in fetal or perinatal complications or congenital anomalies [39]. Martinez and colleagues analyzed pregnancy outcomes from 357 women who underwent oocyte cryopreservation via vitrification before oncologic treatment; 4 of 7 had live births with no congenital anomalies [38]. A large retrospective cohort study examining obstetric and perinatal outcomes between fresh and vitrified oocytes showed no differences in obstetrical complications such as pregnancy-induced hypertension, premature rupture of membranes, cesarean delivery, diabetes, or preterm delivery. Adverse neonatal outcomes including low birth weight, birth defects, and neonatal intensive care unit admission were also similar between fresh and vitrified oocytes [40]. One of the largest studies analyzing the incidence of specific congenital anomalies from 936 live births from both oocyte slow freeze and vitrification cycles showed that the incidence of birth defects of 1.3% is similar to those occurring in naturally conceived infants [41].

Elective Oocyte Cryopreservation

In the United States, the only age demographic that shows an increase in the rate of pregnancies are women ages 35–39 and 40 and older, highlighting a trend of delayed childbearing for reproductive-age women [42]. This corresponds to the ages where both fertility declines and the risk of both miscarriages and birth defects increases [43]. Most women face infertility not from cancer or systemic disease, but rather from the passage of time and age-related fertility decline. Today, multiple social and demographic pressures conspire to encourage women to delay and defer childbearing including education and career aspirations, later marriage, no partner, economic barriers, media images of late-in-life celebrity motherhood, and a host of other factors. Given the above reasons, women may wish to postpone childbearing for social reasons. A recent national representative study also showed that the majority of respondents support elective oocyte cryopreservation [44].

Given the progressive loss of oocyte quantity and quality with aging, the use of oocyte cryopreservation can be used as a strategy by women to defer childbearing to maintain reproductive autonomy. The ASRM endorses oocyte cryopreservation for medically indicated fertility preservation but has not directly endorsed oocyte cryopreservation for the sole purpose of reproductive aging [17]. However, there have been increasing amounts of data suggesting that oocyte cryopreservation is both effective and safe when used for elective deferring of childbearing. The ASRM practice guidelines on mature oocyte cryopreservation summarizes four of the earlier randomized controlled trials showing similar implantation and clinical pregnancy rates when comparing fresh to vitrified warmed oocytes that were cryopreserved [17]. Continued data emerging supports oocyte vitrification as an efficient option for elective fertility preservation [45].

Patient selection, counseling, and informed consent for oocyte cryopreservation are paramount when counseling women on future reproductive choices [46]. Ideally, women should be 38 years old or younger given age-related declines in fertility and increased risk of chromosomal aneuploidy. Evaluation typically starts with an assessment of ovarian reserve to determine if a patient will be a good candidate for oocyte preservation and to give a realistic assessment of the number of oocytes to be retrieved. It is important to stress that there is no guarantee of future success of oocyte cryopreservation and therefore the technology should not be used to encourage women to delay childbearing. Rather, it should be used as a tool for women who wish to electively freeze their eggs as part of their longer-term reproductive goals.

REFERENCES

1. Chen C. Pregnancy after human oocyte cryopreservation. *Lancet* 1986;327:884–6.
2. Levi-Setti PE, Patrizio P, Scaravelli G. Evolution of human oocyte cryopreservation: Slow freezing versus vitrification. *Curr Opin Endocrinol Diabetes Obes* 2016;23(6):445–50.
3. Glujovsky D, Riestra B, Sueldo C, Fiszbajn G, Repping S, Nodar F, Papier S, Ciapponi A. Vitrification versus slow freezing for women undergoing oocyte cryopreservation (Review). *Cochrane Database Syst Rev* 2014.
4. Pelin Cil A, Bang H, Oktay K. Age-specific probability of live birth with oocyte cryopreservation: An individual patient data meta-analysis. *Fertil Steril* 2013;100:492–9.
5. National Cancer Institute. Surveillance Epidemiology and End Results. http://seer.cancer.gov.
6. Howlader N, Noone AM, Krapcho M, Neyman N, Aminou R, Waldron W et al. *SEER Cancer Statistics Review, 1975–2009.* Bethesda, MD: National Cancer Institute. http://seer.cancer.gov.
7. Loren AW, Mangu PB, Beck LN, Brennan L, Magdalinski AJ, Partridge AH, Quinn G, Wallace WH, Oktay K. Fertility preservation for patients with cancer: American Society of Clinical Oncology clinical practice guideline update. *J Clin Oncol* 2013;31:2500–11.
8. Schover LR, Rybicki LA, Martin BA, Bringelsen KA. Having children after cancer. A pilot survey of survivors' attitudes and experiences. *Cancer* 1999;86(4):697–709.
9. Shover LR, Brey K, Lichtin A, Lipshultz LI, Jeha S. Knowledge and experience regarding cancer, infertility, and sperm banking in younger male survivors. *J Clin Oncol* 2002;20(7):1880–9.
10. Quinn GP, Vadaparampil ST, Lee J, Jacobsen PB, Bepler G, Lancaster J, Keefe DL, Albrecht TL. Physician referral for fertility preservation in oncology patients: A national study of practice behaviors. *J Clin Oncol* 2009;27:5952–7.
11. Letourneau JM, Ebbel EE, Katz PP, Katz A, Ai W, Chien AJ, Melisko ME, Cedars MI, Rosen MP. Pre-treatment fertility counseling and fertility preservation improve quality of life in reproductive age women with cancer. *Cancer* 2012;118(6):1710–7.
12. Jeruss JS, Woodruff TK. Preservation of fertility in patients with cancer. *N Engl J Med* 2009;360(9): 902–11.
13. ACOG Committee 607. Gynecologic concerns in children and adolescents with cancer. 2014.
14. Sonmezer M, Oktay K. Fertility preservation in female patients. *Hum Reprod Update* 2004;10:251–66.
15. Kosasa TS, McNamee PI, Morton C, Huang TT. Pregnancy rates after transfer of cryopreserved blastocysts cultured in a sequential media. *Am J Obstet Gynecol* 2005;192(6):2035–9.
16. Wong KM, Mastenbroek S, Repping S. Cryopreservation of human embryos and its contribution to in vitro fertilization success rates. *Fertil Steril* 2014;102:19–26.
17. The Practice Committees of the American Society for Reproductive Medicine. Mature oocyte cryopreservation: A guideline. *Fertil Steril* 2013;99:37–43.
18. Oktay K, Pelin Cil A, Bang H. Efficiency of oocyte cryopreservation: A meta-analysis. *Fertil Steril* 2006;86:70–80.
19. Grifo JA, Noyes N. Delivery rate using cryopreserved oocytes is comparable to conventional in vitro fertilization using fresh oocytes: Potential fertility preservation for female cancer patients. *Fertil Steril* 2010;93:391–6.
20. Garcia JI, Noriega-Portella L, Noreiga-Hoces L. Efficacy of oocyte vitrification combined with blastocyst stage transfer in an egg donation program. *Hum Reprod* 2011;26:782–90.
21. Cobo A, Kuwayama M, Perez S, Ruiz A, Pellicer A, Remohi J. Comparison of concomitant outcome achieved with fresh and cryopreserved donor oocytes vitrified by the cryotop method. *Fertil Steril* 2008;89:1657–64.

22. Trokoudes K, Pavlides C, Zhang X. Comparison outcome of fresh and vitrified donor oocytes in an egg-sharing donation program. *Fertil Steril* 2011;95:1996–2000.
23. Cobo A, Meseguer M, Remohi J, Pellicer A. Use of cryo-banked oocytes in an ovum donation programmed: A prospective, randomized, controlled, clinical trial. *Hum Reprod* 2010;25:2239–46.
24. Doyle JO, Richter KS, Lim J, Stillman RJ, Graham JR, Tucker MJ. Successful elective and medically indicated oocyte vitrification and warming for autologous in vitro fertilization, with predicted birth probabilities for fertility preservation according to number of cryopreserved oocytes and age at retrieval. *Fertil Steril* 2016;105:459–66.
25. Cakmak H, Rosen MP. Ovarian stimulation in cancer patients. *Fertil Steril* 2013;99:1476–84.
26. Reddy J, Oktay K. Ovarian stimulation and fertility preservation with the use of aromatase inhibitors in women with breast cancer. *Fertil Steril* 2012;98:1363–9.
27. Freidler S, Koc O, Gidoni Y, Raziel A, Ron-El R. Ovarian response to stimulation for fertility preservation in women with malignant disease: A systematic review and meta-analysis. *Fertil Steril* 2012;97: 125–33.
28. Cardozo E, Thomson AP, Karmon AE, Dickinson KA, Wright DL, Sabatini ME. Ovarian stimulation and in-vitro fertilization outcomes of cancer patients undergoing fertility preservation compared to age matched controls: A 17-year experience. *J Assist Reprod Genet* 2015;32:587–96.
29. Das M, Shehata F, Moria A, Holzer H, Son W, Tulandi T. Ovarian reserve, response to gonadotropins, and oocyte maturity in women with malignancy. *Fertil Steril* 2011;96:122–5.
30. Robertson AD, Missmer SA, Ginsburg ES. Embryo yield after in vitro fertilization in women undergoing embryo banking for fertility preservation before chemotherapy. *Fertil Steril* 2011;95:588–91.
31. Pavone ME, Hirshfeld-Cytron J, Lawson AK, Smith K, Kazer R, Klock S. Fertility preservation outcomes may differ by cancer diagnosis. *J Hum Reprod Sci* 2014;7(2):111–8.
32. Alvarez RM, Ramanathan P. Fertility preservation in female oncology patients: The influence of the type of cancer on ovarian stimulation response. *Hum Reprod* 2016 Jul 1. pii: dew158.
33. Oktay K, Kim JY, Barad D, Babeyev SN. Association of BRCA1 mutations with occult primary ovarian insufficiency: A possible explanation for the link between infertility and breast/ovarian cancer risks. *J Clin Oncol* 2010;28:240–4.
34. Kim MK, Lee DR, Han JE, Kim YS, Lee WS, Won HJ, Kim JW, Yoon TK. Live birth with vitrified-warmed oocytes of a chronic myeloid leukemia patient nine years after allogenic bone marrow transplantation. *Assist Reprod Genet* 2011;28:1167–70.
35. Yang D, Brown SE, Nguyen K, Reddy V, Brubaker C, Winslow KL. Live birth after the transfer of human embryos developed from cryopreserved oocytes harvested before cancer treatment. *Fertil Steril* 2006;87:1469.
36. Sanchez-Serrano M, Crespo J, Mirabet V, Cobo A, Escriba MJ, Simon C, Pellicer A. Twins born after transplantation of ovarian cortical tissue and oocyte vitrification. *Fertil Steril* 2010;93:268.e11–3.
37. Garcia-Velasco JA, Domingo J, Cobo A, Martinez M, Carmona L, Pellicer A. Five years' experience using oocyte vitrification to preserve fertility for medical and nonmedical indications. *Fertil Steril* 2013;99:1994–9.
38. Martinez M, Rabadan S, Domingo J, Cobo A, Pellicer A, Garcia-Velasco JA. Obstetric outcome after oocyte vitrification and warming for fertility preservation in women with cancer. *Reprod Biomed Online* 2014;29(6):722–8.
39. Setti PE, Albani E, Morenghi E, Morreale G, Piane LD, Scaravelli G, Patrizio P. Comparative analysis of fetal and neonatal outcomes of pregnancies from fresh and cryopreserved/thawed oocytes in the same group of patients. *Fertil Steril* 2013;100:396–401.
40. Cobo A, Serra V, Garrido N, Olmo I, Pellicer A, Remohi J. Obstetric and perinatal outcomes of babies born from vitrified oocytes. *Fertil Steril* 2014;102:1006–15.
41. Noyes N, Porcu E, Borini A. Over 900 oocyte cryopreservation babies born with no apparent increase in congenital anomalies. *Reprod Biomed Online* 2009;18(6):769–76.
42. Ventura SJ, Curtin SC, Abma JC. Estimated pregnancy rates and rates of pregnancy outcomes for the United States, 1990–2008. *National Vital Statistics Reports* 2012;60(7);1–22.
43. Female age-related fertility decline. Committee Opinion No. 589. American College of Obstetricians and Gynecologists Committee on Gynecologic Practice and Practice Committee. *Fertil Steril* 2014 Mar;101(3):633–4.

44. Lewis EI, Missmer SA, Farland LV, Ginsburg ES. Public support in the United States for elective oocyte cryopreservation. *Fertil Steril* 2016 Oct;106(5):1183–9.

45. Cobo A, García-Velasco JA, Coello A, Domingo J, Pellicer A, Remohí J. Oocyte vitrification as an efficient option for elective fertility preservation. *Fertil Steril* 2016 Mar;105(3):755–64.

46. Essential elements of informed consent for elective oocyte cryopreservation: A Practice Committee opinion. Practice Committee of Society for Assisted Reproductive Technology. Practice Committee of American Society for Reproductive Medicine. *Fertil Steril* 2008 Nov;90(5 Suppl):S134–5.

18

The IVF Laboratory

Denny Sakkas, C. Brent Barrett, and Kathryn J. Go

Introduction

The treatment of infertility has been a technological challenge as far back as the fourteenth century when there are accounts of Arab peoples using artificial insemination on horses. Even in the third century AD, records show that Jewish thinkers were discussing the possibility of accidental or unintentional human insemination by artificial means.

The first attempts at human artificial insemination by John Hunter are believed to have occurred in 1785, with a baby born the same year. Early reports of donor insemination were published in the *British Medical Journal* in 1945, and in 1955, four successful pregnancies using previously frozen sperm were reported. In 1944, Rock and Menkin [1] reported the first case of in vitro fertilization (IVF) and embryo development in the human. Interestingly, they made the following description about the developing fertilized embryo: "One of these (embryo), when first seen in cleavage, consisted of one large blastomere and two smaller ones, each of the three containing a round, vesicular nucleus. The second egg from this same patient was in a similar stage, but part of the cytoplasm appeared fragmented, and soon proceeded to undergo rapid degenerative changes."

It took until the 1960s and 1970s for many of the different clinical and laboratory aspects of IVF to be improved for more routine use [2–4]. In 1973, the first IVF pregnancy in the world was reported by a team in Melbourne, Australia, which resulted in early embryo death [5]. Subsequently, in 1977, another IVF pregnancy was reported, but it was an ectopic pregnancy [6]. Finally, in 1978, the culmination of knowledge in the technologies associated with IVF led to the first IVF birth in the world [7].

This chapter will give a broad review of current laboratory technologies and procedures that allow IVF to be a routine clinical procedure.

Laboratory Procedures after Recovery of Oocytes

Routine IVF

Stimulation protocols and oocyte recovery techniques have been reviewed early in this book. Once satisfactory stimulation is achieved, the retrieved oocyte–cumulus complexes are collected from follicular aspirates using the following procedure.

Oocyte Retrieval

All steps are performed using sterile technique. Extra caution and protective equipment should be used for infectious disease patients. Once the patient paperwork or Electronic Record File is verified, the embryologist should check for any special instructions involved with the case. Identifiers, including name, date of birth, clinic or patient number, and so on, should be noted and confirmed on all laboratory items to be used.

The procedure is initiated by providing the retrieval/operating room with medium for egg collection. This can be phosphate-buffered saline or a holding medium normally containing HEPES

(4-(2-hydroxyethyl)-1-piperazineethanesulfonic acid) or sometimes MOPS 3-(*N*-morpholino) propane-sulfonic acid [8]. These are both organic chemical buffering agents that are used in cell culture to assist in maintaining physiological pH. This property allows them to act as a better buffering agent, in particular, when the oocytes are maintained outside of an incubator and at 37°C. The medium may or may not contain heparin to limit clotting of the follicular aspirate.

Before commencing the procedure, it is imperative to verify the patient's name, its spelling, the patient's date of birth, and name-band. A checklist sheet documenting this step should be maintained. Once collection begins, the aspirate is poured from the test tube into a tissue culture dish and the contents are scanned for the presence of a cumulus–oocyte complex. The following procedure should be performed at a controlled temperature of 37°C. The oocyte–cumulus complexes are pipetted into a tissue culture dish containing a buffered medium or an equilibrated culture medium when working in an appropriately gassed environment. This step is repeated for all tubes received from the physician. Ideally, the oocytes should be washed in rinse dishes, containing culture medium under oil, and a predetermined number of oocytes should be placed into each culture medium drop. A commonly used medium to maintain the oocyte–cumulus complexes is HEPES-buffered human tubal fluid (HTF) medium (Irvine Scientific, Santa Ana, California) overlaid by paraffin oil. Many clinics also perform egg retrieval directly into HTF or other egg-handling medium with bicarbonate. In these practices, the retrieval can be performed in a mobile incubator where the eggs are collected and harvested in an enclosed environment of 37°C in 5.0% CO_2, 5% O_2, 90% N_2, or 5% CO_2, in air. This avoids any additional manipulation of the oocyte–cumulus complexes.

The dish or dishes are then placed in an incubator, making sure that all details relating to patient's name on the dish(es) and the correct location in the incubator are verified. Once the retrieval is finished, the number of eggs, timing, who performed the procedure, and so on, must be documented.

Analysis and Preparation of Semen Samples for IVF

Semen samples are routinely obtained from the male by masturbation into a sterile container. The male should generally have not ejaculated for 2–3 days before collection.

Analysis

A previous diagnostic semen analysis is normally carried out according to World Health Organization guidelines [9]. This will help direct the type of treatment a couple may undergo. In general, sperm concentration, motility, and morphology are required parameters. Other diagnostic tests for the male can include an assessment of sperm nuclear DNA. This test has, however, led to some controversy as it is believed to provide useful information in relation to the male's ability to achieve a conception naturally or after intrauterine insemination, but the results relating to IVF are less convincing [10–13]. A cutoff of approximately >30% of sperm exhibiting DNA fragmentation is linked with lower chances of conception [14,15]. Another diagnostic test that can be used is the hyaluronan (HA) binding test [16–19]. This test provides information about the maturity of the sperm. Briefly, human sperm that bind to HA exhibit attributes similar to that of zona pellucida–bound sperm, including minimal DNA fragmentation, normal shape, and low frequency of chromosomal aneuploidies [19–21]. In preliminary results from a multicenter clinical trial, it was shown that when patients with less than 65% binding efficiency are screened and selected before intracytoplasmic sperm injection (ICSI), their success rates are improved by incorporating HA binding in their treatment [22].

Preparation

For the purposes of an IVF cycle, a simple count and motility screen is normally sufficient as the aim is to prepare the sperm for treatment rather than for diagnosis. Once collected, the semen is allowed to liquefy for up to 30–45 minutes. It can then be prepared using either a swim-up technique or, more commonly, density gradient centrifugation. Sperm preparation for assisted conception by density gradient centrifugation routinely uses 0.5- to 1-mL volumes of a 40% suspension layered over 0.5–1 mL of a 90% suspension of a colloidal silica suspension in an isotonic salt solution mixed in HTF. Semen is overlaid on the 40% and 90% layers and then centrifuged for approximately 20 minutes (300 g). Sperm in the 90% pellet are harvested, washed in HTF media, and then stored in an incubator until use. The swim-up method requires centrifugation of the ejaculate to form a pellet followed by layering of clean medium (0.5–1 mL) over the pellet. The sperm are then allowed to swim freely up into the clean portion and are then harvested.

Insemination and ICSI

Once the sample is prepared, the total motile sperm concentration is calculated using the volume and number of motile sperm. Insemination can then be performed by adding a predetermined amount to the droplet of culture medium containing the cumulus-enclosed oocytes. Oocytes can be inseminated in groups or individually in droplets of embryo culture medium with between 50,000 and 500,000 motile sperm per milliliter. Insemination is routinely performed between 1300 and 1500, allowing incubation. There are some indications that embryo quality is improved when clinics have utilized a short insemination period [23,24] whereby the sperm are introduced for a period of 1–4 h only and then the oocytes are removed. With this approach, the oocytes are not exposed to radical oxygen species and other possible harmful factors generated by the large population of sperm overnight.

This step is critical to be witnessed, as verification must be made that the name and other identifiers on the sperm tube match that of the patient's retrieval dish containing the oocytes.

If the sperm preparation is substandard in number or motility, or if the patient has previously been identified to be a candidate for ICSI, the following procedure is followed. In preparation for ICSI, the cumulus–oocyte complexes are first placed in a medium with hyaluronidase for <2 minutes for partial removal of the cumulus cells. The remaining cumulus cells are removed by mechanical manipulation of the oocyte during further rinsing in the medium. Mechanical manipulation consists of passing the oocyte–cumulus complex through a series of pipettes decreasing in size from 250 to 135 µm. The aim is to denude the oocytes of the cumulus cells to allow complete visualization of the oocyte and polar body so that the ICSI procedure can proceed.

ICSI is sometimes now chosen as the standard method of insemination. Current rates of ICSI utilization in the United States are close to 70% of cycles. This has led to investigating whether it is overused. A recent paper showed that routine insemination may actually yield more fertilized eggs on the whole when compared to ICSI [25]. Other concerns with ICSI remain, in particular, with respect to its safety. Current data, however, indicate that children born after ICSI have not shown any differences when compared to children born from routine IVF or natural conception [26–28].

Embryo Culture and Medium Selection

At 16–18 h after insemination (day 1), each oocyte is examined for evidence of fertilization and placed into groups or individual droplets of sequential cleavage stage and blastocyst media for culture throughout the culture phase or in a single-step culture medium [29–32]. The general constituents of the sequential and single-step culture media are shown in Table 18.1. Embryos can remain in the cleavage medium until the morning of day 3 when they are changed over to blastocyst medium (Table 18.1). Embryos are then maintained in blastocyst medium until day 5 or day 6 depending on the day of transfer decided for the treatment of the patient. Even with single-step medium, the embryos can be changed over on day 3 of culture or be maintained throughout the whole culture period in the same droplets. Numerous commercial single-step and sequential culture media exist, which broadly follow the above protocol.

A common constituent of modern embryo culture media are various amino acids. This is in contrast to early media, such as HTF, which were simple salt solutions. The major benefit of the new complete human embryo culture media has been a dramatic improvement in their ability to improve blastocyst culture. Amino acids are important regulators of many cellular functions: chelators, osmolytes, pH buffers, antioxidants, regulators of energy metabolism, and biosynthetic precursors and energy substrates.

TABLE 18.1

Major Constituents and Differences of Days 1–3 Cleavage Stage and Days 3–5 Blastocyst Stage Media

Sequential Cleavage Culture Media	Sequential Blastocyst Culture Media	Single-Step Media
Days 1–3	Days 3–6	Days 1–6
• Low or no glucose	• High glucose	• Glucose
• High pyruvate and lactate	• Low pyruvate and lactate	• Pyruvate and lactate
• EDTA	• Essential amino acids	• EDTA
• Nonessential amino acids	• Nonessential amino acids	• Amino acids

The other main constituent is the protein source. A number of choices are available: human serum albumin (HSA), recombinant HSA, or serum supplements that usually consist of a high percentage of HSA and alpha- and beta-globulins.

Assessment of the Embryo

Numerous methods have been adopted to assess the embryo as it develops from the pronucleate through to the blastocyst stage. The many transformations that take place during the fertilization process make the pronucleate stage a dynamic stage to assess. The human oocyte contains the majority of the developmental materials and maternal mRNA for ensuring that the embryo reaches the 4- to 8-cell stage. The quality of the oocyte, therefore, plays a crucial role for determining embryo development and subsequent viability. Features assessed include the orientation of pronuclei relative to the polar bodies, alignment of pronuclei and nucleoli, the appearance of the cytoplasm, presence of nucleolar precursor bodies, and the timing of nuclear membrane breakdown [33].

The most widely used criteria for selecting the best embryos for transfer have been based on cell number and morphology. This is still the mainstay of the embryologists' tool for selecting which embryo to transfer. Variations on the basic selection of the best cleaving embryo by cell number and morphology have been used. For example, it is believed that by using strict embryo criteria to select "top" quality embryos, one can achieve a high implantation rate [34]. Top quality embryos have the following characteristics: four or five blastomeres on day 2 and at least seven blastomeres on day 3 after fertilization, absence of multinucleated blastomeres, and <20% of fragments on day 2 and day 3 after fertilization. When these criteria were utilized in a small prospective randomized clinical trial comparing single- and double-embryo transfers, it was found that, in single-embryo transfers where a top quality embryo was available, an implantation rate of 42.3% and an ongoing pregnancy rate of 38.5% were obtained [34]. A variation of this methodology has been used for many years at Boston IVF by selecting what is termed as the high implantation potential (HIP) embryo. These embryos show similar prediction outcomes to the top quality embryos and are a good indicator of the potential of an embryo to reach the blastocyst stage (Figure 18.1).

However, assessment of the embryos at either the pronuclear or cleavage stages can, at best, be considered an assessment of the oocyte. The quality of the oocyte is undoubtedly important, as the quality of the developing embryo is ultimately dependent on the quality of the gametes from which it is derived, but this provides limited information regarding true embryo developmental potential. Furthermore, there is the potential of a paternal effect on development that is mainly evident after the 8-cell stage when the embryonic genome is activated. Only by culturing embryos past this stage to the blastocyst does it become possible to assess true embryonic development.

The use of blastocyst culture is becoming a more prevalent tool for embryo selection. A number of reasons have supported its more widespread adoption, in particular in the United States. These include the more effective selection of embryos at the blastocyst stage, cryopreservation by vitrification, and the more recent rise in the use of preimplantation genetic screening using trophectoderm biopsy (covered in Chapter 12).

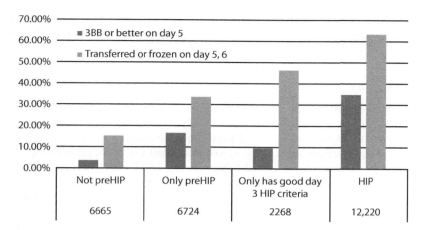

FIGURE 18.1 The developmental potential of embryos assessed on day 2 and day 3 to the blastocyst stage according to their high implantation potential (HIP) criteria. A day 2 embryo is assessed as a preHIP if it reaches the 4- to 6-cell stage with <50% fragmentation and no multinucleation. A HIP embryo is one that has been assessed as a preHIP embryo on day 2 and subsequently reaches the 7- to 10-cell stage with <20% fragmentation and no multinucleation on day 3. The percentages of embryos to reach a high-grade blastocyst (3BB or better on day 5) and those that were either transferred on day 5 or frozen on day 5 or 6 are shown. The number of embryos assessed is shown below each group.

For assessing blastocysts, the simplest criteria are reflected using an alphanumeric scoring system. This takes into account three aspects of blastocyst morphology: degree of blastocoels expansion, inner cell mass (ICM) development, and trophectoderm (TE) development (Figure 18.2).

Recently, a more detailed analysis of the impact that the different assessment criteria have on viability has indicated that the trophectoderm provides greater predictive weight for embryo selection. A study by Ahlstrom et al. [35] concluded that the predictive strength of the trophectoderm grade was greater compared to that for the ICM for selecting the best blastocyst for embryo transfer. It has been suggested that even though ICM is important, a strong trophectoderm layer is essential at this stage of embryo development, allowing successful hatching and implantation. This has subsequently been validated by a

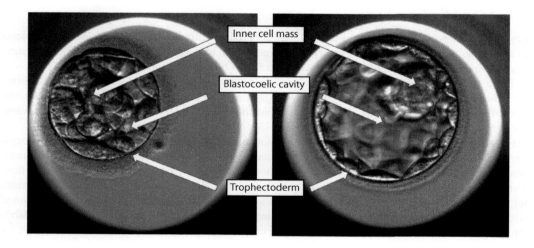

FIGURE 18.2 Blastocyst scoring characterizes the expansion of the blastocoelic cavity and the quality of the trophectoderm (TE) and tightness of the inner cell mass (ICM). The figure on the left shows the blastocoelic cavity just forming and the initial differentiation of cells identifiable by microscopy to the ICM and TE. The figure on the right shows a more advanced expanded blastocyst with clear ICM and TE.

number of studies [36–40], which all highlighted the need for a strong trophectoderm grading in relation to pregnancy. Interestingly, one study found that a poor ICM grading was also related to higher miscarriage rates [41].

Time Lapse Imaging

More recently, the use of time lapse imaging and the use of a morphokinetic scoring system have been examined to predict embryo viability. The majority of published studies have looked at retrospective data analyses, and the algorithms provided have shown usefulness in predicting embryo viability [42,43]. In particular, Meseguer and colleagues have published a series of papers using a triage system. In the first paper, Rubio et al. [44] analyzed 5225 embryos, of which, 1659 embryos were selected for transfer. Using these data, they found that embryos with direct cleavage from 2- to 3-cells, whereby the embryo remains for a prolonged period at the 3-cell stage, had a very low implantation rate (1.2%). On the basis of these findings, the authors suggested direct cleavage from 2- to 3-cells as a novel exclusion criterion for embryo selection. In addition, they combined standard morphological assessment, exclusion criteria, and inclusion criteria using an algorithm for embryo selection, which ranked embryos exhibiting an excellent cleavage pattern as A with a sliding scale down to D, E, and F as embryos that showed anomalies in timing of cleavage at different stages. In this algorithm, they classified embryos into 10 categories (A+/A−, B+/B−, C+/C−, D+/D−, E, and F or discarded) with different percentages of implantation. This algorithm was subsequently validated [45] prospectively, showing that, per treated cycle, the ongoing pregnancy rate was significantly increased from 51.4% (95% CI, 46.7–56.0) for the morphokinetics assessment group compared with 41.7% (95% CI, 36.9–46.5) for the standard incubator (non-morphokinetics) group. One criticism of this study was that the incubator systems were not the same and the difference may have been attributed to the superior incubator system and environment of the morphokinetics group, particularly the gas phase. In a subsequent randomized trial using a time lapse incubator as a control without morphokinetics, Goodman et al. [46] concluded that the addition of time lapse morphokinetic data did not significantly improve clinical reproductive outcomes in all patients and in those with blastocyst transfers. The jury appears to be still out on the utility of the time lapse systems. It may also be that we need to reassess the parameters we are examining [47].

Oocyte and Embryo Freezing

Cryopreservation is now an integral part of many IVF clinics throughout the world, enabling patients to utilize the maximum number of embryos generated from any one oocyte retrieval while protecting against ovarian hyperstimulation syndrome and the risk of higher-order multiple births.

There are a number of different cryoprotectants currently used in cryostorage of the oocyte/embryo, e.g., dimethyl sulfoxide (DMSO), ethylene glycol, glycerol, and propane-1,2-diol, together with numerous different methodologies, i.e., slow freeze–rapid thaw, rapid freeze–rapid thaw, and vitrification. Freezing can be applied at all stages of embryo development and to the oocyte.

For embryos, all the older slow protocols have now been largely superseded by the use of blastocyst vitrification, which appears to provide the most consistent pregnancy results [48]. This recent meta-analysis concluded that data from available randomized controlled trials suggest that vitrification/warming is superior to slow freezing/thawing with regard to clinical outcomes and cryosurvival rates for oocytes, cleavage-stage embryos, and blastocysts. They went on to state that improvements obtained with the introduction of vitrification have several important clinical implications in ART and that laboratories that continue to use slow freezing should consider transitioning to the use of vitrification for cryopreservation.

Most importantly, it is evident that vitrification now has allowed live birth outcomes from frozen embryo transfers to surpass those from fresh transfers [49]. The question now is whether clinically, it makes more sense to transfer only frozen embryos rather than perform transfers in fresh cycles. The data appear to be compelling on two fronts. First, there is the deleterious effect of a stimulated uterine environment, particularly elevated progesterone levels, that appear to harm the chance of pregnancy [50], and second, live birth weights of children born from frozen embryo transfers are consistently better when compared to those from fresh embryo transfers [51,52].

For the oocyte, the majority of data have been collected from donor oocytes whereby success rates of vitrified oocytes versus fresh oocytes have been shown to be equivalent [53]. Oocyte vitrification for donors provides numerous advantages, including being more efficient, more economical, easier for both donors and recipients, and potentially also safer, because eggs can now be quarantined for 6 months (or longer) to retest for infectious diseases in the donors [53]. Oocyte vitrification also provides the opportunity for fertility preservation for social or medical reasons, e.g., in advance of oncologic therapy [54].

Vitrification Procedure

The vitrification procedure consists of three solutions that are used to achieve equilibration of the oocyte or embryo for different times. Commonly used solutions may or may not contain DMSO. One protocol, for example, involves an equilibration solution (containing the cryoprotectants DMSO and ethylene glycol with a serum supplement) and a vitrification solution (containing the same solutions but in a higher concentration). The aim of any freezing or vitrification protocol is to use the cryoprotectants to replace any water in the oocyte/embryo while still providing protection to the cell membrane and other organelles. Removal of water effectively removes any chance of crystals forming within the oocyte/embryo and creating damage.

Routinely, the oocyte/embryo is incubated in the equilibration solution for between 5 and 10 minutes while they are placed in the final vitrification solution for between 30 and 60 seconds. The timings are dependent on specific protocols recommended by manufacturers or used by individual laboratories. When removed from the vitrification solution, the embryo is normally pipetted onto a cryostorage device in minimal volume that just covers the embryo or oocyte. These devices should allow the embryo in its cryoprotectant to be vitrified at very high cooling rates.

To warm embryos before transfer, the reverse process is effectively applied. An initial thawing solution containing sucrose and the serum supplement is used, followed by a diluted form of the same solution that contains less sucrose. Finally, the oocyte/embryo is allowed to recover in the usual culture medium for a period before use.

Conclusion

IVF reproductive technologies have come a long way since the first birth in 1978. The technical progression from ICSI to treat many male infertility patients to the use of preimplantation genetic screening and vitrification, which has allowed dramatic improvements in both oocyte and embryo storage, has shown how laboratory improvements can influence success. Technological advances in the IVF laboratory including improvements in molecular analysis and novel noninvasive assessment profiles using microscopy and revolutionary microfluidic platforms are currently being used in other areas of medicine and will likely affect the IVF laboratory in the near future and further improve the chances of patients having a normal healthy offspring.

REFERENCES

1. Rock J, Menkin MF. In vitro fertilization and cleavage of human ovarian eggs. *Science* 1944;100:105–7.
2. Whittingham DG. Culture of mouse ova. *J Reprod Fert* 1971;14(suppl):7–21.
3. Brinster RL. Embryo development. *J Animal Sci* 1974;38:1003–12.
4. Biggers JD, Borland RM. Physiological aspects of growth and development of the preimplantation mammalian embryo. *Annu Rev Physiol* 1976;38:95–119.
5. De Kretser D, Dennis P, Hudson B, Leeton J, Lopata A, Outch K, Talbot J, Wood C. Transfer of a human zygote. *Lancet* 1973;2:728–9.

6. Steptoe PC, Edwards RG. Reimplantation of a human embryo with subsequent tubal pregnancy. *Lancet* 1976;1:880–2.

7. Steptoe PC, Edwards RG. Birth after the reimplantation of a human embryo [letter]. *Lancet* 1978;2:366.

8. Swain JE, Pool TB. New pH-buffering system for media utilized during gamete and embryo manipulations for assisted reproduction. *Reprod Biomed Online* 2009;18:799–810.

9. WHO. *World Health Organization Laboratory Manual for Examination of Human Semen.* 5th ed., Cambridge: Cambridge University Press; 2010.

10. Bungum M, Humaidan P, Spano M, Jepson K, Bungum L, Giwercman A. The predictive value of sperm chromatin structure assay (SCSA) parameters for the outcome of intrauterine insemination, IVF and ICSI. *Hum Reprod* 2004;19:1401–8.

11. Virro MR, Larson-Cook KL, Evenson DP. Sperm chromatin structure assay (SCSA) parameters are related to fertilization, blastocyst development, and ongoing pregnancy in in vitro fertilization and intracytoplasmic sperm injection cycles. *Fertil Steril* 2004;81:1289–95.

12. Sakkas D, Alvarez JG. Sperm DNA fragmentation: Mechanisms of origin, impact on reproductive outcome, and analysis. *Fertil Steril* 2010;93:1027–36.

13. Carrell DT. Contributions of spermatozoa to embryogenesis: Assays to evaluate their genetic and epigenetic fitness. *Reprod Biomed Online* 2008;16:474–84.

14. Evenson DP, Jost LK, Marshall D, Zinaman MJ, Clegg E, Purvis K, De Angelis P, Claussen OP. Utility of the sperm chromatin structure assay as a diagnostic and prognostic tool in the human fertility clinic. *Human Reprod* 1999;14:1039–49.

15. Evenson DP, Larson KL, Jost LK. Sperm chromatin structure assay: Its clinical use for detecting sperm DNA fragmentation in male infertility and comparisons with other techniques. *J Androl* 2002;23:25–43.

16. Sbracia M, Grasso J, Sayme N, Stronk J, Huszar G. Hyaluronic acid substantially increases the retention of motility in cryopreserved/thawed human spermatozoa. *Hum Reprod* 1997;12:1949–54.

17. Huszar G, Ozkavukcu S, Jakab A, Celik-Ozenci C, Sati GL, Cayli S. Hyaluronic acid binding ability of human sperm reflects cellular maturity and fertilizing potential: Selection of sperm for intracytoplasmic sperm injection. *Curr Opin Obstet Gynecol* 2006;18:260–7.

18. Huszar G, Jakab A, Sakkas D, Ozenci CC, Cayli S, Delpiano E, Ozkavukcu S. Fertility testing and ICSI sperm selection by hyaluronic acid binding: Clinical and genetic aspects. *Reprod Biomed Online* 2007;14:650–63.

19. Jakab A, Sakkas D, Delpiano E, Cayli S, Kovanci E, Ward D, Ravelli A, Huszar G. Intracytoplasmic sperm injection: A novel selection method for sperm with normal frequency of chromosomal aneuploidies. *Fertil Steril* 2005;84:1665–73.

20. Cayli S, Jakab A, Ovari L, Delpiano E, Celik-Ozenci C, Sakkas D, Ward D, Huszar G. Biochemical markers of sperm function: Male fertility and sperm selection for ICSI. *Reprod Biomed Online* 2003;7:462–8.

21. Celik-Ozenci C, Catalanotti J, Jakab A, Aksu C, Ward D, Bray-Ward P, Demir R, Huszar G. Human sperm maintain their shape following decondensation and denaturation for fluorescent in situ hybridization: Shape analysis and objective morphometry. *Biol Reprod* 2003;69:1347–55.

22. Worrilow KC, Eid S, Woodhouse D, Perloe M, Smith S, Witmyer J, Ivani K, Khoury C, Ball GD, Elliot T et al. Use of hyaluronan in the selection of sperm for intracytoplasmic sperm injection (ICSI): Significant improvement in clinical outcomes—Multicenter, double-blinded and randomized controlled trial. *Hum Reprod* 2013;28:306–14.

23. Kattera S, Chen C. Short coincubation of gametes in in vitro fertilization improves implantation and pregnancy rates: A prospective, randomized, controlled study. *Fertil Steril* 2003;80:1017–21.

24. Gianaroli L, Cristina MM, Ferraretti AP, Fiorentino A, Tosti E, Panzella S, Dale B. Reducing the time of sperm-oocyte interaction in human in-vitro fertilization improves the implantation rate. *Hum Reprod* 1996;11:166–71.

25. Boulet SL, Mehta A, Kissin DM, Warner L, Kawwass JF, Jamieson DJ. Trends in use of and reproductive outcomes associated with intracytoplasmic sperm injection. *JAMA* 2015;313:255–63.

26. Bonduelle M, Wilikens A, Buysse A, Van AE, Wisanto A, Devroey P, Van Steirteghem AC, Liebaers I. Prospective follow-up study of 877 children born after intracytoplasmic sperm injection (ICSI), with ejaculated epididymal and testicular spermatozoa and after replacement of cryopreserved embryos obtained after ICSI. *Hum Reprod* 1996;11(Suppl 4):131–55.

27. Leunens L, Celestin-Westreich S, Bonduelle M, Liebaers I, Ponjaert-Kristoffersen I. Follow-up of cognitive and motor development of 10-year-old singleton children born after ICSI compared with spontaneously conceived children. *Hum Reprod* 2008;23:105–11.

28. Belva F, De SF, Tournaye H, Liebaers I, Devroey P, Haentjens P, Bonduelle M. Neonatal outcome of 724 children born after ICSI using non-ejaculated sperm. *Hum Reprod* 2011;26:1752–8.

29. Gardner DK, Lane M. Culture of viable human blastocysts in defined sequential serum-free media. *Hum Reprod* 1998;13(Suppl 3):148–59.

30. Gardner DK, Lane M. Culture of viable human blastocysts in defined sequential serum-free media. *Hum Reprod* 1998;13:148–59.

31. Quinn P. Culture systems: Sequential. *Methods Mol Biol* 2012;912:211–30.

32. Biggers JD, Summers MC. Choosing a culture medium: Making informed choices. *Fertil Steril* 2008; 90:473–83.

33. Scott L. Pronuclear scoring as a predictor of embryo development. *Reprod Biomed Online* 2003;6:201–14.

34. Van Royen E, Mangelschots K, De ND, Valkenburg M, Van de Meerssche M, Ryckaert G, Eestermans W, Gerris J. Characterization of a top quality embryo, a step towards single-embryo transfer. *Hum Reprod* 1999;14:2345–9.

35. Ahlstrom A, Westin C, Reismer E, Wikland M, Hardarson T. Trophectoderm morphology: An important parameter for predicting live birth after single blastocyst transfer. *Hum Reprod* 2011;26:3289–96.

36. Hill MJ, Richter KS, Heitmann RJ, Graham JR, Tucker MJ, DeCherney AH, Browne PE, Levens ED. Trophectoderm grade predicts outcomes of single-blastocyst transfers. *Fertil Steril* 2013;99:1283–9.

37. Chen X, Zhang J, Wu X, Cao S, Zhou L, Wang Y, Chen X, Lu J, Zhao C, Chen M et al. Trophectoderm morphology predicts outcomes of pregnancy in vitrified-warmed single-blastocyst transfer cycle in a Chinese population. *J Assist Reprod Genet* 2014;31:1475–81.

38. Thompson SM, Onwubalili N, Brown K, Jindal SK, McGovern PG. Blastocyst expansion score and trophectoderm morphology strongly predict successful clinical pregnancy and live birth following elective single embryo blastocyst transfer (eSET): A national study. *J Assist Reprod Genet* 2013;30:1577–81.

39. van der Weiden RM. Trophectoderm morphology grading reflects interactions between embryo and endometrium. *Fertil Steril* 2013;100:e23.

40. Honnma H, Baba T, Sasaki M, Hashiba Y, Ohno H, Fukunaga T, Endo T, Saito T, Asada Y. Trophectoderm morphology significantly affects the rates of ongoing pregnancy and miscarriage in frozen-thawed single-blastocyst transfer cycle in vitro fertilization. *Fertil Steril* 2012;98:361–7.

41. Van den Abbeel E, Balaban B, Ziebe S, Lundin K, Cuesta MJ, Klein BM, Helmgaard L, Arce JC. Association between blastocyst morphology and outcome of single-blastocyst transfer. *Reprod Biomed Online* 2013;27:353–61.

42. Meseguer M, Herrero J, Tejera A, Hilligsoe KM, Ramsing NB, Remohi J. The use of morphokinetics as a predictor of embryo implantation. *Hum Reprod* 2011;26:2658–71.

43. Meseguer M, Rubio I, Cruz M, Basile N, Marcos J, Requena A. Embryo incubation and selection in a time-lapse monitoring system improves pregnancy outcome compared with a standard incubator: A retrospective cohort study. *Fertil Steril* 2012;98:1481–89.

44. Rubio I, Kuhlmann R, Agerholm I, Kirk J, Herrero J, Escriba MJ, Bellver J, Meseguer M. Limited implantation success of direct-cleaved human zygotes: A time-lapse study. *Fertil Steril* 2012;98:1458–63.

45. Rubio I, Galan A, Larreategui Z, Ayerdi F, Bellver J, Herrero J, Meseguer M. Clinical validation of embryo culture and selection by morphokinetic analysis: A randomized, controlled trial of the EmbryoScope. *Fertil Steril* 2014;102:1287–94.

46. Goodman LR, Goldberg J, Falcone T, Austin C, Desai N. Does the addition of time-lapse morphokinetics in the selection of embryos for transfer improve pregnancy rates? A randomized controlled trial. *Fertil Steril* 2016;105:275–85.

47. Sakkas D. Cleavage in the preimplantation embryo: It is all about being in the right place at the right time! *Mol Hum Reprod* 2016;22:679–80.

48. Rienzi L, Gracia C, Maggiulli R, LaBarbera AR, Kaser DJ, Ubaldi FM, Vanderpoel S, Racowsky C. Oocyte, embryo and blastocyst cryopreservation in ART: Systematic review and meta-analysis comparing slow-freezing versus vitrification to produce evidence for the development of global guidance. *Hum Reprod Update* 2017;23:139–155.

49. Centers for Disease Control and Prevention, 2014 Assisted Reproductive Technology National Summary Report. https://www.cdc.gov/art/reports/2014/national-summary.html
50. Venetis CA, Kolibianakis EM, Bosdou JK, Tarlatzis BC. Progesterone elevation and probability of pregnancy after IVF: A systematic review and meta-analysis of over 60,000 cycles. *Hum Reprod Update* 2013;19:433–57.
51. Shih W, Rushford DD, Bourne H, Garrett C, McBain JC, Healy DL, Baker HW. Factors affecting low birthweight after assisted reproduction technology: Difference between transfer of fresh and cryopreserved embryos suggests an adverse effect of oocyte collection. *Hum Reprod* 2008;23:1644–53.
52. Maas K, Galkina E, Thornton K, Penzias AS, Sakkas D. No change in live birthweight of IVF singleton deliveries over an 18-year period despite significant clinical and laboratory changes. *Hum Reprod* 2016;31:1987–96.
53. Cobo A, Remohi J, Chang CC, Nagy ZP. Oocyte cryopreservation for donor egg banking. *Reprod Biomed Online* 2011;23:341–6.
54. Cobo A, Garcia-Velasco JA, Domingo J, Remohi J, Pellicer A. Is vitrification of oocytes useful for fertility preservation for age-related fertility decline and in cancer patients? *Fertil Steril* 2013;99:1485–95.

19

Tools for Effective Nursing in the Care of the Infertile Patient

Sharon Edwards, Susan Gordon-Pinnell, and Kristin MacCutcheon

Introduction

Reproductive Endocrinology and Infertility (REI) or Assisted Reproductive Technology (ART) nursing is a relatively new field that began in the 1970s with hospital-based infertility clinics where nurses were considered the doctor's "assistant." The field has expanded considerably from those days into a complex and unique specialty requiring a high level of skill, compassion, understanding, and patience. The REI nurse is the crucial link between the patient and physician as an advocate, giving support, education, and help in navigating the complicated system she has just entered. On any given day, he or she may discuss the areas of reproductive anatomy, laboratory procedures, genetics, insurance, law, and ethics. The REI nurse is also the "glue" that holds the rest of the team together by being the liaison for the medical staff, embryology, endocrinology, financial services, clinic and surgical procedures, and mental health practitioners. Since the REI nurse is such an integral part of the patient's journey, he or she must be well trained and understand that the role played has a far-reaching impact on each patient encountered. There truly is an "art" to ART nursing.

Acquiring a Knowledge Base

What brings someone to REI nursing? For some, it is personal experience, either themselves, a family member, or a friend. Experiencing the emotional struggle and stress of infertility has a profound effect on many nurses and leads to a desire to help others. For many, it represents a change from the typical hospital-based practice on a floor or critical care unit, allowing a better life/work balance and a field that is constantly changing and growing. For most, it is having a background in Women's Health nursing and the interest and challenge of a specialty practice. Whatever the reason or past experience, REI is a new field that requires intensive training and learning from a variety of sources. It takes about 6 months to understand all the mechanics of infertility and up to a year to feel competent and knowledgeable as an REI nurse.

Sources of Education

- There are multiple resources for a nurse new to infertility to access. The American Society for Reproductive Medicine (ASRM) (www.asrm.org) has dozens of modules for both new and seasoned nurses, from basic infertility to embryology for the nursing professional. The nursing arm of ASRM, the Nurses' Professional Group, has developed a certificate course acknowledging nursing excellence in the field, which is the gold standard for REI nursing. Several pharmaceutical companies have PhDs on staff who provide one-on-one training in the clinic setting for nurses in basic infertility and a variety of specialty subjects. In addition, there are annual conferences that offer courses on many topics needed to acquire a solid knowledge base for infertility.

- On-the-job training is an important and crucial aspect of nursing education as it deals with day-to-day, real-life situations that are important to develop a "feel" for what the patient experiences. Seasoned REI nurses can mentor the new nurse on the nuts and bolts of the specialty, offering experience and wisdom in a practical application. The best training method is to have a comprehensive orientation schedule over the course of 2 to 3 months with specific elements that gradually progress the new nurse from observation to fielding calls with the seasoned nurse as mentor. An effective tool during this training period is role playing. The seasoned mentor nurse pretends to be a patient, asking questions in different ways. Doing this ensures the new nurse understands the content and is not just memorizing what was taught and is an effective teaching method. A checklist to "sign off" the new nurse as having been exposed to and understand all the necessary elements rounds out the educational experience.

What the REI Nurse Needs to Know

- *Infertility 101*: This comprises the "basics" of infertility, explaining to the patient male and female reproductive anatomy, the menstrual cycle, endocrine hormones, and how they interact.
- *The infertility workup*: Many tests are needed to evaluate the cause of infertility, and it is the REI nurse's responsibility to order and explain this testing to the patient. The basics include a cavity study (hysterosalpingogram, saline sonohysterogram, office hysteroscopy), endocrine hormone assay (cycle day 3 testing and can include follicle-stimulating hormone, antimullerian hormone, and estradiol levels), ultrasound (basal antral follicle count), and semen analysis for the male.
- *Abnormalities and what they mean*: Sometimes abnormalities can interfere with cycle timing, so understanding and explaining how this affects a patient is important. Things such as fibroids, ovarian cysts, or polyps can negatively affect implantation and carrying a fetus to term. The REI nurse must be able to assist with explanation on courses of treatment to resolve these issues.
- *Treatment options*: The variety of options can be overwhelming for a patient to grasp, and the decision-making process can be stressful. Understanding the many protocols, medications, and regimens is a key ingredient for successful REI nurse–patient interactions. Patients often do not understand everything being said in the follow-up visit with their physician and look to the nurse to explain what had just been discussed. They may be nervous, don't want to appear unknowledgeable, and therefore don't ask questions of their physician. Because of the strong bond formed with their nurse, patients feel safe and cared for, and are able to look to their nurse to go through the treatment options again to come to an informed decision. It is therefore imperative that an REI nurse be adept at treatment options. These can include timed intercourse, intrauterine insemination (IUI) with clomiphene citrate/letrozole, IUI with gonadotropins, natural cycles, in vitro fertilization (IVF) cycles, natural insemination versus intracytoplasmic sperm injection (ICSI), preimplantation genetic screening/preimplantation genetic diagnosis, as well as third-party reproduction (donor egg and/or gestational carrier services). In the end, the REI nurse is the one who takes the information given to a patient, breaks it down step by step in a way that can be understood, and implements it in a way so the patient doesn't feel so overwhelmed. Quite an impressive amount of knowledge to master!

Elements for Effective REI Nursing

Once the REI nurse has learned the medical and scientific basis of her craft, she must follow through on the other necessary elements needed as part of the care team. Communication and attention to detail are critical components of effective nursing for both the patient and other members of the team. As the primary liaison for the patient, the REI nurse must have good documentation practices, must have detailed notes for all team members to easily access, must communicate to all parties, and must be articulate in those communications.

- *Attention to detail*: This is imperative owing to the multifactorial aspect of the patient's care. As the "go to" member of the team, the REI nurse is the "quarterback" for the team and must be meticulous in detailing all aspects of treatment. Decisions are made that must be coordinated, from the physician to the embryologist to the financial counselor to the appointment scheduler, and all are fed through the REI nurse. Attention to every detail must be noted and acted on, whether it is to the team or to the patient. Treatment plans are modified, patients change their minds, and many things happen on a daily basis requiring the quarterback to monitor and ensure these details are attended to and implemented.

- *Communication and Documentation*: Nurses learn early on in their education, "if it wasn't documented, it wasn't done." Every interaction with the patient must be clearly and concisely written. It is the REI nurse's obligation to ensure that the next health care team member who accesses the patient chart is aware of all that has transpired, and that all interactions with the patient are documented. It is also imperative that the nurse is clear and concise with the patient, whether it is in person, by phone, or by e-mail. Patients hang on to every word expressed and give great value to what is said and great value to anything said that may be expressed differently or perceived as contradictory. For this reason, every interaction must be documented in objective terms with precise language to prevent misinterpretation and provide clarity to both patient and team members.

  Timely and effective communication can be accomplished through a variety of means, and infertility nurses may field 50–80 calls a day. E-mail, texting, and an EMR patient portal are a few of the ways nurses communicate in the new paradigm. Patients are anxious and stressed, and if they are unable to speak to their nurse live, they expect a return call quickly. A policy should be in place that all calls are returned by the end of that day, regardless of whether there is a solution or not. While all issues may not be resolved, the patient will understand that their issue is being addressed and reassured that their concerns are taken seriously. The patient experience involves not only good medical care but good customer service care as well.

- *Informed Consent*: While informed consent is ultimately the responsibility of the physician, the process begins with a discussion of the proposed treatment plan with the physician and ultimately involves multiple staff across departmental lines. After the initial discussion, the nursing team provides educational materials and consent forms for the patient to review. When the patient and partner (if applicable) are ready to move forward, they meet with the nurse to review the consent forms and obtain signatures. If any issues arise from the wording of the consent or it appears the patient requires clarification of the treatment plan that the nurse has already addressed, the nurse will arrange for the patient to meet again with the physician. Informed consent is a shared responsibility that the REI nurse contributes to in a meaningful way, and the patient looks to her nurse as a guide through understanding the elements.

- *Triage*: The nurse plays an important role in the triage of medical and emotional issues that need to be addressed during the course of treatment and brought to the attention of the physician. For example, ectopic pregnancies can be more common in the infertile population who undergo IVF treatment. A patient who calls with a menses that is lighter than usual, has bleeding at an anticipated time of the menstrual cycles, has abnormal rising human chorionic gonadotropin (hCG) titers, or complains of pain should be considered at risk of having an ectopic pregnancy. Ovarian hyperstimulation syndrome (OHSS) complicates any fertility treatment but is more common in the patient undergoing IVF and being triggered with hCG. Symptoms can occur any time from the time of the egg retrieval until the pregnancy test. Initial symptoms include abdominal distention and pain. Symptoms of more advanced OHSS include shortness of breath, nausea and vomiting, and severe pain—these patients need to be brought in for evaluation expeditiously. These are examples of why REI nurses must have a thorough understanding of complications and know the signs and symptoms of many nuances presented by patients. Since the nurse is in frequent contact with the patient, the nurse is the person fielding these important calls—if not properly triaged, these patients can be at risk for serious consequences.

- *Patient Education*: It begins the moment a patient walks into the clinic and lasts through the entire journey. REI nurses encounter women and men on a daily basis who need accurate and compassionate information about the process of infertility treatment. There are many ways to provide the necessary information, and a formal patient education program should be in place not only to teach patients the details of their treatment plan but also to guide patients through all the steps along the way.

  The nurse guides the patient through many medical and nonmedical aspects, such as financial implications, insurance benefits, appointment setting, consenting, medications and treatment. A comprehensive system is set up to teach and instruct patients with each new step encountered, and there are two main elements of a good patient education program:

  - Instruction by the primary nurse each time the patient meets with the physician
  - A formal education consultation with an experienced nurse each time the patient has a new treatment he or she hasn't done before (such as the first time a patient does IUI or IVF)

  When the patient has a consult with the physician, there is usually a "next step" that the primary nurse helps to explain—comprehensive testing after the initial consult, the results of that testing after the follow-up consult, discussion about progress once treatment begins, to name a few. This is ongoing throughout the patient experience.

  The second, and very important, patient education interaction is when a first-time regimen is ordered, such as an IUI or IVF cycle. There are several ways clinics set up education forums—large group teaching sessions, one-on-one in-person sessions, and online programs. Large group sessions are difficult to teach as they involve multiple treatment plans and medications and are not individualized to the patient. They tend to be ineffective and often create more questions than they answer. One-on-one in-person sessions are very individualized and effective but terribly inefficient and not practical for the primary nurse to do as each session is an hour-long process. The most efficient and beneficial method is to do an online program that involves computer-based information, real-time medication video, and a follow-up phone consultation with the Nurse Educator. This allows the patient to review the literature and instructions at home at a time of their choosing. It is less stressful as the patient can do this over a period of time and review the information as many times as needed. The key part of this type of program is the follow-up phone call by the nurse to make sure that the patient has read the material and understands it—a short "quiz" can take place during the conversation. If the nurse feels that the patient does not fully understand the treatment plan or what is involved, she brings the patient in to the clinic to go over it in person. This method has a high patient satisfaction index, respects the patient's time, and can be easily managed by the clinic. The vast majority of patients will successfully complete their patient education process in this manner; those who don't are those with no access to a computer, those who experience a language barrier, or those who prefer to learn medication injection "hands on."

- *Being a Patient Advocate*: REI nurses are in a unique position to help guide the patient experience since patients identify their nurse as their most important contact, and see or speak to their nurse more often than their physician. The inability to conceive or maintain a pregnancy often creates a crisis for women and their partners and they look to their nurse for care, compassion, and help. Many patients put on their best faces in front of the physician but confide in the nurse how they are truly feeling, and it is a special role that nurses take on to reduce the patient's anxiety and validate their feelings. Nurses guide patients through the grief of failed treatment, provide empathy after a loss, and allow the patient to feel safe in expressing their loss of control. Because nurses are often closely involved with the emotional aspects of what the patient experiences, they may be the first to recognize anxiety and depression in patients they work with. When this happens, it is crucial the nurse speak to the physician and formulate a plan of care that includes a mental health professional—most patients will deny they have an issue but prolonged depression will affect all aspects of the patient's life and must be addressed. A clinic should have access to a list of qualified professionals who are experienced in patients undergoing infertility. The ideal would be to have a social worker or psychologist on site to meet with patients or intervene if there is an urgent need.

Conclusion

The scope of REI nursing practice continues to expand as new developments in science, treatment protocols, medication, and laboratory procedures evolve, along with the ever-changing norms of society. The scientific, emotional, legal, and changing patient population provides an exciting environment with many opportunities for a nurse to grow. Every day, we learn something from our patients and from each other, and this makes our field amazing. Strong, qualified nurses will always be needed to provide a foundation for the patient struggling with infertility—they are a critical link when a patient is successful and an empathic friend when it isn't. The role is complex but the rewards are many, and it is a privilege to be a part of the journey.

20

The Mind/Body Connection

Alice D. Domar

Introduction

Every woman who is experiencing infertility has been told at some point to "just relax," "go on vacation," "quit your job," "stop trying so hard," or the old favorite, "just adopt and then it will happen." The assumption behind all of these comments is that the woman's stress level is in some way preventing conception. But is that true? Are infertile women more stressed than fertile women? And if so, does their stress level preclude pregnancy? Can it truly prevent infertile women from benefiting from the advances in reproductive technologies? And will relaxing indeed lead to conception? Why not simply offer medication to treat symptoms of anxiety and/or depression? These are the questions that will be answered in the following pages.

The Psychological Impact of Infertility

One of the problems with assessing the distress levels of infertile women, or many other kinds of patients facing medical treatment for that matter, is that the typical way to assess distress is with self-report psychological questionnaires. And in order to get accurate data, one needs to collect accurate responses. However, many patients feel an intense need to come across as a "good patient"; they, in effect, "fake good" and may thus underestimate their level of distress. This phenomenon was highlighted in a study in Sweden on in vitro fertilization (IVF) patients [1]. Women were psychologically assessed several times during an IVF cycle and their well-being scores were in the normal range and consistently comparable with Swedish reference values. The authors theorized that the reason why patients tested so well is that they ... "kept their worries and anxieties to themselves because they had great expectations regarding both themselves and the anticipated treatment. Perhaps they also wanted to show how well they felt and that they could handle the treatment." Several other studies with infertility patients have come to similar conclusions; self-report measures in the infertile population may well underestimate the level of distress.

Despite this concern, there have been numerous studies using self-report measures that have shown that infertile women have more symptoms of depression and anxiety than the general population. Research has shown that the prevalence of depressive symptoms in the infertile population is twice that of the general population [2]. In addition, infertile women have comparable levels of anxiety and depression as women with heart disease, HIV+ status, or metastatic cancer [3].

However, the gold standard in psychological testing is not a self-report measure but instead a structured psychiatric interview conducted by a mental health professional. An innovative study on 112 patients presenting to an infertility clinic for the first time included such an interview [4]. A total of 40.2% of the women met the criteria for a psychiatric disorder; the most common was anxiety disorder (23.2%), followed by depressive disorder (17%). This compares with a community sample prevalence of 3%.

It is obvious that infertile women are suffering. If almost half of new infertility patients report significant psychological symptoms, since the level of distress tends to rise as duration increases, and to intensify as treatment becomes more complex, it is reasonable to theorize that more than half of patients actively receiving treatment are experiencing a diagnosable level of anxiety and/or depression.

In one of the most recent studies [5], 39.1% of the infertile women and 15.3% of their male partners met the criteria for major depressive disorder (MDD) over an 18-month study period. MDD must be taken seriously since it can be associated with suicidal risk. In fact, suicidal risk is not insignificant in infertile women. In a cross-sectional study of 106 infertile women, the rate of women who were determined to be at risk for suicide was 9.4% [6], which is shockingly high. In addition, recent long-term research indicates that some patients remain distressed for many years, even ones whose treatment was successful. Ten percent of women who underwent IVF treatment 11–17 years previously continued to experience heightened levels of distress [7]. And a Swedish study that assessed women 20–23 years after IVF treatment had similar findings: previous IVF treatment was associated with a significantly increased risk of depression, obsession–compulsion, and somatization [8]. Women who never conceived were at the highest risk for depression and phobic anxiety.

There are many reasons why infertile women experience such high levels of distress—the process affects their relationship with their partner, their sex life, their relationships with family and friends, their job, their financial security, and their relationship with God. Men and women do not react to infertility in the same way, at the same time, or with the same level of commitment. In most cases, the infertile couple is surrounded by the fertility of their siblings, friends, neighbors, and coworkers. Imagine the couple who starts trying the same time as a sibling or close friend and then find themselves 2 or 3 years later still childless when the other couple announces their second pregnancy. Many jobs involve structured meetings and travel, neither of which is conducive to invasive and unexpected infertility treatments. Money is already an issue for most couples; the thought of spending $15,000 on a treatment that has less than a 40% chance of succeeding will force many couples into conflict. Finally, the issue of religiosity needs to be addressed. The majority of individuals in this country pray and believe in a higher power. For many, this is the first time that God has not answered their prayers, leading many to question either their own level of goodness, or the existence of God.

Whether a particular couple experiences conflict in one of these areas or more likely in all seven, it is not surprising that infertility can cause such emotional upheaval. To top it off, the comments from well-meaning family and friends, such as the ones that introduced this chapter, can contribute to a "blame the victim" mentality.

Unfortunately, the mental health needs of this patient population are not currently being met. In a recent study of 352 women and 274 men receiving treatment in one of five infertility clinics, 56.5% of women and 32.1% of men scored in the clinical range for depressive symptoms [9]. A total of 75.9% of women and 60.6% of men scored in the clinical range for anxiety. Only 21% of women and 11.3% of men reported receiving mental health services; 26.7% of women and 24.1% of men reported that mental health support information had been made available to them. However, those patients who reported high levels of depression and/or anxiety, even those who had experienced the symptoms for long periods, were no more likely to be offered information than the nondistressed patients.

The Impact of Stress on Treatment Outcome

Since IVF involves a relatively similar protocol throughout the world, research on the impact of stress on reproductive outcome has focused mainly on IVF patients. There have been numerous studies that have investigated the relationship between stress before or during an IVF cycle and subsequent pregnancy rates [10]. Most, although not all, of these studies show a significant relationship between distress and pregnancy (i.e., the most distressed patients have the lowest pregnancy rates). It is possible that there may be cultural issues that are contributing to the conflicting results. For example, a large study from the Netherlands [11] did not find a relationship between distress and IVF outcome, but the authors noted that there was a floor effect—few of the patients in the study reported any distress at all. It is apparently common in some cultures to underreport distress on self-report scales. It is also possible that some women are more reproductively sensitive to stress than others.

One of the best-designed studies was on 151 women before beginning an IVF or GIFT cycle [12,13]. The strength of this study was the fact that they collected numerous psychological factors, including not only how stressed the patients reported feeling, but what factors about the treatment were the most stressful, as well as a number of physical factors, such as number and quality of oocytes retrieved, pregnancy outcomes, and birthweight. The baseline level of stress was significantly related to outcome; stress levels were correlated to number of retrieved oocytes, percentage fertilized, pregnancy rates, live birthrate, and birthweight. The strength of the correlation between distress and pregnancy was strong—the subjects who expressed the least baseline level of distress were 93% more likely to give birth than the patients who reported the highest baseline level of distress.

Research to date supports the hypothesis that stress can hamper reproduction in couples trying naturally [14]. In a study of 501 couples attempting to conceive naturally, women with the highest levels of salivary alpha-amylase, a biomarker of stress, had a twofold increased risk of infertility. The mechanism of action, however, is unknown.

The Impact of Psychological Distress on Dropout Rates

Until recently, it was assumed that patients would pursue infertility treatment until one of two events occurred—their physician told them that further treatment was unadvisable (so-called active censoring) or they ran out of money. This theory was well accepted by most health care professionals in the infertility field, simply because the patients they saw on a day-to-day basis were the ones who chose to continue treatment. The ones who dropped out of treatment came to no one's attention and were thus forgotten. However, research conducted in the past decade reveals a completely different scenario— patients drop out in large numbers. And since the research is coming from countries or states where IVF is covered by insurance, money was clearly not the motivation to terminate treatment. Anywhere from 40% to 65% of insurance-covered nonpregnant patients discontinue treatment before completing their covered cycles.

As it turns out, active censoring is relatively rare—a study from the Netherlands, in which there was a cumulative dropout rate of 62% after three cycles, found that only 14% of the patients who dropped out of treatment did so because of physician recommendation [15]. The most recent research shows that the primary reason why patients drop out of IVF treatment is psychological stress. In a Swedish study of 974 couples, the patients reported that "psychological burden" was the reason they discontinued treatment [16]. An Australian study showed the same results—66% of couples who dropped out of IVF cited the emotional strain as their reason for terminating treatment [17]. In a study of 211 couples who dropped out for reasons other than active censoring, the most commonly cited reason was psychological burden, followed by the perception of a poor prognosis [18]. This study also revealed that the couples who dropped out of treatment were as satisfied with their care as couples who remained in treatment, so the quality of care does not seem to be a contributing factor in patients' dropout decisions.

In a study on insured couples in the United States [19], stress was once again the most common reason cited in couples who dropped out of treatment. In addition, age was a factor in terms of dropout behavior; 34% of women aged 40 and below who were insured for six IVF cycles did not begin a third cycle, while for women aged 40–42 years, the percentage of those who dropped out was 68%.

Obviously, couples who drop out of treatment are likely to sacrifice their chance of pregnancy. A retrospective German study on 2130 IVF patients analyzed the cumulative pregnancy rate and found that 31.4% of couples achieved pregnancy after three cycles; however, if couples had undergone one more cycle, the rate would have increased to 41% [20]. If a couple had undergone the six insurance-covered cycles, the rate would have climbed to 60%.

Finally, it appears to be possible to predict which patients are more likely to drop out of treatment. In a prospective study of women beginning IVF, it was determined that pretreatment levels of depression were significantly predictive of patient treatment termination after only one cycle [21].

Two studies indicate that the impact that stress can have on treatment retention is actually determined before even seeking out medical intervention. In a study of couples in California who did not pursue any treatment after an initial consultation [22], it was discovered that depressive symptoms played an important role; depressed women were less likely to pursue treatment. An Australian study noted that women who reported depressive symptoms were unlikely to have sought out medical advice for the treatment of their infertility [23].

A recent systematic review on the reasons and predictors of treatment discontinuation included 22 studies that sampled 21,453 patients [24]. The most common reasons for discontinuation were postponement of treatment, physical and psychological burden, relational and personal problems, treatment rejection, and organizational and clinic problems.

Thus, it is obvious that psychological distress plays a large role in IVF retention. Patients who are depressed before treatment are more likely to drop out after only one cycle, and throughout the IVF process, patients cite psychological burden as the primary reason for dropping out of treatment. Obviously, premature termination limits a couple's ability to get pregnant. However, in one recent study, a simple psychological intervention was associated with a significant decrease in treatment termination [25]. In a randomized controlled trial that included 166 women about to begin their first IVF cycle, women who received a stress reduction packet in the mail, which included both relaxation and cognitive coping components, had a 5.5% dropout rate during the 1-year study period, compared to a 15.2% rate in the routine care control patients. In addition, the intervention patients reported significantly less psychological distress.

The Impact of Psychological Interventions on Infertile Women

If one does accept the theory that distress is associated with lower pregnancy rates in infertile women, then interventions designed to decrease distress should lead to higher pregnancy rates. And in fact, the majority of the research to date supports this notion. In the most recent meta-analysis of the literature, which included 39 studies [26], the authors concluded that... "statistically significant and robust overall effects of psychosocial intervention were found for both clinical pregnancy... and combined psychological outcomes." In addition, the larger the reduction in anxiety, the greater the improvement in pregnancy rates. Finally, interventions that focused on cognitive–behavior therapy (CBT) were particularly recommended.

Psychological interventions can take many forms, ranging from individual therapy to stress management programs. The term *counseling* can take many forms. Most would assume that would involve treatment for an individual or couple. But counseling can apply to many forms of intervention. For example, a randomized, controlled, prospective study was performed on 60 IVF patients in Turkey to assess the impact of "counseling" on IVF patients [27]. In this case, counseling was provided by the IVF nurses and included several hours of personal attention and support. The couples who received this intervention reported lower anxiety and depression scores as well as a 43% pregnancy rate, compared to a 17% rate in the control group who received routine nursing care.

There have not been solid data to support the use of brief psychotherapy with infertile individuals or couples. And in fact, research does not show any benefit [28]. In a study of 265 couples in the Netherlands, 84 of the couples agreed to be randomized to either a routine care control group or to an intervention that included three sessions with a social worker. There were no differences in psychological parameters or pregnancy rates between the two groups. This is the most recent of several studies that have not shown any definitive benefit of brief counseling.

Research on other interventions has shown more promise. In one randomized, controlled prospective study, 185 infertile women were assigned to either the 10-session Mind/Body Program for Infertility, a 10-session support group, or a routine care control group [29]. The mind/body intervention included instruction in relaxation techniques, stress management strategies, and lifestyle modifications. The support group included time for members both to voice their concerns about the impact that infertility was having on their lives and to provide support to each other. All subjects continued to receive routine infertility care. During the 1-year follow-up study period, 55% of the mind/body patients and 54% of the support group patients experienced a live birth, compared to only 20% of the control subjects. In addition, there were differences in psychological health [30]. The mind/body patients experienced a decrease in negative symptoms such as anxiety and depression, the support patients remained the same, while the control patients experienced a worsening of symptoms.

In a subsequent study in Japan, 74 subjects were randomized to either a five-session mind/body group or a routine care control group [31]. The mind/body subjects experienced a significant decrease in psychological distress and natural killer cell activity while the control subjects experienced no change. In addition, 38% of the mind/body subjects became pregnant during the study period compared to 13.5% of the control subjects.

In research performed at Boston IVF [32], 143 women who were about to begin their first IVF cycle were randomized to either the 10-session Mind/Body Program group or to a control group. Only 9% of the mind/body patients attended at least half of the program before their first IVF cycle, but 76% were able to before their second cycle. Clinical pregnancy rates for cycle 1 were 43% for both groups, but for cycle 2, they were 52% for the mind/body patients and 20% for the controls.

Psychological interventions that can be offered online are increasing in popularity. The Mind/Body Program for Infertility was recently modified into an online program in a randomized controlled study [33]. Seventy-one women experiencing infertility were randomized to either participate in the online program or routine care. The intervention group had significantly lower levels of depressive symptoms than the controls and a pregnancy rate of 42%, compared to a 17% rate in the control group.

The data thus far on the effectiveness of psychological interventions point to a longer-term stress-management kind of approach, rather than the more traditional use of individual or couples' counseling or brief therapy. There have been two less recent meta-analyses on psychological interventions. One [34] concluded that skills-based interventions were more effective than more traditional therapy, and the other [35] concluded that interventions of at least six sessions are more effective than shorter ones.

Mind/body interventions have been well researched; their effectiveness has been established with a variety of medical and psychological conditions, including hypertension, menopausal symptoms, premenstrual symptoms, insomnia, chronic pain, anxiety, cardiac arrhythmias, chemotherapy side effects, depressive symptoms, and gastrointestinal problems. The application of mind/body techniques to infertility began in 1986 and the clinical use is increasingly rapidly.

The Mind/Body Program for Infertility

The Mind/Body Program for Infertility was founded by the author and first offered in 1987. It was designed to teach relaxation and cognitive strategies to infertile women. The goal of the program was psychological symptom reduction, not pregnancy, and this message was disseminated to all interested patients. After the first 50 women completed the program, it was noted that they were experiencing significant psychological symptom reduction as well as a higher-than-anticipated pregnancy rate [36]. The program was first offered within the division of behavioral medicine at Beth Israel Deaconess Medical Center in Boston but was moved to Boston IVF in 2002.

At this point in time, after 29 years of clinical practice, pregnancy rates within 6 months of program completion average 45%–50%, and every psychological parameter measured, including anxiety, depression, hostility, and confusion, decreases significantly. In addition, patients report significant reductions in physical symptoms such as insomnia, headaches, abdominal pain, and gastrointestinal symptoms. Health care professionals from around the world have been trained as group leaders and uniformly report the same positive changes.

All potential participants must attend an intake appointment with the group leader. Participants are mailed a lengthy questionnaire that they are instructed to bring to the intake. There are multiple goals for this session. It provides an opportunity for the group leader and patient to get to know each other better; the group leader obtains a comprehensive medical, psychological, social, and lifestyle history; the group leader can explain how the program is run; and it gives the patient an opportunity to ask questions.

Groups are led by a PhD psychologist with extensive knowledge of infertility. Each group leader is supported by two "peer counselors" who are graduates of the program; peer counselors are chosen because, as program participants, they experienced excellent symptom relief and successfully incorporated the mind/body skills into their lives. They serve as role models and as a liaison between the leader and the patients. The Mind/Body Program also includes a buddy system. Patients are paired with another patient the first night. If there are two patients with similar circumstances (for example, secondary infertility, recurrent miscarriages, or a history of a stillbirth), they are paired up; otherwise, it is done on a geographical basis. Buddies are asked to speak to one another at least once per week and each buddy pair brings in a snack for the group once.

Patients with any kind of infertility diagnosis, including endometriosis, ovarian dysfunction, advanced age, male factor, premature ovarian failure, recurrent miscarriage, tubal blockage, and unexplained infertility, may attend. The groups include married heterosexual women, single women, lesbian women, and women with secondary infertility (although secondary patients may only have one child, women with more than one child are referred for individual counseling since their presence would be likely to upset the primary patients).

Table 20.1 outlines each session of the program and every session follows a similar schedule, as can be seen in Table 20.2. Each session incorporates relaxation training, social support, and a new stress management strategy. Despite the fact that the first half-hour of social support is optional, virtually all participants choose to attend. This is their time to share their stories, compare experiences, and complain about their husbands/mothers-in-law/doctors.

The program is designed to treat patients' anxiety first, so the first two sessions are dedicated to relaxation training. The next one is focused on self-nurturance, after which lifestyle habits are addressed. The current research on the impact of lifestyle behaviors is presented, such as the impact of smoking on IVF outcome, and participants are encouraged to discontinue smoking, limit their alcohol and caffeine intake, maintain a moderate exercise routine and healthy weight, and avoid alternative medicine methods such as herbs. The next sessions are dedicated to cognitive approaches to stress reduction, such as cognitive restructuring, journaling to express negative emotions, and effective communication strategies.

TABLE 20.1

Sessions of the Mind/Body Program for Infertility

1. Group leader and peer counselor introductions, research on the stress/infertility connection, the physiology of the relaxation response, participant and partner introductions, program mechanics[a]
2. Physiology of diaphragmatic breathing, mini-relaxation exercises, effective communication
3. The art of self-nurturance, how to reintroduce joy into one's life
4. The impact of lifestyle behaviors on fertility: weight, smoking, alcohol, exercise. The safety and efficacy of alternative medicine approaches
5. Introduction and experiential exercise of hatha yoga
6. Introduction to cognitive restructuring
7. All day Sunday session—couples yoga, the use of humor to reduce stress, goal setting, couples communication[a]
8. Completion of cognitive restructuring
9. The impact of emotional expression on health, journaling. Guest lectures from prior participants who went on to adopt or do donor egg[a]
10. Assertiveness, goal-setting, summary, goodbyes

[a] Husbands/partners attend these sessions.

TABLE 20.2

Outline of Each Mind/Body Session

30 minutes	Optional sharing support time
15 minutes	Relaxation exercise (different one each week)
10 minutes	Patients pair up to discuss individual progress
30 minutes	Group discussion on how members are doing incorporating mind/body skills into their lives, review of previous week's assignment
10 minutes	Brief lecture by the group leader on the topic of the evening
30 minutes	Experiential exercise on evening's topic
20 minutes	Group discussion on topic, Q&A
5 minutes	Mini-relaxation exercise

One of the sessions includes guest lectures by prior participants who moved on to either adoption or egg donation.

Husbands/partners attend 3 of the 10 sessions; the first introductory session, the Sunday session that is focused on couples' communication and bonding, and the ninth session where the men meet as a group with a male therapist to discuss how they are handling the crisis of infertility.

At the first session, each participant is asked to describe what they hope to get out of the program, i.e., where they hope to be by the 10th session. Then, at the 10th session, patients are asked whether or not they reached their goal. This tends to be a very emotional time, since each patient recounts her emotional state a mere 10 weeks ago and thanks the group, and group leader, for helping her get to such a much healthier place.

At the 10th session, participants complete a similar but shorter questionnaire to the one they completed before the intake. Each patient is offered an appointment with the group leader to review their progress, compare their pre- with their post-program status, and set goals for their continued improvement.

Patients consistently experience statistically significant reductions in all measured physical and psychological symptoms. But perhaps more important, their attitude toward their infertility changes. As opposed to their sole identity as an infertile woman at the intake, they leave being a healthy active woman who happens to be experiencing infertility. They don't cry for days when they start to menstruate, they tolerate pregnancy announcements from others, and they feel more comfortable meeting their own needs, such as skipping baby showers or not visiting friends with newborns. Perhaps one of the most unexpected side effects of the program is the participant's willingness to try avenues that did not feel tolerable before participation, such as undergoing IVF or deciding to pursue donor egg or adoption.

Mind/Body Approaches versus Pharmacotherapy

The most common treatment for depressive symptoms is medication. However, there is no direct evidence that pharmacological treatment of depressive symptoms in infertile women provides benefit, and there is some preliminary evidence that women taking selective serotonin reuptake inhibitors (SSRIs) may have lower pregnancy rates from assisted reproductive technology (ART) treatment [37]. Recent research has shown that antidepressant medication is associated with a reduced probability of conceiving in women attempting to conceive naturally [38] and a negative impact on semen parameters in men [39]. Given that SSRI use during pregnancy may increase the risk of autism spectrum disorder in the offspring [40], alternatives to medication to treat depressive symptoms in infertile individuals is needed. Since approximately 11% of infertile women take an SSRI (although far fewer report this use to their infertility specialist [37]), it is vital to investigate nonpharmacological approaches.

In one study of 89 infertile women with depressive symptoms, participants were randomized to receive 20 mg of fluoxetine for 90 days, CBT plus relaxation for 10 sessions, or routine care [41]. The CBT group had significantly more improvements in their stress scores than both the fluoxetine and control groups. Thus, CBT should be considered a first-line course of treatment in infertile women with mild to moderate depressive symptoms.

Summary

Women experiencing infertility report significant levels of emotional distress. Their distress can make them difficult to treat, may make treatment less effective, and increases their tendency to drop out of treatment, which might have been successful. Psychological interventions can decrease symptoms of anxiety and depression and are associated with increases in pregnancy rates. A mind/body approach can satisfy the numerous needs of patients, including decreasing distress, increasing social support, increasing the chance of pregnancy, and helping them move on to alternative treatments, including ART and third-party reproduction.

REFERENCES

1. Anderheim L, Holter H, Bergh C, Moller A. Does psychological stress affect the outcome of in vitro fertilization? *Hum Reprod* 2005;20:2969–75.
2. Domar AD, Broome A. The prevalence and predictability of depression in infertile women. *Fertil Steril* 1992;58:1158–63.
3. Domar AD, Zuttermeister PC, Friedman R. The psychological impact of infertility: A comparison to women with other medical conditions. *J Psychsom Obstet Gynaecol* 1993;14:45–52.
4. Chen TH, Chang SP, Tsai CF, Juang KD. Prevalence of depressive and anxiety disorders in an assisted reproductive technique clinic. *Hum Reprod* 2004;19:2313–8.
5. Holley SR, Pasch LA, Bleil ME, Gregorich S, Katz PK, Adler NE. Prevalence and predictors of major depressive disorder for fertility treatment patients and their partners. *Fertil Steril* 2015;103:1332–9.
6. Shani C, Yelena S, Reut BK, Adrian S, Sami H. Suicidal risk among infertile women undergoing in vitro fertilization: Incidence and risk factors. *Psychiatry Res* 2016;240:53–9.
7. Gameiro S, van den Belt-Dusebout A, Smeenk J, Braat D, van Leeuwen F, Verhaak C. Women's adjustment trajectories during IVF and impact on mental health 11–17 years later. *Human Reprod* 2016; Epub ahead of print.
8. Vikstrom J, Josefsson A, Bladh M, Sydsjo G. Mental health in women 20–23 years after IVF treatment: A Swedish cross-sectional study. *BMJ Open* 2015;5:e009426.
9. Pasch LA, Holley SR, Bleil ME, Shehab D, Katz PP, Adler NE. Addressing the needs of fertility treatment patients and their partners: Are they informed of and do they receive mental health services? *Fertil Steril* 2016; Epub ahead of print.
10. Domar AD. Infertility and the mind/body connection. *The Female Patient* 2005;30:24–8.
11. Lintsen AME, Verhaak CM, Eijkemans MJC, Smeenk JMJ, Braat DDM. Anxiety and depression have no influence on the cancellation and pregnancy rates of a first IVF or ICSI treatment. *Hum Reprod* 2009;24:1092–8.
12. Klonoff-Cohen H, Chu E, Natarajan L, Sieber W. A prospective study of stress among women undergoing in vitro fertilization or gamete intrafallopian transfer. *Fertil Steril* 2001;76:675–87.
13. Klonoff-Cohen H, Natarajan L. The Concerns During Assisted Reproduction Technologies (CART) scale and pregnancy outcomes. *Fertil Steril* 2004;4:982–8.
14. Lynch CD, Sundaram R, Maisog JM, Sweeney AM, Buck Louis GM. Preconception stress increases the risk of infertility: Results from a couple-based prospective cohort study—The LIFE study. *Hum Reprod* 2014;29:1067–75.
15. Land JA, Courtar DA, Evers JL. Patient dropout in an assisted reproductive technology program: Implications for pregnancy rates. *Fertil Steril* 1997;68:278–81.
16. Olivius K, Friden B, Lundin K, Bergh C. Cumulative probability of live birth after three in vitro fertilization/intracytoplasmic sperm injection cycles. *Fertil Steril* 2002;77:505–10.
17. Hammarberg K, Astbury J, Baker H. Women's experiences of IVF: A follow-up study. *Hum Reprod* 2001;16:374–83.
18. Olivius C, Friden B, Borg G, Bergh C. Why do couples discontinue in vitro fertilization treatment? A cohort study. *Fertil Steril* 2004;81:258–61.
19. Domar AD, Smith K, Conboy L, Iannone M, Alper M. A prospective investigation into the reasons why insured United States patients drop out of in vitro fertilization treatment. *Fertil Steril* 2010;94:1457–9.
20. Shroder AK, Katalinic A, Diedrich K, Ludwig M. Cumulative pregnancy rates and drop out rates in a German IVF programme: 4102 cycles in 2130 patients. *Reprod Biomed Online* 2004;5:600–6.
21. Smeenk JM, Verhaak CM, Stolwijk AM, Kremer JA, Braat DD. Reasons for dropout in an in vitro fertilization/intracytoplasmic sperm injection program. *Fertil Steril* 2004;81:262–8.
22. Eisenberg ML, Smith JF, Millstein SG, Nachtigall RD, Adler NE, Pasch LA, Katz PP. Predictors of not pursuing infertility treatment after an infertility diagnosis: Examination of a prospective US cohort. *Fertil Steril* 2010;94:2369–71.
23. Herbert DL, Lucke JC, Dobson AJ. Depression: An emotional obstacle to seeking medical advice for infertility. *Fertil Steril* 2010;94:1817–21.
24. Gameiro S, Boivin J, Peronace L, Verhaak CM. Why do patients discontinue fertility treatment? A systematic review of reasons and predictors of discontinuation in fertility treatment. *Hum Reprod Update* 2012;18:652–69.

25. Domar AD, Gross J, Rooney K, Boivin J. Exploratory randomized trial on the effects of a brief psychological intervention on emotions, quality of life, discontinuation, and pregnancy rates in in vitro fertilization patients. *Fertil Steril* 2015;104:440–51.
26. Frederiksen Y, Farver-Vestergaard I, Skovgard NG, Ingerslev HJ, Zachariae R. Efficacy of psychosocial interventions for psychological and pregnancy outcomes in infertile women and men: A systematic review and meta-analysis. *BMJ Open* 2015;28:1–18.
27. Terzioglu F. Investigation into effectiveness of counseling on assisted reproductive techniques in Turkey. *J Psychosom Obstet Gynaecol* 2001;22:133–41.
28. de Klerk, Hunfeld JA, Duivenvoorden MA, Fauser BC, Passchier J, Macklon NS. Effectiveness of a psychological counseling intervention for first-time IVF couples: A randomized controlled trial. *Hum Reprod* 2005;20:1333–8.
29. Domar AD, Clapp D, Slawsby EA, Dusek J, Kessel B, Freizinger M. Impact of group psychological interventions on pregnancy rates in infertile women. *Fertil Steril* 2000;73:805–11.
30. Domar AD, Clapp D, Orav J, Kessel B, Freizinger M. The impact of group psychological interventions on distress in infertile women. *Health Psychol* 2000;19:568–75.
31. Hosaka T, Matsubayashi H, Sugiyama Y, Izumi S, Makino T. Effect of psychiatric group intervention on natural-killer cell activity and pregnancy rate. *Gen Hosp Psychiatr* 2002;24:353–6.
32. Domar AD, Rooney KL, Wiegand B, Orav EJ, Alper MM, Berger BM, Nikolovski J. Impact of a group mind/body program on pregnancy rates in IVF patients. *Fertil Steril* 2011;95:2269–73.
33. Clifton J, Parent J, Worrall G, Seehuus M, Evans M, Forehand R, Domar AD. An internet-based mind/body intervention to mitigate distress in women experiencing infertility: A randomized pilot trial. Oral presentation, ASRM, October 2016, Salt Lake City, Utah.
34. Boivin J. A review of psychosocial interventions in infertility. *Soc Sci Med* 2003;57:2325–41.
35. Hammerli K, Znoj H, Barth J. The efficacy of psychological interventions for infertile patients: A meta-analysis examining mental health and pregnancy rates. *Hum Reprod* 2009;15:279–95.
36. Domar AD, Seibel MM, Benson H. The mind/body program for infertility: A new behavioral treatment approach for women with infertility. *Fertil Steril* 1990;53:246–9.
37. Domar AD, Moragianni VA, Ryley DA, Urato AC. The risks of selective serotonin reuptake inhibitor use in infertile women: A review of the impact on fertility, pregnancy, neonatal health and beyond. *Hum Reprod* 2013;28:160–71.
38. Casilla-Lennon MM, Meltzer-Brody S, Steiner AZ. The effect of antidepressants on fertility. *Am J Obstet Gynecol* 2016; Epub ahead of print.
39. Norr L, Bennedsen B, Fedder J, Larsen ER. Use of selective serotonin reuptake inhibitors reduces fertility in men. *Andrology* 2016; Epub ahead of print.
40. El Marroun H, White T, van der Knaap N, Homberg J, Fernandez GF, Schoemaker NK, Jaddoe V, Hofman A, Verhulst F, Hudziak J, Stricker B, Tiemeier H. Prenatal exposure to selective serotonin reuptake inhibitors and social responsiveness symptoms of autism: Population-based study of young children. *Br J Psychiatr* 2014;205:95–102.
41. Faramarzi M, Pasha H, Esmailzadah S, Kheirkhah F, Heidary S, Afshar Z. The effect of the cognitive behavior therapy and pharmacotherapy on infertility stress: A randomized controlled trial. *Int J Fertil Steril* 2013;7:199–206.

21

Infertility Counseling and the Role of the Infertility Counselor

Jeanie Ungerleider, Terry Chen Rothchild, and Lynn Nichols

Infertility as a Crisis

Infertility is a medical condition that can affect every part of an individual's or couple's life. It may challenge the ways in which people feel about themselves and their relationships with their partner, family, and friends. It often affects their work environment and general outlook on life. Few situations in life are as challenging and overwhelming. Because of this, infertility is considered a life crisis.

For those going through infertility, this often is the first time that an experience in life may feel totally beyond their control. Most people assume that if they only work hard enough, they will succeed and achieve their goals, including when to become parents. Being faced with infertility often runs counter to individuals' and couples' experiences and expectations about life. Not being able to get pregnant when they want to and feeling a lack of control in this area can be frustrating and frightening. These feelings can then get amplified by the disappointment of repeated failed treatment. Indeed, the uncertainty as to whether they will ever conceive and have a healthy baby can create mounting anxiety. The infertile couple is surrounded by peers who are pregnant with their first, second, or third child, while they struggle with infertility treatments and feeling increasingly resentful, angry, and isolated from their usual supports.

Infertility is a crisis of identity that can challenge one's sense of self and self-worth. It can impair one's definition of who they are and whether they will ever have a meaningful place in the world. For women, infertility challenges their long-held assumptions of being mothers someday. The more that a woman's self-identity is defined by being a mother, the more at risk is she for psychological distress and feelings of inadequacy. The longer that infertility continues, the more a sense of helplessness and hopelessness can take over, which can lead to greater depression. A diagnosis of male factor problem can feel devastating for the man. This finding can challenge his sense of masculinity, potency, and identity.

Factors contributing to different people's coping styles include personality differences, family history, and life experiences. These factors can shape how people experience and handle this particular life crisis. Moreover, women and men can demonstrate very different ways of coping with the diagnosis of infertility. Women often feel anxious and depressed because they are mindful of the limits of their biological clock. There is the heightened awareness of the urgency of time and a painful reminder of disappointment each month when there is no pregnancy. Women are sometimes angry with themselves or their partners for not starting to build their family sooner. They are burdened with feelings of guilt and regret about their delay. In some cases, for women who had a prior termination of pregnancy, they may come to feel that their infertility is a punishment for having had an earlier abortion.

Women who are faced with infertility often want to discuss their feelings and concerns with their partners, which can dominate their conversations when the couple spends time together. Generally speaking, men may tend to respond with optimism, assuring their partner of a positive outcome. Not wanting to fuel or add to their partner's distress, they may wish to limit or avoid conversation about infertility. The couple's growing sense of feeling disconnected from each other can add to an already sense of isolation and alienation from the outside world.

Tensions such as these often interfere with the couple's sexual relationship. No longer is their lovemaking pleasurable and intimate. Sex becomes a task to accomplish the goal of conception. When the woman's and man's styles are in such contrast, it can interfere with their going forward with infertility treatment as a couple.

> A couple was referred to the infertility counselor by their physician because they expressed conflict over how aggressive they wanted their infertility treatment to be and showed difficulty with decision making. The husband, age 36, was annoyed by his wife's insistence on seeking infertility treatment just 6 months into their marriage. His wife, age 39, was convinced that she would have problems conceiving because of her history of erratic menstrual cycles. The husband complained that his wife had become totally obsessed and preoccupied with having a baby to the exclusion of his needs. The counselor met weekly with the couple, helping them to communicate more effectively with each other. Their increased ability to partner together and to appreciate each of their different coping styles allowed this couple to proceed more effectively with infertility treatment.

The Role of the Counselor in an Infertility Practice

Most major infertility practices have licensed independent clinical social workers or psychologists available who specialize in infertility counseling. Many of these clinicians are members of the American Society for Reproductive Medicine (ASRM) and the Mental Health Professional Group of ASRM that offer practice guidelines and guidance for the mental health professionals. The role of the infertility counselor is multifaceted and ever-changing depending on the request of the physician, the expressed needs of the individual or couple, and the level of distress and crisis in their life. The counselor can serve the role of a clinical evaluator, a consulting member of the health care team, a supportive counselor, a bereavement counselor, a patient advocate, or, more broadly, a psychotherapist. Furthermore, the infertility counselor can make referrals to resources in the community and be a liaison to other mental health professionals, such as psychopharmacologists and psychotherapists, on behalf of the health care team. The roles of the infertility counselor can shift with the individual or couple over time and reflect the complex process of infertility treatment as well as people's responses to their treatment and changing needs.

Counseling can offer support in dealing with the unique stresses of ongoing medical treatments and the uncertainty of outcome, including the possibility of unsuccessful treatment cycles. If an individual or couple is having a difficult time going through the medical process, seeing a counselor one on one can help address the issues that are specific to the individual or couple and provide the needed support and strategies.

Counseling is helpful for those who are having difficulty making informed treatment decisions or choosing treatment options. It is also useful for those who have experienced a miscarriage and are grieving this very powerful and real loss. The counselor can offer acute bereavement counseling in response to the immediate loss as well as assist them in the resolution of their grief over time. The counselor can also provide resources to bereavement support groups, readings, and websites. Being able to do some grief work initially will help those who have faced loss move forward with the medical process with more emotional resiliency.

Counseling is also recommended for people who are facing the end of medical treatment and are having difficulty making this decision, or wishing to discuss other options and alternatives, such as the use of donor egg or donor sperm, gestational care arrangement, adoption, or childfree living. Some of these issues will be covered later in this chapter.

If the individual or couple is experiencing stress, depression, or anxiety to a degree that is significantly affecting their life or making it hard to enjoy life, it is advisable to refer them to a counselor before any medical treatment begins. As outlined in the ASRM Fact Sheet on Infertility Counseling and Support, signs and symptoms to consider include the following:

- Persistent feelings of sadness, guilt, or worthlessness
- Loss of interest in usual activities and relationships
- Agitation and anxiety
- Constant preoccupation with infertility
- Difficulty concentrating and remembering
- Change in appetite, weight, or sleep patterns
- Social isolation
- Increased use of alcohol or drugs
- Increased mood swings
- Marital conflicts
- Other current or past stress that heightens infertility distress

In making a clinical assessment of the individual's or couple's needs, the counselor can determine the most appropriate treatment modality. This can be in the form of individual counseling, couples counseling, a support group, a Mind/Body program, or a combination of these options. In individual and couples counseling, the counselor can help sort out feelings of how their infertility has affected them and their partner as well as help them deal with family, friends, and the fertile society. Couples learn ways to strengthen their relationship and develop skills to navigate the emotional roller coaster of infertility. A peer support group can help reduce the feelings of isolation and provide a support network, and additionally, a Mind/Body Program can teach self-care skills and address lifestyle changes that can have beneficial effects for a lifetime. It is generally agreed that the outcome for those people who seek out professional help in some form is much better than those who choose to remain socially isolated and grieve alone, especially if infertility treatment is prolonged and disappointing.

The following case demonstrates the various roles that an infertility counselor can provide over time in helping a person with their emotional needs and assisting as part of the health care team:

> A 37-year-old married woman presented with depression and crying whenever she got her period. She was obsessed about getting pregnant for the last 1½ years. While quite motivated, she stated that she was very anxious about the medical process and reported a history of panic reactions based on childhood fears. There were "worriers" in her family, and her own anxiety had worsened as each treatment cycle was met with failure. The counselor offered her opportunities to safely talk about and examine her fears, helped her gain perspective on overwhelming feelings and issues, helped her identify what resources and assistance she needed most at each stage of her cycle, and shared relevant information with her physician and nurse coordinator so that she felt well cared for by her whole team. Based on ongoing discussions and increasing trust with the counselor, this woman was able to see how unable she was at advocating for herself in the initial stages of medical treatment given her overwhelming level of distress, which was in sharp contrast to her effectiveness as a manager at her job. During counseling sessions, she also gained insight into how by not allowing her husband to participate in her treatment, it served to protect her husband but, consequently, provided inadequate care to herself. She recognized this as a pattern that was counterproductive to them both. After undergoing four in vitro fertilization (IVF) cycles with the needed emotional support from her whole health care team and husband, she went on to have a successful pregnancy and delivery.

A woman can bring a complicated history, such as a trauma history or other past stress, which can heighten infertility distress. In the counselor's understanding of the cause of her distress, the counselor can effectively help to facilitate the woman's care with her health care team and intervene when necessary in a particular area of concern in order to assist her in going forward with treatment.

A woman presented with anxiety and stress as her first IVF procedure approached and questioned whether she could go forward. She was increasingly having difficulty sleeping and concentrating at work. In the assessment with the counselor, she revealed a history of emotional and sexual abuse. She realized that she was terrified of having the procedure done by a physician whom she would not know and was not scheduled to meet until the day of the procedure. She was also fearful of having anesthesia, which she never experienced. The counselor was able to advocate on behalf of the woman and arranged for her to meet briefly with the physician, O.R. nurse, and anesthesiologist before the day of her IVF procedure. This helped diminish her anxiety considerably and made her feel well cared for. The staff also benefited from the advanced meeting and understanding of this special situation.

The Role of the Infertility Counselor in Assisted Conception

Newer ways of having a family with the use of donor egg, donor sperm, gestational carrier arrangement, preimplantation genetic diagnosis (PGD) for gender selection, and embryo donation have become increasingly successful for individuals and couples to have a child. These choices of family building raise unique social, emotional, and ethical issues. As part of most IVF programs, it is considered invaluable for people to meet with an infertility counselor to discuss these complex issues.

Donor Egg or Donor Sperm Consultation

When the use of a third party in the reproductive process (donor egg or donor sperm) is recommended to infertile individuals and couples, new sets of concerns and feelings arise. This includes feelings about the medical condition that necessitated the use of a donor. Additionally, the loss of the genetic tie to the prospective mother or father and its meaning may become central. Practical issues such as disclosure must also be addressed. While the decision to tell the child about its genetic origins is a personal one, it is an issue that should be explored with the couple before treatment begins. Those coming into infertility clinics with the hopes of creating their own child have often gone through and continue to go through a multitude of emotional experiences from positive anticipation to frustration, disappointment, and continued loss. Here, the counselor can continue to assist couples manage the emotional roller coaster associated with infertility treatment.

The topics covered in the psycho-educational consultation of third-party reproduction may include transitioning from a traditional form of treatment to the use of a third party; the feelings involved in making this decision; choosing an anonymous or known donor and the benefits and challenges associated to either choice; issues of disclosure, including when and how to tell the child, the notion of privacy versus secrecy, and how to discuss disclosure with family and friends; transitioning to parenthood and parenting at an older age, if applicable; and the possibility of treatment failure and alternatives for future planning.

In her role as clinical evaluator and consulting member of the health care team, the counselor also participates in the screening of the anonymous and known egg donor. While the donor undergoes a thorough medical screening, it is the responsibility of the counselor to conduct a psychosocial evaluation. The purpose of this portion of the donor screening is to have an understanding of the donor's current life situation as well as assess her personal and family psychiatric history. It is also to determine whether or not she is aware of and prepared to meet the responsibilities and demands present in an egg donation cycle. The counselor follows the ASRM general guidelines for the Psychological Assessment of Oocyte Donors and Recipients to help determine if a donor is an appropriate candidate. It is also the responsibility of the counselor to inform the donor about the potential emotional benefits and risks associated with egg donation and help her determine if the decision to serve as a donor is well thought out and in her best interest, thus helping her make a psychologically informed consent.

In instances where a known donor is considered, it is important for the infertility counselor to explore and discuss with the recipients and donor together their feelings about the relationship and future expectations between all parties, including with the future child. It is essential that everyone involved meet at the time of the medical screening and be in agreement with decisions that have the potential to affect a future family.

Gestational Carrier Arrangement Consultation

The use of gestational carrier arrangement is rarely the first choice for family building in assisted conception. More often the case, people come to this after exhausting other options, such as intrauterine insemination and IVF. Medical conditions on the part of the woman, such as the loss of or impaired uterus, can also determine the use of gestational carrier arrangement in some cases. The most common gestational carrier arrangement these days is for the intended or prospective mother or an egg donor to provide the egg and the intended or prospective father or sperm donor to provide the sperm. The resulting embryo is transferred to the gestational carrier, who has no genetic connection to the child.

> After multiple attempts with assisted conception, including several IVF cycles and two recent miscarriages, a couple was recommended gestational carrier arrangement as another option. The woman showed diminished egg quality and quantity so egg donation was also recommended to increase the couple's chance of success. Counseling was provided to them at this point to help them accept having another woman carry their child and understand the various psychological issues related to both gestational carrier arrangement and egg donation. The couple went on to secure a gestational carrier, and after two attempts, their gestational carrier got pregnant and delivered a term child for this couple, who had gone through many years of trying on their own.

The role of the professional counselor in gestational carrier arrangement consultation is to determine what is best for all the participants involved, including the existing children, and to foresee the range of psychological issues that occur in third-party reproduction and pregnancy and address these to the individualized, psychosocial situations of the participants. The standard practice is for the counselor to have the first consultation with the intended parents to discuss the psychological issues related to gestational carrier arrangement and to assist them in assessing their readiness to take part in a gestational carrier arrangement. This consultation is followed by one evaluative consultation with the prospective gestational carrier and her husband or partner to assess their psychological readiness to participate in a gestational carrier arrangement. Last, a joint consultation is provided to the intended parents and gestational carrier and husband or partner together to discuss and assess their readiness to take part in a gestational carrier arrangement with one another. This joint meeting is an important opportunity to define everyone's mutual expectations with regard to the nature of their relationship during the medical process, pregnancy, and after the delivery as well as to discuss their agreement on potential decision-making ahead, such as twin pregnancy, selective reduction, or circumstances for the termination of a pregnancy.

The counselor will also either provide or make arrangement for standardized psychological testing of the prospective carrier as part of the screening process. This typically includes a personality test, such as the Minnesota Multiphasic Personality Inventory-2 or the Personality Assessment Inventory, as well as another psychological assessment instrument, such as the Rorschach Comprehensive System, or measurements assessing the gestational carrier's capacity to cope with stress and the quality of her interpersonal relationships.

The evaluation of the carrier by the counselor is an in-depth process and also involves evaluation of her husband or partner as well. Many factors go into the selection of an appropriate gestational carrier, including understanding her motivation or underlying reason to be a gestational carrier for someone. It is important that she has had positive experiences with previous pregnancies and be raising a child of her own. It is critical to assess her psychosocial history and current life situation as well as her psychological history and emotional well-being. It is also important for the gestational carrier to have an adequate support system, in particular her husband or partner, who supports her wish to be a gestational carrier and helps her and her children during a pregnancy, especially should she require bed rest or hospitalized bed rest. She must be at peace about the relinquishment of the child to the intended parents. The goal is for the prospective gestational carrier to leave the program whole and unharmed and feel satisfied with the process and her relationship with the intended parents.

It is important for all participants involved to have legal, medical, and psychological consultations. Once the medical process is underway, ongoing psychological counseling for the intended parents on an as needed basis as well as follow-up with their gestational carrier can be an option offered in an effort to help facilitate the gestational carrier process and support their relationship during the pregnancy and afterward. If participants are well matched and invested in the psychological preparedness and considerations, the experience can be mutually fulfilling and satisfying. Additionally, it is a wonderful opportunity to create a positive legacy for the forthcoming child.

In contrast to this group of infertile couples, there are also single adults and gay and lesbian couples who are entering infertility practices and looking to the donor process or gestational care arrangement as a way of becoming parents. These groups of people, who have not experienced problems with infertility by and large, may not necessarily go through the same emotional experiences as the infertility group. The issue of loss, mourning, and grief work may be quite different depending on their reason for treatment. Nonetheless, the use of a third party in the reproductive process does raise certain unique social, emotional, and ethical issues for all recipients, donors, and children. Additionally, with both of these groups, the infertility counselor has an opportunity to address concerns about how to raise these children as healthy and wholesome beings and help children deal with information about their assisted conception in their various life stages.

PGD for Gender Selection Consultation

PGD is a technology used in conjunction with IVF to test for healthy embryos before transfer to the woman's uterus. One indication for performing PGD is when the couple is at risk for having a child with an inherited genetic disorder (i.e., cystic fibrosis, Tay–Sachs disease). A single cell is removed from each embryo and can be tested for the specific genetic disorders. Only embryos free of genetic abnormalities are selected for implantation. Before the advent of PGD, testing for genetic disorders was limited and could only be done during the first trimester of pregnancy. The woman would have to endure the stress of waiting for the results. If carrying a genetically abnormal fetus, she would be faced with the psychological trauma associated with decision making around pregnancy termination. PGD now offers individuals the opportunity to determine healthy embryos before transfer, which also reduces much emotional distress with pregnancy.

PGD can also be performed to determine the chromosomal makeup of the embryo including an assessment of the sex chromosomes. There are now some IVF centers that offer PGD to determine the gender of the embryo. Gender selection can be used to eliminate those embryos of a certain gender with a transmittable genetic disorder. Some prospective parent(s) may have a strong gender preference so may request use of PGD for gender selection. Still others may choose PGD for family balancing. For example, the couple already has a child or children of one gender and expresses the desire to have another child of the opposite gender. In this situation, all the embryos would be tested to determine their gender, and then the healthy embryos of the preferred sex would be transferred to the woman's uterus.

Sex selection raises various psychosocial, ethical, and controversial issues, such as if a couple has not yet had a child, should they be allowed to select the sex of their offspring? Just because the technology exists, should it be used in this way? Some IVF centers will only offer sex selection for family balancing.

It is important for counseling to be available to individuals and couples who are considering PGD for gender selection to allow them to think through the unique psychosocial and ethical questions that are inherent in this technology. For example, if a person wants to have a female child, and they undergo IVF with PGD, and there are no healthy female embryos, would they transfer the healthy male embryos instead? If they decide not to transfer the healthy male embryos, then what would be the disposition plan of these newly created embryos? The possible options would be to consider freezing the embryos and postpone making any decisions, donating them for medical research, or donating the embryos to another couple or individual. They could also choose to discard the embryos. Thorough discussion of each of these choices needs to be carefully explored before commencing the IVF cycle. If there is a difference of opinion between the couple, they will need assistance in reaching a decision that they can both agree upon.

Embryo Donation Consultation

When a couple or individual has created embryos through infertility treatment with IVF and successfully completed their family building, they need to consider the disposition of the extra embryos that they no longer need. They could decide to continue to keep them frozen, paying a yearly storage charge until they are ready to make a final decision on disposition. With the success of IVF, there are now more than 600,000 extra frozen embryos stored in laboratories across the United States. The majority of recipients choose to dispose of their extra embryos or donate them for medical research. Still a few recipients will consider the option of donating their excess frozen embryos to others who are infertile and in need of embryos to build a family. Donated embryos can offer these people another viable way for family building. This can also be a practical way for single women or same-sex couples to create their families. In addition to some IVF centers, there are also a few agencies, such as the National Embryo Donation Center, that will help facilitate the donation of embryos.

There are several reasons for considering embryo donation. Recipients may not have been able to create healthy embryos with their own gametes, or be faced with a male or female factor problem, or wish to avoid transmitting a genetic disease to their offspring. In some instances, recipients may favor embryo donation instead of one partner having a genetic link to the child and not the other. This would be a way for each parent to have an equal connection to their child. For some recipients, the cost is another major factor in their decision to use donated embryos. It is considerably less than paying for an IVF cycle with donor gametes. Becoming a recipient of embryo donation takes considerably less time than going through an adoption process. Finally, it gives the prospective mother the opportunity to experience pregnancy and bond with her baby from the beginning.

There are many more recipients who want donated embryos than there are people willing to donate. Often when an infertile couple finally achieves a successful pregnancy and then has a baby, they may initially consider donating their extra embryos to another couple or individual who is struggling to conceive. However, once they have their own child or children and become parents, the reality of donating their unused embryos takes on a very different meaning. Parents begin to think about the fact that their frozen embryos would become full genetic siblings to their children if they were to donate them to another person. Anticipating this possible reality raises a host of emotions, questions, and thoughts to consider.

Counseling for embryo donors and recipients is extremely helpful in thinking through the psychosocial, ethical, and legal issues unique to embryo donation. The Practice Committee of the ASRM and the Practice Committee of the Society for Assisted Reproductive Technology provide explicit 2012 Guidelines for Gamete and Embryo Donation. The complex and often charged emotions that embryo donation raises need to be thoroughly explored and understood. It is useful for both embryo donors and recipients to completely understand the implications of their decision in order to make a psychological informed consent. Before recipients can move forward with considering embryo donation, they need time to work through their loss of ever having a biological and genetic child with their partner.

The following are some of the issues to consider: Will they choose a known donor/known recipient situation? What kind of relationship would the donor family have with the recipient family? What would be the expectations of the relationship with the child who was created through embryo donation? Would the recipient's children and donor's children know about each other? And if so, when and how do they explain this unique situation to their children? In an anonymous embryo donation, the donors and recipients will independently decide how much information to share about each other's family and if they would want the option to have contact with the child at 18 years or older.

Parents choosing to donate their extra embryos to an infertile couple or individual often feel tremendous empathy and identification with those who are struggling to conceive. Donating can be an opportunity to help another family in a very powerful way, and at the same time, it may be compatible with the donating couple's values and religious beliefs. For the donating couple, it can be a welcomed solution if disposing of extra embryos or donating their embryos to medical research feels ethically and morally unacceptable to them.

Egg Freezing

The advances in reproductive technology, particularly the success in freezing and thawing, have made it possible for women to preserve their eggs for future use. For women in their 30s who are not ready to start a family or do not yet have a partner, egg freezing can be a viable option. Because these procedures are not covered by insurance, they are only available to women who can afford the expense. There are additional costs of yearly fees for cryopreservation of their eggs.

Summary

The journey through infertility treatments is often uncertain and may be fraught with intense emotions and expectations. The role of the counselor can make a significant difference in how individuals and couples navigate the emotional stresses of infertility. The team focuses attention on the individual's medical, physical, emotional, and psychosocial well-being. Patients appreciate the value of this personalized interdisciplinary approach.

The assisted reproductive technologies continue to be more successful and sophisticated, with the availability of ovum freezing and more extensive use of preimplantation genetic testing. These advances raise complex ethical, emotional, and psychosocial issues, which need to be addressed. The expanding array of individuals involved in making a baby may include an ovum donor, sperm donor, gestational carrier, and the intended parents who will be raising the child. Such complex relationships necessitate careful understanding of the issues and exploration of their implications for the individual, couple, and future child. The infertility counselor's role is increasing as more people make use of these pathways to parenthood.

BOX 21.1   WHERE TO FIND AN INFERTILITY COUNSELOR?

Mental health professionals, including social workers, psychologists, and psychiatrists, are trained to evaluate and treat individuals and couples who are in crisis. Because of the complexities of infertility and the treatment options that are available, individuals and couples would benefit most from a referral to a mental health professional with expertise in the field of infertility. Besides getting a referral from their own physician who specializes in infertility treatment, people can turn to ASRM, Path 2 Parenthood, and RESOLVE, as valuable resources for seeking out qualified mental health professionals in their community as well as information.

American Society for Reproductive Medicine (ASRM)
205-978-5000
www.asrm.org

Path 2 Parenthood
888-917-3777
www.path2parenthood.org

RESOLVE: The National Infertility Association
703-556-7172
www.resolve.org

How to learn more about adoption?
The first step is to talk with a mental health professional about the emotional and practical issues related to adoption. There are various types of adoption, including open/identified or closed adoption as well as domestic and international. The following resources are provided for additional information:

National Council for Adoption
703-299-6633
www.adoptioncouncil.org

RESOLVE: The National Infertility Association
703-556-7172
www.resolve.org

22

Medical Ethics in Reproductive Medicine

Steven R. Bayer and Kim L. Thornton

The introduction of in vitro fertilization (IVF) more than 30 years ago is one of the most significant advancements in the field of reproductive medicine. More than 5 million babies have been born worldwide as a result of this technology. IVF has benefited many couples, but has also resulted in the emergence of ethical dilemmas that continue to challenge IVF centers today. The specialty is ethically charged since its primary focus is on reproduction. The goal of reproduction is to produce an offspring and nurture that offspring. While this is not refuted, the societal concerns are the means that may be undertaken to produce this offspring. In the traditional sense, the act of reproduction is a private, natural, and conjugal act between two people. However, treatment with the available technologies does everything but meet these criteria. Nevertheless, the right to procreate or reproduce is a liberty that is held sacred by all of us. As caregivers, we must respect this right, yet at the same time it is our responsibility to use the available technologies in a responsible manner. This is the role of ethics in reproductive medicine.

Definition

Ethics is defined as a code of moral principles derived from a system of values and beliefs that helps define the correctness of our actions.

Ethics in Medicine and Nursing

The practice of medicine and nursing is founded on ethics. Physicians take the Hippocratic Oath, where it is stated, "*...I will follow that system of regimen which, according to my ability and judgment, I consider for the benefit of my patients, and abstain from whatever is deleterious and mischievous.*" A similar statement is present in the nursing code of ethics, The Nightingale Pledge, "*...I will abstain from whatever is deleterious and mischievous and will not take or knowingly administer any harmful drug.*" In society, it is implicit and expected that physicians and nurses practice ethically within the bounds of their profession and always do what is in the best interest of their patients. This is understood but whose interests do we need to protect? It is complicated in the field of reproductive medicine considering that there can be many participants involved in the treatment. Obviously, we have to look out for the interests of the woman undergoing treatment who is assuming the immediate risks of the treatment and the risks associated with the pregnancy. We also have to protect the rights of her partner who is not exposed to any risks of the treatment, but this individual must first desire to become a parent and also be willing to help care for any offspring(s) that result from the treatment. As providers, we must also determine the impact of our decisions on the yet unborn child. To further complicate matters, there are other participants to be considered in cases of egg donation and gestational surrogacy. Therefore, before any treatment is started, it is imperative that all participants are adequately informed and closely evaluated to ensure that their interests are not compromised as a result of the treatment and its outcome.

Integration of Ethics into Clinical Practice

In every center, there should be an opportunity to examine the ethical issues that arise during patient care. To this end, there are four key components that must be in place, including open dialogue, an ethics committee, available resources, and ethical analysis.

Open Dialogue

When compared to most other medical problems, the treatment of the infertile couple is unique because it can only be accomplished through a coordinated effort of a comprehensive team made up of physicians, nurses, scientists, mental health professionals, and other key personnel. Every member of the team deserves equal respect considering that each plays an important role in the treatment of the couple. Each team member interacts with the couple at a different level, which gives each a unique perspective of the couple and the treatment that is being rendered. Each member must feel comfortable with the treatment plan; if not, they must be able to voice their concern freely, which is taken seriously and addressed by the team.

Ethics Committee

Every center should have a committee in place and a forum to discuss ethical issues. The committee can simply include a physician, a nurse, a mental health professional, and a representative from the laboratory. Depending on the topic that is being discussed, input from an ethicist, lawyer, or member of the clergy may also be helpful. While it is optimal to have periodic committee meetings, it may be necessary to assemble the committee on short notice to resolve an urgent issue. One role of the committee is to review the ethical issues concerning a specific treatment (i.e., egg donation, gestational carrier treatment). If a decision is made to offer the treatment, the next step is to develop a comprehensive policy detailing how the treatment will be administered. A final role of the committee is to discuss ethical issues concerning individual cases.

Available Resources

An important part of an ethical analysis is utilization of available resources. The resources come from the knowledge of individual committee members and from outside resources as well. The Ethics Committee of the American Society for Reproductive Medicine (ASRM) was formed in the mid-1980s and has been proactive in addressing ethical issues of the technologies as they are developed. The committee has published reports and statements entitled *Ethical Considerations of Assisted Reproductive Technologies* as supplements to the journal *Fertility and Sterility*. Position papers and statements are available at the ASRM website (www.asrm.org).

A sampling of position papers published in the past few years are as follows:

- Access to fertility treatment by gays, lesbians, and unmarried persons
- Child-rearing ability and the provision of fertility services
- Defining embryo donation
- Fertility preservation and reproduction of patients facing gonadotoxic therapies
- Fertility treatment when the prognosis is very poor or futile
- Financial compensation of oocyte donors
- Human immunodeficiency virus and infertility treatment
- Ooctye or embryo donation to women of advanced age
- Use of reproductive technology for sex selection for nonmedical reasons

Ethical Analysis

The framework that is used to perform an ethical analysis is based on several fundamental ethical principles. These principles are used when performing a formal ethical analysis and used by the physician in day-to-day patient care. Before an ethical analysis can be performed, one must first have underlying values and the proper perspective. John Gregory (1724–1773) was instrumental in advancing the concept of medical ethics through his invention of "*professionalism*," which changed the focus of medical ethics from being physician-based to patient-based. He described virtues that a physician must exhibit to provide ethical care of patients. Others including Thomas Percival (1740–1804) expanded Gregory's professional virtues. While these virtues apply to the physician–patient relationship, they are also applicable to all of those who participate in an ethical analysis.

- *Integrity*: A commitment to the practice of medicine in accordance with the standards of intellectual and moral excellence
- *Compassion*: Sympathetic awareness of a patient's distress along with a desire to diminish the distress
- *Self-effacement*: Putting aside and not acting on irrelevant differences between oneself and the patient (i.e., religion, race, sexual orientation, socioeconomic status, etc.)
- *Self-sacrifice*: The sacrifice of one's interests to protect and promote the interests of others

Therefore, to perform an ethical analysis, it must be done with compassion and integrity and must be devoid of any bias or prejudice. The important ethical principles and concepts that are used to perform an ethical analysis are discussed below.

Principle of Respect for Patient Autonomy

Patient autonomy is one of the most powerful and prevailing ethical principles. Autonomy is synonymous with independence or freedom. This ethical principle implies that it is the right of the patient to choose his or her treatment and that this choice must be respected. However, it is the obligation of the physician to truthfully inform the patient of the consequences of any action including the benefits, risks, complications, and alternatives. This principle is founded on the concept of informed consent.

Principle of Double Effect

The principle of *double effect* is in essence a compromise of two other important ethical principles: *beneficence* and *non-maleficence*. The principle of beneficence is the driving force of patient care. This principle refers to the ultimate goal of any treatment, which is to do something good for the patient. The principle of non-maleficence is to do no harm to the patient. If we strictly adhere to the non-maleficence principle, then no treatment would be offered to our patients because there is always the possibility of a bad outcome. The decision to move forward with a treatment occurs when there is a greater balance between good and bad outcomes. While it is important that the harm or risk of any treatment be recognized, the absolute avoidance of harm should not take more importance over the potential benefit of any treatment.

Principle of Distributive Justice/Public Stewardship

The principle of justice mandates fair and equitable treatment for all. Society has a responsibility to adhere to this principle and is in accordance with support of human dignity and human rights. Therefore, there should be no prejudice in the administration of treatment to the populace and equal access for all. It also applies to the individual physician as well; the physician should not in any way be prejudicial in regard to who is offered treatment and who is not.

Paternalism

Paternalism is not an ethical principle, per se, but can play a role in the ethical analysis. Paternalism refers to the action of a physician who in an authoritative and directive fashion influences the decision-making process. If this action is based on clinical knowledge and absent of any bias or prejudice, it is consistent with the principle of double effect, but at the same time, it counters patient autonomy. As fertility specialists, we feel obligated to carry out our patient's request; however, in some circumstances, an alternative treatment or no treatment at all may be the indicated course of action.

Standard of Care

Before a physician offers any type of treatment to a patient, it is important to make sure the treatment falls within the standard of care. Standards of practice have been established by ASRM, a national organization, and standards of practice may exist in the city or region where the IVF center is located. This may hold special importance if the treatment under consideration has never been offered—a situation where more critical assessment of all potential outcomes should be discussed before proceeding. On the other hand, even if a treatment is considered the standard of care, it does not necessarily mean that it is guaranteed to be safe. An example of this is the complications that were realized after the administration of diethylstilbestrol to pregnant women in the 1960s.

Impact on the Community

While any treatment may be ethically sound, it is important to step back and assess the impact of its potential effect on the community. The size of the community can vary. A narrow definition of community can be the IVF center itself. Within any center, there may be staff members who have strong opinions for or against a proposed treatment. For instance, after careful analysis and deliberation, it may be determined that gender selection is ethical. However, if team members are uncomfortable with this treatment, then there should be reconsideration whether to offer gender selection at all or only offer it under certain conditions. The broadest definition of community can be society at large. The pursuit of human cloning by a small group of scientists several years ago drew worldwide attention. There was public outcry that cloning crosses ethical boundaries and some countries enacted laws against this practice.

Case Presentations

Case #1

A 35-year-old G0 P0 female presents with a history of infertility. The standard fertility workup confirmed the diagnosis of unexplained infertility. The workup also included routine genetic screening, which confirmed that both she and her husband were carriers of *cystic fibrosis* (CF).

> Cystic fibrosis, an autosomal recessive disease, is one of the most commonly inherited diseases. It results in thickened mucus production that can alter pulmonary and pancreatic function. The median life expectancy of affected individuals is 37 years.

The couple was seen in consultation, and they were informed that they had a one in four chance of having a child that would be affected by CF. Treatment options to avoid this genetic risk were discussed, including prenatal genetic testing after pregnancy was established, IVF with preimplantation genetic diagnosis, and the use of donor gametes. The couple was not interested in any of the options and basically stated they were not overly concerned about having a child with the disease in part because they had a friend who had a 3-year-old daughter with CF and "she was doing just fine." To provide further counseling, the couple was referred to a CF specialist at a local children's hospital to learn more details about the disease. The couple was then seen in follow-up and again they restated the lack of concern for the risk and they wanted to try for a pregnancy with intrauterine insemination (IUI) treatment. According to the couple, if pregnancy is achieved, they most likely would not do prenatal genetic testing.

The case was presented in front of the ethics committee. The committee recognized that those born with CF undergo suffering and have a shortened lifespan. Further, the couple had options to avoid having an affected offspring. While the couple can continue to try on their own, a decision was made that the center would not be a participant in any treatment (IUI or IVF alone) that would put the offspring at risk for having the disease. The decision not to treat counters patient autonomy but it was felt that the potential for harm to the offspring far outweighed any benefit to the couple.

The introduction of genetics has caused the emergence of new ethical dilemmas and challenges for all IVF centers. Many couples, fertile and infertile, are presenting with genetic risks. There is a spectrum of severity of genetic disorders—at one end of the spectrum is Tay–Sachs disease, which is fatal and children don't live beyond the age of 4–5 years, and at the other extreme is polycystic kidney disease whereby affected individuals do not become symptomatic many times until they are in their 50s to 60s. There is no easy answer, but all IVF centers need to establish a threshold risk whereby treatment is not offered.

Case #2

A 40-year-old G1 P1 woman presents with her husband with unexplained infertility. The couple has one daughter and they inquired about gender selection in their quest for a male offspring. They were told that it was the policy of the center that gender selection can only be done when there is another indication to do preimplantation genetic screening (PGS). In addition, a visit with a social worker is mandatory and the couple had to agree to transfer embryos of the undesired gender if they were the only ones available. The topic was never brought up again by the couple, and they underwent several cycles of insemination treatments that were unsuccessful. They then pursued IVF treatment and requested that because of the woman's age, they would like to have PGS performed to rule out aneuploidy. The couple underwent their first cycle of treatment. Eight embryos were biopsied and only two were found to be chromosomally normal. The couple presented for the embryo transfer; when they found out that both embryos were female, they chose to forego the transfer and discard the embryos. During the follow-up visit, the couple was informed about the center's policy regarding gender selection. They never returned for another cycle.

A couple's desire for an offspring of a certain sex has been present since antiquity, and for most, it is for family balancing purposes. There has been speculation that a woman's diet or the frequency or timing of intercourse can affect whether she has a male or female infant. Over a decade ago, sperm washing techniques were developed to select out the X- or Y-bearing sperm. In retrospect, all of these techniques did little to help the couple achieve their goal. The advances in IVF and PGS have provided the opportunity to determine the gender of the embryo.

There is ongoing debate as to whether gender selection is an ethical practice. At one end of the spectrum is the couple who presents, stating that they have three sons at home and would like to have a female offspring for family balancing. They would also transfer embryos of the undesired gender if they were the only ones available. This is a scenario that many would agree is an acceptable situation to consider gender selection. At the other extreme is the couple who requests gender selection for their first born and also indicate that if the PGS testing demonstrates no embryos of the desired gender, under no circumstances would they consider transferring embryos.

At Boston IVF, there has been an evolution in our approach to gender selection over the past decade. Initially, we were concerned about whether offering gender selection was an ethical practice and we elected not to offer this option to couples. Over time, the clinicians, nurses, and embryologists in the laboratory handling these embryos became more comfortable with the concept of gender selection for family balancing purposes for the infertile couple who was undergoing IVF plus PGS for aneuploidy screening. Further, if only embryos of the undesired sex were available, then it was requested that the couple agree to transfer them. Presently, we have modified the policy once again such that any couple (fertile or infertile) can undergo gender selection for the purposes of family balancing or for their first born. In addition, the disposition of embryos of the undesired gender will be left up to the couple. This policy was developed by a subcommittee who reviewed the position paper written by the American Society for Reproductive Medicine on gender selection [1]. After the policy was developed, it was presented and approved by the laboratory staff, nursing staff, and medical staff at Boston IVF. An *important part of the written policy is that all couples desiring gender selection must meet with a social worker to discuss. After this visit, the social worker and treating physician review the case and make a determination as to whether it is appropriate to move forward with the treatment.*

Case #3

A 40-year-old G1 P0010 woman presents with a 5-year history of unexplained infertility. She was diagnosed with cerebral palsy at birth and is a paraplegic confined to a wheelchair. She had medical problems including hypertension and obesity. At another fertility center, she underwent treatment with clomiphene citrate plus IUIs, which were unsuccessful. She now presents for consideration of more aggressive treatment. Because of her medical state, she was referred to a maternal fetal medicine expert for counseling about the risks and complications associated with a future pregnancy. There was added concern that the treatment may result in a multiple pregnancy that could further heighten any risks. She was given medical clearance to proceed. During the workup, a hysterosalpingogram confirmed the presence of polyps in the uterine cavity. A decision was made to proceed with a hysteroscopy. A preoperative echocardiogram was ordered by the anesthesiologist and confirmed that she had pulmonary hypertension. During pregnancy, pulmonary hypertension poses a significant medical risk and results in a 50% rate of maternal mortality. The patient was seen in consult and the implications of her condition were discussed. However, she was not concerned and stated that *"I am a survivor and always beat the odds."* She wanted to move forward with the surgery and then ultimately treatment. A decision was made by the physician not to treat this patient based on medical reasons and the high likelihood of a bad outcome during a future pregnancy—*maternal death.*

This case illustrates an example of paternalism and how it influenced the decision not to move forward. The decision not to treat this patient was made in an unbiased fashion and was based on medical fact. It was determined that the severity of a bad outcome as a result of the treatment far outweighed the benefit of the treatment—the principle of double effect. The decision not to treat countered patient autonomy.

Case #4

A 45-year-old G2 P2 woman presents with a history of a tubal ligation. She is in a new relationship and requests IVF treatment. She has regular menstrual cycles and is in good health. The ovarian reserve testing was normal and suggested an adequate ovarian reserve. The physician had a long discussion about the impact of age on treatment success. Despite the adequate ovarian reserve, the chance of an IVF cycle being successful in a woman of this age is 0%–1%. Other treatment options were discussed with the couple, including egg donation and adoption. The couple would consider egg donation but they wanted to try one cycle of IVF. The physician counseled the couple on the risks of IVF including OHSS, complications associated with the anesthesia and the egg retrieval, and the increased rate of miscarriage and chance of having a child with Down syndrome (1:30) if a pregnancy continues. They were encouraged to follow up with a social worker. The physician agreed with the couple's request. The patient underwent an IVF cycle—eight eggs were retrieved, five embryos were transferred, and the pregnancy test was negative.

One of the important ethical principles is patient autonomy. This principle is founded on the concept of informed consent whereby there is a discussion of the treatment success, potential risks and complications, and treatment alternatives. The chance of pregnancy after treatment in this case was extremely low. However, for many patients in this situation, there may be a psychological benefit in undergoing an IVF cycle even if it fails.

The Ethics Committee of the ASRM published a position paper addressing the role of treatment in the infertile patient when the prognosis is considered very poor or futile [2]. The committee defined a very poor and futile prognosis when the anticipated success rate is 1%–5% and <1%, respectively. They concluded that the physician has the right to refuse to initiate treatment in these cases; however, treatment may be considered when it is determined that the couple would receive a psychological benefit. Before the treatment is pursued, the couple must be thoroughly counseled as to the low odds of success, and they should meet with a mental health professional.

Case #5

A 56-year-old woman presents with her husband for consideration of egg donation. Their 18-year-old daughter, their only child, recently died from complications of leukemia. She has been menopausal for 5 years. She is in excellent health and was recently provided medical clearance from her internist to proceed with egg donation and an eventual pregnancy. The reproductive endocrinologist referred to the center's policy that the upper age limit for egg donation was 50 and therefore the patient could not undergo the treatment. After continued discussion, it was clear that the couple was still grieving the loss of their daughter. They were referred to a social worker for grief counseling. After the counseling sessions, the couple decided not to pursue treatment.

There are well-publicized reports of older women including the 72-year-old woman who achieved pregnancy after egg donation, which gives many a level of discomfort. Should there be an upper age limit for egg donation? There are medical concerns about the documented increased risks of pregnancy in older women. There are also ethical concerns for children being born to older women. An untimely death of the mother could place the potential offspring in jeopardy.

Boston IVF developed a policy setting the age limit at 50 for women undergoing egg donation. This decision was based on the documented medical risks to the older woman during pregnancy and ethical concerns for the unborn child. It was also determined this age cutoff is the standard in the community after other IVF centers in the Boston area were polled.

Case #6

An unmarried, female, same-sex couple presented for consideration of treatment. Their desire was that one partner would donate eggs to the other partner and a known sperm donor would be used. At Boston IVF, this treatment is termed "Partner Assisted Reproduction (PAR)." The first woman is a 35-year-old G1 P1 female in good health and meets all criteria to be an egg donor and the recipient is a 43-year-old G0 P0 female who is also a suitable recipient. Therapeutic donor insemination was offered to the latter patient, but there was concern that her advanced age would significantly decrease the chance of success. The couple was offered PAR treatment and the recipient conceived after the first cycle of IVF treatment.

In simple terms, this case involves a woman who achieved pregnancy after known egg and known sperm donation. ASRM guidelines were used to determine the suitability of both the egg and sperm donor. It is also important to explore anticipated roles and responsibilities of each participant in the upbringing of a future offspring. Therefore, all parties met with a social worker and a lawyer. As a result of the legal counseling, a contract was developed and signed by all participants detailing their rights and any responsibilities.

The LGBT community is accessing fertility services for family building with greater frequency. Female same-sex couples are pursuing donor insemination and PAR treatment. Male same-sex couples are starting families with egg donation and gestational surrogacy. Whether the couple is heterosexual or homosexual, the protocols for administering these treatments are the same. All parties should meet with a social worker. Legal counseling is important for all same-sex couples who are not married. With the advent of egg freezing for fertility preservation, medical specialists are counseling their transgender patients before hormonal or surgical treatment that they should consider preserving their fertility with either eggs freezing or sperm banking.

How to Stay Out of Trouble

The reproductive endocrinologist deals with ethical issues on a daily basis, which can be time consuming and stressful. Being proactive will help avert some of the ethical dilemmas. Some tips are as follows:

Written Policies and Procedures

It is important that every center has written policies and procedures in place for every treatment that is offered. These written documents should be developed by the team and represent a consensus of the group. These guidelines should be reviewed and updated on a regular basis. It is important that patients are made aware of specific treatment criteria elaborated in these policies that affect their treatment options. Individual cases that fall outside of the guidelines can be reviewed by the treatment team.

Stop Them at the Gate

When an ethical issue involving a couple is encountered, it is of paramount importance that treatment is not initiated until the issue has been thoroughly investigated and resolved. If treatment has been started, it is much more difficult to halt the treatment, and from the patient's perspective, the physician has already given approval for the patient to undergo. As a physician, we want to please our patients, but in some situations, the issue of concern must be investigated before proceeding.

Don't Be the First

The field of reproductive medicine is a highly competitive field and there is motivation to set your center apart from competitors in offering a new treatment. In most cases, it is better to be cautious and not offer the treatment until it has been thoroughly researched and confirmed to be effective and safe.

Get Legal Input

Many of our treatments have legal implications. There are lawyers who are well versed in reproductive law and are also helpful in the development of policies and consent forms.

Take a Stand

As physicians, we have the right to refuse treatment in situations where we feel uncomfortable or where there is concern about the consequences of treatment. The decision made not to treat has to be based on medical fact and not from any inherent bias. In these situations, it is important that the physician maintain the high ground and do what is right. When discharging a patient from a practice, it is important not to abandon the patient. An appropriate level of care must be provided that falls within the guidelines of the practice for a certain period of time, which allows the patient to establish care with another provider.

REFERENCES

1. Ethics Committee of the American Society for Reproductive Medicine. Use of reproductive technology for sex selection for nonmedical reasons. *Fertil Steril* 2015;103:1418–22.
2. Ethics Committee of the American Society for Reproductive Medicine. Fertility treatment when the prognosis is very poor or futile: A committee opinion. *Fertil Steril* 2012;98:e6–e9.

23

Integrating Quality Management into a Fertility Practice

Michael M. Alper

What is a Quality Management System (QMS) and what does it have to do with an infertility practice? If you have never heard the term QMS, you are not alone. I had not a clue what it meant just a few years ago and I certainly had no idea of its relevance to medicine. The purpose of this chapter is not to give a detailed analysis of a QMS, but rather to understand how it relates (in simple terms) to what we do every day in our practice of medicine.

The underlying purpose of a QMS is simple—*"Say what you do and do what you say."* A QMS provides the tools to clearly delineate what everyone's responsibility is within your organization. It gets down to the core of your corporate essence—what you are about, why you do what you do, how you do it, and how you can do things better. The system is derived from the organization itself and it is not something that is imposed from the outside. Therefore, part of the fun of developing a QMS is the creation of it. Sure, it is work. But it is also worthwhile as I hope to explain in this chapter.

Why Is Quality Management Important?

Let me illustrate an example for the need of a QMS. I was visiting a highly respected in vitro fertilization (IVF) practice in the northeast United States. I asked the medical director what protocol they followed to replace frozen embryos. He precisely and carefully reviewed their technique to accomplish this. I then asked him for a written summary so I could discuss his technique with my colleagues back in Boston. After shuffling through his files, he came up with an over-photocopied and illegible summary of the protocol. He apologized and commented that *"most of what we do is in our heads."* So, what is wrong with this picture? How are residents and fellows and new colleagues supposed to learn existing protocols at this IVF center? How do the nurses know what is expected of them? How can one keep track of changes in the protocol to observe subsequent changes in outcome? Documentation is the cornerstone of a QMS, and this example illustrates the dire need for QMS in any infertility practice.

IVF centers are complex organizations. They involve the integration of many specialized professionals including physicians, nurses, scientists, administration, and others. In fact, it is a "mini-hospital." These different entities have to work well as a team (Figure 23.1). They need to communicate well since a change in one area can quickly affect the others. The organization falls apart if any one area fails. A QMS ensures that the infrastructure is set for all the players in the organization to communicate and achieve the common goals of the organization. Failure of an organization to function properly results in potentially serious errors at the very worst or corporate dysfunction at the very least.

ISO—An Example of QMS

The International Standard Organization called "ISO" is the most recognized standard for a QMS. This is a global organization with regional organizations in most countries to represent the international

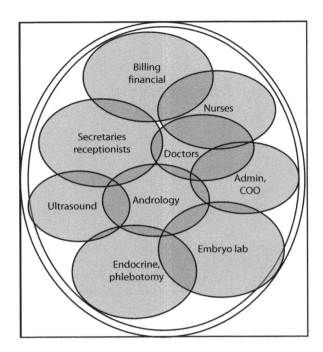

FIGURE 23.1   The IVF team must be a coordinated effort of many disciplines that must all communicate with one another.

standard. ISO governs thousands of standards. For example, the standards for making a part such as a bolt need to be standardized so that a particular sized bolt from one Company A could replace another from Company B. So, these standards exist for several thousand products to keep some uniformity. Another important ISO function is to develop manufacturing standards. For example, if you are designing an aircraft for Boeing and wanted to install a particular aircraft part, you would purchase it only from a manufacturer that was ISO-certified. This is one way to govern that the part comes from a company that meets certain manufacturing standards. Similarly, ISO standards exist for service industries. These standards are the "ISO-9001" standards. It is these standards that can be applied to the health care industry and IVF in particular.

There are several steps for becoming ISO certified (Figure 23.2). For any service company to become "ISO-certified," it must first understand the standards that must be met. Typically, consultants with QMS experience work with the organization to understand and apply the standards. The time and expense for this process vary with the organization and its size but typically takes several months. The consultant must work with the employees to develop a QM system according to ISO standards. It must then be

---

How to get ISO-certified:

1. Know the ISO standard
2. Document a quality management system
3. Implement the system
4. Be surveyed (assessed) by an accredited registrar
5. Be issued a certificate of conformity
6. Be listed in the register of certified companies

FIGURE 23.2   Steps required for ISO certification.

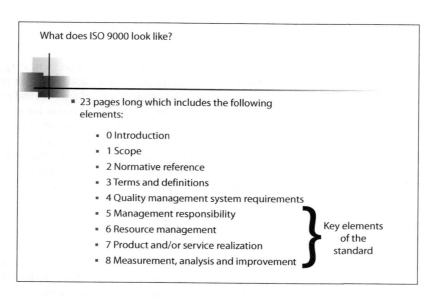

What does ISO 9000 look like?

- 23 pages long which includes the following elements:
  - 0 Introduction
  - 1 Scope
  - 2 Normative reference
  - 3 Terms and definitions
  - 4 Quality management system requirements
  - 5 Management responsibility
  - 6 Resource management
  - 7 Product and/or service realization
  - 8 Measurement, analysis and improvement

} Key elements of the standard

FIGURE 23.3 Elements required for ISO certification.

implemented to be sure it functions properly. A survey is conducted and, if successful, the certificate of conformity is issued. In order to maintain ISO certification after initial certification, an annual inspection from an outside certification body must occur.

The ISO standard is clearly laid out in a 23-page document of the elements required (Figure 23.3). These requirements are readily available from the ISO organizations (see http://www.asq.org/). These must be applied to the particular organization.

I have interpreted what ISO does for an organization to make them more understandable. A more detailed account can be found in the references at the end of the chapter. So, what does a QMS such as ISO teach us? Here are the main points: (1) documentation, (2) a process approach, (3) setting expectations for staff, (4) never be happy with the status quo, (5) leadership, (6) communication, and (7) focus on the customer.

Documentation

Before implementing a QMS at Boston IVF, we asked all employees to collect every single document that they have seen in the organization no matter how old it was. These documents could include anything from the organization including protocols, handouts, marketing materials, and so on. To my astonishment, we had close to 3000 documents at Boston IVF! Some were older versions of documents (e.g., consent forms), instructions that few people ever knew existed, and so on.

A QMS requires a company to organize and maintain its documents. All documents need to be clearly identified and assigned to someone in the organization to control. All revisions made to any document must be authorized and recorded. All employees must know where to find the latest version of the document. It sounds simple but it requires considerable effort to identify which items are important and forces the organization to revamp and revise outdated materials. The exercise of identifying and managing organizations' documents is an important part of "cleaning house," resulting in a more organized and "neat" approach. Our company found it extremely useful.

Documentation goes beyond collecting and organizing materials. Virtually everything that goes on in the organization that involves a process should be written down. What should happen when a potential patient calls requesting information? How are patient complaints handled? All these instructions should be clearly laid out.

A Process Approach to Problem Solving

So often in life and in business, we make decisions based on emotions and not on facts. A QMS should develop an organization's tools to solve problems based on the analysis of facts. Sure, gut feelings are often important, but both major and minor corporate decisions require careful analysis and process. For example, what happens if an employee has an idea for improving a procedure? He may tell his supervisor, but the idea could die if not carefully evaluated. There needs to be a method developed for suggestions to be heard and analyzed. This would be a process for improvement within the organization. Another simple example is ordering. Who can order what within the organization? What process exists for purchasing that covers all departments? All this must be documented and flow charts must be developed for certain processes so that all employees can clearly understand how things are done.

Setting Expectation for the Staff

It is typical for employees to want to succeed at their work. Human nature is to do a good job. Experience dictates that when an employee is failing at their work, it is commonly the result of a failure of the supervisor to clearly delineate the expectations, or the lack of training and tools that the employee receives.

It is vital for a clear job description and expectation be presented to the employee. Also, we often fall short training staff on how to accomplish what we expect of them. And training does not start and end at the orientation. A QMS forces us to clearly identify how we manage staff training and competency. After all, a company's greatest asset is its employees and it is imperative that performance is constantly measured and accountability is delineated.

Never Be Happy with the Status Quo

A fundamental requirement of a QMS system is to foster continual improvement. There is a rare task in any organization that cannot be done better. So, how does one foster the notion that continual improvement is critical for the future of any company? This corporate personality trait starts from the top and continues to the bottom of the company. Every employee with an idea for improvement must be encouraged to share their ideas and know the steps to take when presenting their suggestions. It is the employees on the front line who often know how to make their jobs more effective or efficient.

Leadership

The mission of any organization needs to be developed and followed. For that to occur, management must take leadership. Physicians receive no instruction in leadership training. In fact, I would say that it is uncommon for physicians who spend most of their career learning how to care for individual patients to also have the skills to motivate and lead an organization. These skills are typically developed in business (and not medical) schools. Typical fertility practices consist of several physicians practicing under one roof. A common frustration is bringing the group together to develop common practice patterns. It actually is not hard to accomplish this, but there needs to be one person driving the process.

Books have been written on the skills required to be a leader. Some of these include, among others, good communication skills, belief in people, leading a balanced life, possessing a willingness to continually learn, and radiating positive energy. Leaders establish unity of purpose and direction. Leaders create an environment where people are fully involved in achieving the organizations' objectives. Every manager needs to lead their department and a QMS focuses on responsibilities of management.

Communication

Proper communication both within the IVF center and with the outside world is of paramount importance. In fact, miscommunication can result in significant medical errors that are costly and can hurt the name of the IVF center. There must be an established method to handle patient complaints or suggestions.

IVF centers involve many disciplines. A change in one area typically affects another. For example, if the physicians decide to order an extra three blood tests during an IVF cycle, then nursing, phlebotomy, billing, and other physicians must all be aware of the change. How do these changes in procedure get communicated and followed?

Physicians are often perceived as having their own way of doing things and unwilling to change to develop a more uniform method of treatment. This is not the case when physicians have a way to discuss and debate their views. There must be an effective process to discuss protocols through meetings and discussions. We find that retreats away from the office are the perfect venue to review clinical matters.

The key to delivering optimal service to our patients is through effective communication. Do patients have trouble speaking to the nurse? Is voicemail preventing a patient from having the human touch? Frustration from inability of our patients to speak to the clinical staff in a timely manner is a frequently distressing issue for them.

Focus on the Customer

A QMS refocuses the organization on improving quality. But quality is not a vague concept or dream. If it cannot be measured, then it cannot be quality. The organization must be able to quantify and measure performance. Customer satisfaction is the tool that determines the ultimate success of an IVF center.

So, who are our customers? Certainly our patients are our primary customer. But for us to know if we are doing a good job, we must ask our patients how we are doing. Our product is not babies, but rather the resolution of infertility. Some patients leave our IVF centers with a baby but are dissatisfied with their experience with us. Is that a success? And vice versa, we have many patients without success who are extremely appreciative of the efforts of our staff in helping them deal with and resolve their fertility issue. Our business is to provide a service, not a product. Since we cannot control whether the service will ultimately be successful in achieving a pregnancy, we must direct our efforts to helping our patients build their families by whichever means, or resolving their goals with comfort with child-free living.

We should not ask ourselves how we do at treating our patients; we must ask them. The best method is to survey them and follow the responses over time. Our surveys must be detailed enough to uncover deficiencies. All areas of the organization must be analyzed. Sometimes the results are surprising. How does a doctor know that he or she is effective at what they do? Ask the customer and you will find out.

But an IVF center has many customers beyond the patients. We have relationships with pharmacies, pharmaceutical companies, vendors, and insurance companies. These companies are also our customers and they must be managed as well.

Our employees are our internal customers. No company is effective with unhappy employees. The employees are one of the best marketing tools that a company has. These ambassadors must be satisfied to project the positive, excellent service provided.

SUGGESTED READING

Alper MM, Brinsden P, Fischer R, Wikland M. Is your IVF program good? *Hum Reprod* 2002;17:8–10.

Alper MM. Experience with ISO quality control in assisted reproductive technology. *Fertil Steril* 2013; 100(6):1503–8.

Carson B, Alper M, Keck C. *Quality Management Systems for Assisted Reproductive Technology.* London: Taylor and Francis; 2004.

Keck C. *Quality Management in Assisted Reproduction.* KAP CZ: Czech Republic; 2003.

24

The True ART: How to Deliver the Best Patient Care

Derek Larkin

Have you defined what the patient experience should look like in your practice, or has it evolved from tradition, clinical protocol, and patient workflow?

Ensuring an optimal patient experience is a desire of practitioners and administrators alike. Often, however, the patient experience is a by-product of the evolution of one's clinical workflow rather than a careful and strategic synthesis.

Recent shifts in the U.S. health care marketplace have changed the delivery of care from an operations-centered model to a patient-centered model. In a traditional operations-centered model, decisions regarding patient care are determined by cost, efficiency, and operational flow. With increasing deductibles and health care expenses, U.S. patients are now consumers of health care and, as such, have developed consumer demands of health care service levels. This is particularly true in the US assisted reproductive technology (ART) market, where the majority of fertility treatment is self-pay.

> *Patient centered care is care based on a partnership between the patient, their families, and the health care provider that is focused on the patient's values, preferences and needs* [1].

Whether paying for genetic testing, medications, or in vitro fertilization (IVF)—almost all patients have out-of-pocket expenses with fertility treatment. As such, today's world-class health care organizations have purposefully shifted the health care delivery model from operations-centered and have moved the patient into the center of care. Thus, meeting the needs of your ART patients will require a critical, objective view of your patient care delivery model, as well as an understanding of how to shift from an operations-centered to a patient-centered model.

The Eight Dimensions of Patient-Centered Care grew out of decades of research conducted by the Picker Institute, Harvard Medical School, and the Commonwealth Fund (Figure 24.1). The goal of this research was to identify elements of care that are instrumental in creating a positive patient experience [2]. After studying for years about patient needs, researchers defined patient needs in these eight dimensions.

It may seem like a daunting task to think broadly about what you would like every patient to experience—but working through the process of designing the best patient experience is a worthwhile investment of your time that will yield true, positive results. Consider your patients' environment (clean facilities, friendly greeters), outcomes (data-driven, evidence-based, success rates), and experiential (feelings, attitudes, interactions) aspects of care within your ART center—in light of the eight dimensions of patient-centered care identified.

Delivering the best patient care begins at the top, above the organization, with your vision. At Boston IVF, our vision is: *To become the global leader in fertility care that best understands and meets the needs of patients.* It is imperative for every practice, no matter what size, to have a vision. If the vision is not shared frequently with employees, the result will be *corporate disconnect*—where the goals of employees at different levels will vary, resulting in misalignment and vastly different patient experiences throughout the organization. Ensuring an optimal patient experience is about understanding the needs of your infertile patients, communicating promises and in doing so—setting expectations, and then meeting those promises.

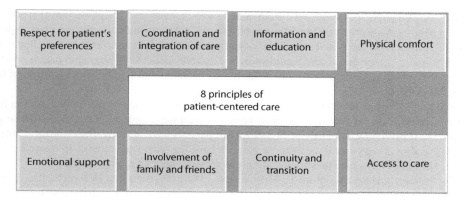

FIGURE 24.1 Picker's eight principles of patient-centered care.

Understanding Patient Needs

Understanding the needs of patients and their communication preferences is key to establishing a relationship of trust while providing improved service and patient care (Table 24.1). Where success means the difference between a life they have dreamed of and something far less, the needs of infertile patients are heightened throughout the treatment. The emotional spectrum is much broader than with patients in other medical specialties, and as such, your goal should be to mitigate the emotional stressors on infertile patients by designing the experience around the concept of hope and increasing control at the patient level. Oftentimes, the decision to see a reproductive endocrinologist is associated with a feeling of admission of failure. Unable to achieve an ongoing pregnancy, patients can present at an IVF center disheartened and disillusioned.

Understanding the psychological burden on patients is critical in understanding the needs of infertile patients, as this patient burden can often result in discontinuation of treatment. In a systematic review of reasons and predictors of discontinuation of treatment of 22 studies that included 21,453 patients [3]—the most common reasons included the following:

- Postponement of treatment (39%)
- Physical or psychological burden (19%)
- Relational and personal problems (17%)
- Treatment rejection (13%)
- Organizational (12%)
- Clinic issues (8%)

TABLE 24.1

Understanding Patient Needs

Patients Feel	Looking to Preserve
Uncertainty	Self-esteem
Vulnerability	Dignity
Powerless	Control
Scared about the consequences of failure	Hope
Shame	Confidentiality
Isolated	Acceptance

In 2011, van Empel et al. conducted a study among 925 patients and 227 physicians that showed that while pregnancy rates were most important to physicians, patient-centered care was most important to patients [4]. Further, the study revealed that a lack of patient-centered care was the most cited reason for switching clinics. The evidence here would suggest a disconnect between physician priority and patient priority; perhaps failing to meet the patient needs results in patients switching clinics and loss of business and possible opportunity of success with those patients.

In 2015, Lande et al. conducted a survey among 134 couples and showed that the top reason for treatment termination included the psychological burden of treatment, and in particular that these patients lost hope [5]. At Boston IVF, we have seen that 25% of patients who fail their first cycle drop out of treatment. Presumably, some percentage of those patients have the means to continue in treatment but have lost hope. How does any practice work toward preserving the hope of their patients?

Fertility patients are eternal optimists. They believe, going into their first IVF cycle, that they will be successful—no matter what the odds. Shifting the clinical conversation to a patient's "cumulative success rate" versus the individual cycle success rate will better set expectations of the overall chance of success with continued treatment in the event of a failed cycle. Crafting these conversations around hope will increase control at the patient level and likely result in higher retention rates/lower dropout rates in the event of an unsuccessful cycle.

One of your corporate brand elements should focus exclusively on hope and family building. Your patients should see success stories; they should understand the treatment process—and know what success looks like. At Boston IVF, The Women's Hospital location in Evansville, Indiana, if you walk through the doors of the reception area, you will see baby footprints up and down the wall, celebrating our many success stories. Our patients have renewed hope when they see those footprints. By renewing hope in our patients, we are meeting a core need.

By identifying emotional stressors, responding quickly to these emotions, increasing patients' control and training staff to understand our patients' needs to communicate respectfully, we can help to positively influence the patient experience.

Measuring Patient Feedback

Part of delivering quality care and building trust between the patient and the organization is developing a system of communication between the IVF center and their patients. Peter Drucker was famous for saying "You cannot manage what you cannot measure—and if you cannot manage it, you cannot improve it."

Two methods for gathering feedback on your patients' experience include (1) self-reporting through patient feedback tools: patient satisfaction survey or verbal and written reports by the patient to a patient advocate, and (2) third-party reporting—the staff reports an incident on behalf of a patient via an incident reporting system. Developing these feedback loops will allow your center to better understand your operation, the quality of your service, and identify areas of opportunity for improvement.

Every IVF center should incorporate a patient satisfaction survey into their standard operations. At Boston IVF, we measure patient satisfaction daily through a third-party company and incorporate the patient responses into a monthly Continuous Quality Improvement (CQI)/Risk Management meeting for review.

The elements that we measure with our patient satisfaction survey include the following:

1. Appointment and access
   a. Reaching a live person over the phone
   b. Ease of scheduling an appointment
   c. Convenience of office hours
   d. Check-in process
   e. Information clearly communicated

2. Comfort and facility
   a. Courtesy of reception staff
   b. Comfort of waiting room
   c. Communication regarding delays
   d. Wait time
   e. Cleanliness of facility
   f. Privacy
3. Financial and billing
   a. Explanation of insurance benefits and financial options
   b. Response time to questions
   c. Estimated costs and fee schedule
   d. Resolution of questions
   e. Adequacy of information before cycle start
4. Overall patient satisfaction
   a. Overall satisfaction
   b. Likelihood to recommend
   c. My expectations were met
   d. Based on my experience, I would choose Boston IVF again
   e. Boston IVF offers the most up-to-date treatments and technology
5. Patient-centered care
   a. Provider and care team were respectful and courteous
   b. Provider gave clear explanations about my condition
   c. Care team was responsive to my needs
   d. Provider spent enough time
   e. RN provided clear understanding of next steps
6. Provider and care team expertise
   a. Follow-up instructions were easily understood
   b. Medication instruction
   c. What to expect during cycle
   d. Instructions of self-administration of medications
   e. RNs are knowledgeable and skillful
   f. Anesthesiologist was knowledgeable and skillful
   g. Staff made sure I felt comfortable in the exam room
   h. Staff made sure I felt comfortable in the recovery room
   i. The ultrasound monitoring staff was friendly and respectful
   j. My provider seemed familiar with my medical history

Third-Party Reporting

Who Owns the Patient Experience?

If a physician and patient are standing at the administrative assistant's desk—each waiting for information, ask yourself… how will the administrative assistant react? Will they ask the physician to wait until answering the patient, or will they ask the patient to wait while answering the physician? At Boston IVF, we have developed a culture where "patients come first"—and throughout our organization, at all levels, we have fostered the understanding that our patients' needs really come first.

Shaping the corporate culture so that everyone feels ownership of the patient experience requires transparency of patient satisfaction results; it also requires a nonpunitive, curiosity-rewarding approach to issues that may arise with patient care.

We implemented an incident reporting feedback system on our company intranet that allows any employee to report a patient incident where they felt an opportunity for improvement exists. Employees are encouraged to fill out the incident report forms, which are then sent to the appropriate managers, with a copy sent to the CQI committee. If we had rolled out this program without first establishing a patient-centric, quality improvement culture—the initiative would have fallen flat for fear of the tool being used punitively. What has made this system so successful, however, has been a culture that is committed to improving the patient experience. There is a natural curiosity that occurs when something goes awry, and a desire to determine why the unexpected outcome occurred—without placing blame on any individual. The culture reveals an organizational commitment to the collective success regarding the patient experience. So, if an individual creates an error—the questions are as follows: Where did the process break down? What information did the employee have or not have when the error was made? What operational processes can we implement to ensure the employee's future success?

An incident report gives us a unique opportunity to improve operations and communication and ultimately to improve the patient experience (Figure 24.2).

Meeting Patient Needs

Successfully meeting patient needs requires a broad understanding of those needs: emotional, physical, and experiential. Oftentimes, clinicians will emphasize outcomes, nursing staff will emphasize operational excellence and care, and administrators will focus on the business aspects, including access and branding. While different roles can better meet specific patient needs—what matters most to patients, and how you define it, should be understood by everyone within your organization.

Moving to a patient-centered care model may require thinking outside of the "operations" box and investment of resources. Some examples of patient-centered care we have implemented include the following:

- Tours and evening hours
- Post-anesthesia care unit bays designed for privacy
- Concierge programs
- Financial cost estimator tools
- Online portals and apps
- Injection training modules and hands-on training
- Collaborative team approach
- Mind/body integration
- Expanded monitoring options

Each of these "investments" we have chosen to make has required us to enhance our level of customer service and change the status quo. I call them investments because each has come with a cost; however, the return on these investments has yielded better patient retention, lower dropout rates, and positive patient reviews.

Our team approach to patient care has allowed the company to grow dramatically, but the patient remains at the center—with individualized care and a small dedicated team.

The Boston IVF and Domar Center integrated model of care provides patients with a comprehensive mind/body program for infertility, on-site individual and couples counseling, acupuncture, nutritional

INCIDENT/NONCONFORMANCE REPORT FORM

INCIDENT STATUS	Draft
REPORT ID#:	Will Be Auto Generated

INCIDENT DATE:	10/31/2016 📅
REPORTED BY:	Derek Larkin 👤📇
YOUR DEPARTMENT:	* ⌄
YOUR LOCATION:	* ⌄
REPORT TYPE:	Select... * ⌄
PRIORITY:	Select... * ⌄

Please indicate the TYPE of incident by checking all of the appropriate boxes:

- ☐ Clinical Error
- ☐ Consent/Consent Form
- ☐ Deviation from Policy
- ☐ Documenting Problem
- ☐ Equipment Problem
- ☐ Financial/Billing Issue
- ☐ HIPAA/Privacy
- ☐ Internal Audit Finding
- ☐ IT/System Issue
- ☐ Lab (Bloods) Order Issue
- ☐ Miscommunication
- ☐ Out of Range Value
- ☐ Patient Sample Problem
- ☐ Patient Satisfaction/Complaint
- ☐ Product Delivery Problem
- ☐ Quality Objective Nonconformance
- ☐ Scheduling/Registration
- ☐ Other (Please describe)

PATIENT INFORMATION (IF APPLICABLE)

FULL NAME:	
EIVF #:	
DOB:	📅
DESCRIPTION OF INCIDENT:	

FIGURE 24.2 Incident/nonconformance report form.

counseling, yoga, a free cycle failure consultation with a psychologist, as well as crisis intervention. For example, patients with a prenatal scan resulting in no heartbeat, or disappointing egg retrieval or fertilization results can see a psychologist within an hour at the expense of the Center. These high-touch, stress-reducing programs are designed to alleviate a patient's level of stress and pain at critical times in their cycle, within moments of a traumatic experience.

In a recent survey of Boston IVF patients, 7.3% reported that the presence of an onsite integrative care center influenced their decision to come to Boston IVF. Thus, investing in the patient experience may not only reduce dropout but as we have seen it can attract new patients to your center as well.

Continuous Quality Improvement

Our goal is to achieve a ≥95% overall patient satisfaction score. We publish the results to our employees monthly via our company intranet because we want the patient experience to be front-of-mind for all of staff.

At the CQI meeting, we review the patient satisfaction results and look at trends from the quantitative responses as well as areas of opportunity for improvement from the qualitative responses. Once we have identified issues, we commit to conducting a root-cause analysis—the results of which are presented at the subsequent monthly meeting. When root-cause analyses are presented at the CQI committee meeting, the results are discussed and often changes are implemented to improve clinical workflow and communication.

The CQI committee consists of an interdepartmental group of employees ranging from the senior management team to medical directors and laboratory management staff. It is an integrated, continuous effort to measure, monitor, and improve patient safety and the performance of infertility and ART services.

The goals of the CQI Committee are to

- Support the organization's mission and strategic plan
- Systematically plan, monitor performance, analyze current performance, and improve and sustain improvements in processes and outcomes of patient care through interdisciplinary teams, clinical service, and department activities and peer review
- Minimize or reduce opportunity for adverse impact on patients, visitors, and staff
- Develop performance measures consistent with the organizational strategic plan
- Measure the organization's key outcomes, activities, and processes to support safety, improvement, and innovation and learning
- Integrate organization-wide performance improvement activities
- Promote interdepartmental and interdisciplinary communication with an integrated approach to problem solving
- Develop an environment that encourages and empowers staff to identify and address issues through the performance improvement process
- Support compliance with accreditation standards and regulatory agency requirements

Mapping Patient Touchpoints

A valuable exercise is to map the entire patient workflow, from a patient's first phone call to the practice to their last interaction with the billing department. Together with an interdepartmental team, including clinicians and staff from each department, preferably at an off-site location (as not to be distracted with the day-to-day business), list on a whiteboard every single patient interaction. These interactions are called touchpoints. During this exercise, you should determine what communication occurs at each

TABLE 24.2

Ten Challenges with Implementing a Patient-Centered Care Model

Cost	Changes will likely come with investments that need to be included in the annual budget
Commitment	From senior management and shareholders
Lack of alignment	Up, down, and across the organization
Size	Of organization might cause delays, increase expense
Branding	Improper messaging of the value proposition
Protocol drift	Different protocols, no standardized training
Silos	Launching pricing/programs without involving all stakeholders
Feedback	Inconsistent or blocked; not understanding true patient needs
Communication	Of the corporate vision and mission toward patient-centeredness
Not part of plan	Not considered a strategic driver

touchpoint, what information is presented, and in what format (brochures, conversations, training sessions, or media). This information and material should be collected in advance of the exercise.

- Are there any information gaps along the patient flow?
- What are the most frequently asked questions from patients at each touchpoint?
- What is the overall "tone" of the communication to patients? Does the tone of your practice convey hope, or is it cold and didactic?
- Are patients' expectations properly set with the materials and communication you currently have?

While one of the goals of this exercise is to ensure that the information patients receive will prepare them for a seamless clinical experience, another objective is to assess the "brand" of your practice. What images are you conveying to your patients? Once you have completed this exercise, you should make modifications to improve communication gaps and brand issues that have been revealed (Table 24.2).

Every single patient encounter matters. Almost every communication I send to my staff includes that sentence. The level of care your patients receive—as well as their ultimate success—go hand in hand in their journey to parenthood. One uplifting smile, hopeful comment, act of kindness, or "extra mile" can change a patient's entire experience. Further, as an organization, you have created expectations, which are viewed as promises by your patients. Every interaction with staff will either reinforce or contradict the promises you have made. Whether you deliver on those promises or fail to deliver will, in some manner, affect your business.

Accenture conducted a study that showed a direct correlation between patient experience and profit margin growth in hospitals [6]. The study revealed that hospitals delivering superior customer experiences saw net increases that were 50% higher than average performers.

Alignment of the organization around the patient is critical to the business of any ART center. The patient experience needs to align with patient expectations [7]—and these expectations need to be carefully and thoughtfully developed.

REFERENCES

1. Boykins D. Core communication competencies in patient-centered care. *ABNF Journal* 2014; 25(2):40–5.
2. National Research Corporation. *Eight Dimensions of PCC.* http://www.nationalresearch.com/products-and-solutions/patient-and-family-experience/eight-dimensions-of-patient-centered-care/; accessed September 5, 2016.
3. Gameiro S, Boivin J, Peronace L et al. Why do patients discontinue fertility treatment? A systematic review of reasons and predictors of discontinuation in fertility treatment. *Hum Reprod Update* 2012; 18:652–69.

4. van Empel IW, Dancet EA, Koolman XH et al. Physicians underestimate the importance of patient-centeredness to patients: A discrete choice experiment in fertility care. *Hum Reprod* 2011 Mar;26(3): 584–93.
5. Lande Y, Seidman DS, Maman E et al. Why do couples discontinue unlimited free IVF treatments? *Gynecol Endocrinol* 2015 Mar;31(3):233–6.
6. Accenture: Insight Driven Health Report. *Patient Engagement: Happy Patients, Healthy Margins*; 2015.
7. Kirkland A. The culture of patient experience. *Healthcare Finance*, July 25, 2015.

Index